SEVENTH EDITION

LANGE Q&A™

PEDIATRICS

Mary Anne Jackson, MD
Chief, Section of Pediatric Infectious Diseases
Children's Mercy Hospital & Clinics
Professor of Pediatrics
University of Missouri, Kansas City School of Medicine
Kansas City, Missouri

Sara S. Viessman, MD
Former Director, Pediatric Residency Program and Associate Professor
Former Director, Med-Peds Residency Program
University of Missouri-Columbia School of Medicine
Columbia, Missouri
Former Associate Dean for Medical Education at Lehigh Valley Hospital
Penn State College of Medicine
Allentown, Pennsylvania

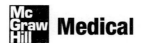

McGraw Hill **Medical**

New York   Chicago   San Francisco   Lisbon   London   Madrid   Mexico City
Milan   New Delhi   San Juan   Seoul   Singapore   Sydney   Toronto

Lange Q&A™: Pediatrics, Seventh Edition

1 2 3 4 5 6 7 8 9 0   QWD/QWD   14 13 12 11 10 9

ISBN 978-0-07-147568-6
MHID 0-07-147568-0

WS
18.2
L872p
2010

Notice

This book was set in Palatino by International Typesetting and Composition.
The editors were Kirsten Funk and Cindy Yoo.
The production supervisor was Catherine Saggese.
Project management was provided by Preeti Longia Sinha, International Typesetting and Composition.
The cover designer was the Gazillion Group.
Quebecor World was printer and binder.

This book is printed on acid-free paper.

Library of Congress Cataloging-in-Publication Data

Lange Q & A pediatrics / [edited by] Mary Anne Jackson, Sara S. Viessman.—7th ed.
    p. ; cm.
  Rev. ed. of: Appleton & Lange review of pediatrics / [edited by] Sara S. Viessman. 6th ed. 2004.
  Includes bibliographical references and index.
  ISBN-13: 978-0-07-147568-6 (pbk. : alk. paper)
  ISBN-10: 0-07-147568-0 (pbk. : alk. paper)
  1. Pediatrics—Examinations, questions, etc.   I. Jackson, Mary Anne.   II. Viessman, Sara S.
 III. Appleton & Lange review of pediatrics.   IV. Title: Lange Q and A pediatrics.   V. Title: Q and A pediatrics.
 VI. Title: Pediatrics.
  [DNLM: 1. Pediatrics—Examination Questions. WS 18.2 L274 2009]
 RJ48.2.L67 2009
  618.9200076—dc22

                                                                            2009027431

McGraw-Hill books are available at special quantity discounts to use as premiums and sales promotions, or for use in corporate training programs. To contact a representative please e-mail us at bulksales@mcgraw-hill.com.

Contents

Contributors

Joseph Y. Allen, MD, FAAP
Assistant Professor of Pediatrics
Baylor College of Medicine
Texas Children's Hospital
Houston, Texas

Joseph T. Cernich, MD
Assistant Professor of Pediatrics
Section of Pediatric Endocrinology and Diabetes
Children's Mercy Hospitals & Clinics
University of Missouri—Kansas City School
    of Medicine
Kansas City, Missouri

Jason W. Custer, MD
Fellow
Department of Pediatric Critical Care
Johns Hopkins University
Baltimore, Maryland

R. Blaine Easley, MD
Assistant Professor
Department of Pediatrics, Anesthesiology
    and Critical Care
Johns Hopkins Medical Institutes
Baltimore, Maryland

Sarah E. Hampl, MD
Assistant Professor of Pediatrics
Children's Mercy Hospitals & Clinics
University of Missouri—Kansas City School
    of Medicine
Kansas City, Missouri

Catalina M. Kersten, MD
Assistant Clinical Professor
Department of Child Health
University of Missouri School of Medicine
Columbia, Missouri

William J. Klish, MD
Professor of Pediatrics
Baylor College of Medicine
Texas Children's Hospital
Houston, Texas

Mary Stahl-Levick, MD, FAAP
Practicing General Pediatrician
ABC Family Pediatricians
Lehigh Valley Hospital and Health Network
Allentown, Pennsylvania

Jennifer A. Lowry, MD
Assistant Professor
Division of Clinical Pharmacology and Medical
    Toxicology
University of Missouri—Kansas City School
    of Medicine
Children's Mercy Hospitals & Clinics
Kansas City, Missouri

Richard J. Mazzacarro, PhD, MD
Pediatric Hospitalist
Department of Pediatrics
Lehigh Valley Hospital
Allentown, Pennsylvania

Angela L. Myers, MD, MPH
Associate Director, Infectious Diseases
    Fellowship Program
Assistant Professor of Pediatrics
University of Missouri—Kansas City School
    of Medicine
Children's Mercy Hospitals & Clinics
Kansas City, Missouri

Eugenia K. Pallotto, MD
Associate Medical Director
Neonatal Intensive Care Unit
Children's Mercy Hospital & Clinics
Assistant Professor of Pediatrics
University of Missouri—Kansas City School
   of Medicine
Kansas City, Missouri

Kristine A. Parbuoni, PharmD, BCPS
Pediatric Clinical Pharmacy Specialist
University of Maryland Medical Center
Clinical Assistant Professor
University of Maryland School of Pharmacy
Baltimore, Maryland

Emily Thorell, MD
Visiting Instructor
Department of Pediatric Infectious Disease
University of Utah School of Medicine
Salt Lake City, Utah

Angela L. Turpin, MD
Associate Medical Director of Diabetes Program
Assistant Professor of Pediatrics
University of Missouri—Kansas City School
   of Medicine
Children's Mercy Hospitals & Clinics
Kansas City, Missouri

Gary S. Wasserman, DO
Chief, Section of Medical Toxicology
Professor of Pediatrics
University of Missouri—Kansas City
Children's Mercy Hospitals & Clinics
Kansas City, Missouri

Student Reviewers

Joseph A. Bart
Lake Erie College of Osteopathic Medicine
Class of 2009

Steven Cohen
University of Missouri, Kansas City School of Medicine
Class of 2009

Rose Ann Cyriac
University of Missouri, Kansas City School of Medicine
Class of 2009

Joshua Lynch, DO
Resident, Emergency Medicine
University at Buffalo

Lisa A. Nowell, MD
Resident, Morgan Stanley Children's Hospital
New York Presbyterian, Columbia University

Crick Watkins
Kansas City University of Medicine and Biosciences
Class of 2009

Preface

If you are reading this book, you are likely engaged in one of the most important responsibilities of your career—caring for a child. Pediatric practitioners fulfill a unique role in medicine in that they see the patient across a continuum of time, often seeing the patient and their family for the first time in the first few minutes of life. As you look into the eyes of a parent and child, you recognize that the responsibility is beyond measure and the balance between providing comprehensive preventative health care and recognizing the need for more in-depth system-specific investigation or treatment can turn on a dime. It requires practitioners to have a solid knowledge base, be thorough in their assessments, be insightful regarding preventative care approaches, and, most importantly, be able to recognize when an urgent treatment plan is needed.

This book should serve as an assessment tool for students, residents, and practitioners who wish to evaluate their pediatric knowledge base and clinical deductive skills. The question focus and organization of chapters were chosen to cover topics, by and large, consistent with the American Board of Pediatric general pediatric core competencies. Chapters cover a range of topics spanning ages from newborn, including the premature infant through adolescence. Comprehensive dedication to issues related to growth and development, feeding and nutrition, fluids, electrolytes, and metabolic disorders are included. The infectious disease chapter covers both common outpatient infection as well as life-threatening infections which occur in the healthy and immunocompromised host. The chapter on injuries, poisoning, and substance abuse provides review of clinical problems which may be seen on both outpatient and emergency care encounters. Critical care and pediatric therapeutic questions target distinctive clinical scenarios and require the clinician to make prompt, evidence-based medical decisions. The answers and discussion which follow each question include reference to key pediatric textbooks and American Academy of Pediatrics guidelines.

To those who use this book, I hope you find it useful and that you are fueled throughout your career by the excitement of discovery stirred by your clinical experiences.

Mary Anne Jackson, MD

Acknowledgements

Many thanks to Sara Viessman for trusting me to complete this labor of love, and to Dr. Martin Loren who first envisioned the text and brought the first five editions to fruition. It has been a pleasure to work with all of the authors that gave of their time and who represent expertise from pediatric centers across the United States.

It has been my pleasure to work with Catherine Johnson, Cindy Yoo, and Kirsten Funk from McGraw-Hill. Their patience, advice, guidance, and encouragement have been invaluable.

I would be remiss if I did not recognize my partners at work who daily remind me how lucky we are to do what we do. To Lindsay and Nick, seeing you challenge yourself throughout life, be it at work or play, has inspired me to broaden my own horizons. And to Jay, your unwavering love has energized me every day for 37 years.

Warm-Up Questions and Exam-Taking Skills

Mary Anne Jackson, MD

Welcome to the Pediatrics Review! In this book, you will find eleven chapters that will prepare you to answer questions on topics that pertain to common diseases in the infant and child. Most questions are introduced with a clinical stem and multiple choice answers are provided. The content covers basic concepts for the beginning medical student as well as more advanced concepts for the senior student or resident training in pediatrics.

The question structure utilizes the single-best-answer format that is widely used for most formalized testing in pediatrics. This format is considered especially appropriate for tests that examine your clinical decision-making skills. A patient-based scenario is used and in most cases appropriate laboratory and other diagnostic findings are included. The question is followed by five answer options. The options include the correct answer and four distractors that represent plausible but incorrect options. The correct answer is evidence based and the critique provides appropriate references if you want to read more about a topic.

Some tips to consider before embarking on the practice test:

1. Utilize the cover test; that is, do not look at the answers initially and read through the entire question. Decide what you believe the correct answer to be before looking at the five options.
2. If you do not know the correct answer, attempt to eliminate those answers you believe are incorrect. If you can narrow down to two answers, you will have a better chance of choosing the correct option.
3. Go with your gut! That is, in most cases, your first instinct is correct so while reviewing your answers is an option (mainly to ensure that you have not omitted any questions), think carefully before you change your first answer.
4. Read the answer section carefully and in the context of the question you just completed.

Questions

DIRECTIONS (Questions 1 through 24): Each of the numbered items or incomplete statements in this section is followed by answers or completions of the statement. Select the one lettered answer or completion that is best in each case.

Clue: Questions 1 and 2 are simple and straightforward, each with only one possible correct answer. For this type of question, you can actually answer the question before looking at the choices. Then read the choices to verify that your answer is there. Finally, review all the other choices to be sure that none is better than the one you selected.

1. You have just confirmed the diagnosis of cystic fibrosis in a 3-year-old child. The parents are concerned about future pregnancies. You explain to them that the pattern of genetic transmission of cystic fibrosis is

   (A) autosomal dominant
   (B) autosomal recessive
   (C) X-linked recessive
   (D) X-linked dominant
   (E) autosomal recessive in some families and X-linked in others

2. A 12-year-old boy just returned from Boy Scout Camp in Wisconsin. He now has fever, myalgia, and a 10-cm skin lesion which looks like a target. You suspect Lyme disease, most likely contracted by which of the following?

   (A) ingestion of unripe fruit
   (B) ingestion of spoiled fruit
   (C) drinking of contaminated water
   (D) the bite of a tick
   (E) the bite of a mosquito

Clue: Unlike the preceding two questions, the answer to Question 3 cannot be anticipated before viewing the list of suggested answers, because there are many possible completions to the statement. Nevertheless, the question is simple and straightforward.

3. A 2-year-old boy presents with extremity swelling and proteinuria and is found on urine analysis. Minimal-change disease is suspected and you explain to the child's parents that this diagnosis

   (A) is the most common cause of nephrotic syndrome in childhood
   (B) has a peak incidence in children between 10 and 15 years of age
   (C) usually results in end-stage renal disease in 5–10 years
   (D) is characterized by normal serum lipids and cholesterol
   (E) typically has a poor response to corticosteroid treatment

Clue: Pay attention to key words when you read a question. Question 4 contains the key words "most likely."

4. You have just prescribed phenytoin for a 12-year-old boy with new onset of epilepsy. Of the following side effects, which is most likely to occur in this patient?

   (A) lymphoma syndrome
   (B) Raynaud phenomenon
   (C) acute hepatic failure
   (D) gingival hyperplasia
   (E) optic atrophy

5. A term infant is born to a mother who has been using crack cocaine. This infant is at increased risk for which of the following?

   (A) anemia
   (B) intrauterine growth retardation
   (C) hypercalcemia
   (D) macrosomia
   (E) postmaturity

6. You examine an 18-year-old male college student with a 5-day history of fever, sore throat, and fatigue. Physical examination reveals an exudative tonsillitis and bilateral enlarged and slightly tender posterior cervical lymph nodes. The spleen is palpable 3 cm below the rib cage. Which agent is most likely responsible for this patient's illness?

   (A) Group A β-hemolytic streptococcus
   (B) Adenovirus
   (C) *Toxoplasma gondii*
   (D) Epstein-Barr virus
   (E) *Corynebacterium diphtheriae*

7. A term infant requires intubation in the delivery room after aspiration of thick meconium and is brought to the neonatal intensive care unit. Which of the following is the most likely risk factor for meconium aspiration syndrome in this infant?

   (A) chromosomal anamoly
   (B) congenital heart disease
   (C) cystic fibrosis
   (D) fetal distress
   (E) tracheoesophageal fistula

8. A newborn infant with stigmata of Down syndrome has a heart murmur. Which of the following cardiac lesions is most likely in this baby?

   (A) hypoplastic left heart syndrome
   (B) total anamolous venous return
   (C) coarctation of the aorta
   (D) anamolous coronary artery
   (E) atrioventricular defect

9. A mother of a 2-month-old wants more information about immunizations. Which of the following statements regarding immunization against *Haemophilus influenzae* type b (Hib) is correct?

   (A) It is indicated for high-risk children only.
   (B) Hib vaccine can be administered effectively as early as 2 months of age.
   (C) Hib vaccine should not be given to children who have had allergic reactions to eggs.
   (D) Hib vaccine should not be administered to children with a history of reaction to DTaP immunization.
   (E) Hib vaccine should be deferred for infants with history of febrile seizures.

10. Acellular pertussis vaccine is recommended for infants, children, adolescents, and adults. Compared to the previously available whole cell vaccine, which of the following best describes these products?

    (A) they are more immunogenic
    (B) they are less expensive
    (C) they are associated with fewer side effects
    (D) they require fewer doses
    (E) they can be combined with the varicella vaccine for the infant under age 1 year

11. It is recommended that young infants should sleep in the supine rather than in the prone position. This is based on data suggesting that the prone position is associated with an increased incidence of which of the following?

    (A) delayed eruption of the first deciduous teeth
    (B) gastroesophageal reflux and aspiration
    (C) macrognathia
    (D) strabismus
    (E) sudden infant death

12. The feeding of honey to infants less than 6 months of age has been associated with which of the following?

    (A) anaphylaxis
    (B) hypernatremia
    (C) botulism
    (D) jaundice
    (E) listeriosis

13. A 1-month-old infant presents with fever of 39°C and vomiting. He was born at term vaginally to an 18-year-old mother who did not have prenatal care. On examination, he is alert but fussy and cries with palpation of his abdomen. He is uncircumcised and both testes are descended. An evaluation for sepsis and meningitis is performed. Urine analysis shows 50–100 WBC/HPF with positive leukocyte esterase and nitrites. CSF examination is normal and cultures from blood, urine, and CSF are pending. You tell his mother that he has urinary tract infection and she asks why this happened. Which of the following is correct in explaining this infant's most likely risk for urinary tract infection?

(A) The mother was colonized with Group B streptococcus and did not receive intrapartum prophylaxis.

(B) The infant is uncircumcised.

(C) The infant has prune belly syndrome.

(D) The infant has galactosemia.

(E) There is a family history of vesicoureteral reflux.

14. A 3-month-old infant presents with poor growth and inadequate weight gain. There is no history of vomiting or diarrhea. Except for the appearance of malnutrition and lack of subcutaneous fat, the physical examination is normal. What is the most likely cause of this child's failure to thrive?

(A) renal disease

(B) a metabolic disorder

(C) tuberculosis

(D) an endocrine disorder

(E) a nonorganic cause

15. A 2-year-old child is being evaluated because the mother notes that her right eye has been turning in. Physical examination documents strabismus with a right esotropia. Attempts to visualize the fundi are unsuccessful, but it is noted that the red reflex is replaced by a yellow-white pupillary reflex in the right eye. This child most likely has which of the following?

(A) retinitis pigmentosa

(B) retinoblastoma

(C) rhabdomyosarcoma

(D) severe hyperopia

(E) severe myopia

16. A 2-year-old child is admitted because of weakness proceeding to coma. According to the parents, he had been well until several hours prior to admission, when they noted diarrhea, cough, wheezing, and sweating. Physical examination reveals a comatose child with diffuse weakness and areflexia. Pupils are pinpoint and unresponsive. Examination of the chest reveals generalized wheezing. Oral secretions are copious. Which of the following should you administer at this time?

(A) adrenaline

(B) atropine

(C) cefotaxime

(D) methylprednisolone

(E) edrophonium

17. A 3-week-old infant is admitted with vomiting of 5 days' duration. Physical examination reveals a rapid heart rate, evidence of dehydration, and ambiguous genitalia. Serum electrolytes are Na^+ 120 meq/L, K^+ 7.5 meq/L, HCO_3^- 12 meq/L, BUN 20 mg/dL. In addition to intravenous fluid replacement with normal saline, administration of which of the following would be most important?

(A) diuretics

(B) potassium exchange resin

(C) glucose and insulin

(D) antibiotics

(E) hydrocortisone

18. A previously well 12-year-old girl presents to clinic because of painful swellings on the front of the legs of about 3 days' duration. Examination reveals tender erythematous nodules, 1–2 cm in diameter, on the extensor surfaces of the lower legs. The remainder of the physical examination is unremarkable. Which of the following is most likely to confirm the cause of this condition?

(A) stool smear and culture

(B) urine analysis and BUN

(C) throat culture

(D) slit-lamp examination of the eye

(E) echocardiogram

19. An 18-year-old boy presents with cough, chest pain, and low-grade nightly fevers of several weeks duration. He has a 4-year history of smoking two packs of cigarettes per day. Chest x-ray reveals a large mass in the mediastinum with extension into the right upper chest. Which of the following is the most likely diagnosis?

    (A) adenocarcinoma
    (B) squamous cell carcinoma
    (C) small cell carcinoma
    (D) lymphoma
    (E) metastatic Wilms tumor

20. A 12-year-old child is seen because of a rash and severe headache which began 2 weeks after returning from vacation in Massachusetts. The skin lesion began as a red macule on the thigh, which gradually expanded over 1 week to reach approximately 15 cm in diameter with red borders and central clearing. The lesion is slightly painful. A few days after the onset of the skin manifestation, the child developed severe headache, myalgias, arthralgias, and malaise. Low-grade fever was present. The mother recalls that the child was bitten by a tick about 1 week prior to the onset of symptoms. This patient's disorder is probably best treated with which of the following?

    (A) corticosteroids
    (B) diphenhydramine
    (C) methotrexate
    (D) nonsteroidal anti-inflammatory drugs
    (E) doxycycline

21. An 8-year-old child is hospitalized because of paroxysms of severe colicky abdominal pain which does not radiate to the back or the groin. Physical examination is unremarkable except for generalized abdominal tenderness. An exploratory laparotomy reveals an edematous intestine without specific lesions. The appendix appears normal but is removed. Postoperatively the abdominal pain persists, and hematuria develops. Values for BUN and creatinine are normal. On the second postoperative day, tender swelling of both ankles and knees is noted. Which of the following additional findings would most likely be present in this child?

    (A) shock
    (B) meningitis
    (C) hepatitis
    (D) a purpuric rash
    (E) hemorrhagic pancreatitis

22. A 10-year-old boy has been having episodes of repetitive and semipurposeful movements of the face and shoulders. The parents believe these movements are worse when the child is under emotional stress. They also volunteer that they have never noted the movements while the patient is asleep. The movements have been present for more than 6 months. The parents are now especially concerned because the child has developed repetitive episodes of throat clearing and snorting. Physical and neurologic examinations are entirely normal. During the examination you note that the child has some blinking of the right eye, twitching of the right face, and grimacing. You ask him to stop these movements, and he is temporarily successful in doing so, but the movements recur. The home situation, social history, and child's development and social adjustment appear normal. A head CT scan is normal. Of the following, which would be the most appropriate next step?

    (A) order an electroencephalogram
    (B) prescribe carbamazepine
    (C) prescribe corticosteroids
    (D) prescribe haloperidol
    (E) refer the child to a psychiatrist

23. A 3-month-old infant is hospitalized because of recurrent right focal seizures that are now generalized in nature. Birth and perinatal history are unremarkable. You note that the child has a flat, purplish-red skin lesion on the left side of the face extending onto the forehead. The remainder of the examination including a complete neurologic examination is within normal limits. The results of a lumbar puncture are normal. You order a CT scan of the head and anticipate seeing which of the following?

    (A) agenesis of the corpus callosum
    (B) a porencephalic cyst
    (C) gyriform calcifications
    (D) hydrocephalus
    (E) normal findings

24. On routine examination of the children of a migrant farm worker, you notice that a 12-year-old child who has received little previous medical care is short and mentally retarded. Physical examination reveals that the liver is enlarged to 5 cm below the right rib cage, and the spleen is enlarged 6 cm below the left rib cage. Lumbodorsal kyphosis is prominent. The child has a peculiar facies with thick lips and a large tongue. Attempts to visualize the retina are unsuccessful because of clouding of the corneas. You expect that examination of this child's urine will reveal which of the following?

    (A) dermatan and heparan sulfate
    (B) galactose
    (C) mannose
    (D) the odor of maple syrup
    (E) the odor of sweaty feet

DIRECTIONS (Questions 25 through 30): Each set of matching questions in this section consists of a list of several numbered items introduced by 5–26 lettered options. For each numbered item select the one lettered option with which it is most closely associated. Each lettered option may be selected once, more than once, or not at all.

Selection of answers for Questions 25 through 27

    (A) miliaria rubra
    (B) verrucae vulgaris
    (C) condyloma acuminatum
    (D) molluscum contagiosum
    (E) pityriasis rosea

25. Small (pinhead to 1 cm), pearly papules with translucent tops and waxy, whitish material inside, distributed on the face and anterior trunk; some lesions are umbilicated

26. Soft, flesh-colored papular or pedunculated lesions around the genitalia and rectum

27. Oval, maculopapular lesions oriented with the long axis along skin tension lines

Selection of answers for Questions 28 through 30

    (A) ABO incompatibility
    (B) α₁-antitrypsin deficiency
    (C) biliary atresia
    (D) breastfeeding jaundice
    (E) breast milk jaundice
    (F) choledochal cyst
    (G) cholelithiasis
    (H) Crigler-Najjar syndrome
    (I) cystic fibrosis
    (J) Dubin-Johnson syndrome
    (K) erythroblastosis (Rh incompatibility)
    (L) galactosemia
    (M) glucose-6-phosphate dehydrogenase deficiency
    (N) hepatitis
    (O) hereditary spherocytosis
    (P) hypothyroidism
    (Q) physiologic hyperbilirubinemia
    (R) sepsis

28. A 3-day-old term, healthy infant is noted to be jaundiced. Physical examination is otherwise normal. Laboratory values: Hb 16.8 g/dL; reticulocytes 1.0%; bilirubin unconjugated 8.5 mg/dL, conjugated 0.8 mg/dL.

29. A 5-week-old infant has been jaundiced for about 2 weeks. He has been asymptomatic and physical examination is otherwise normal. Laboratory values: Hb 14.2 g/dL; reticulocytes 1.2%; bilirubin unconjugated 4.5 mg/dL, conjugated 5.5 mg/dL; ALT 25 IU/L, AST 75 IU/L. Abdominal ultrasound examination reveals a normal-size liver; gallbladder is not visualized.

30. An otherwise well 4-week-old infant has remained jaundiced since day 3 of life despite two exchange transfusions and continuous phototherapy. Laboratory values: Hb 14 g/dL; reticulocytes 1.0%; bilirubin unconjugated 16 mg/dL, conjugated 0.2 mg/dL; ALT 15 IU/L, AST 40 IU/L. A Coombs test prior to the first exchange transfusion was negative. Ultrasound examination reveals a normal liver and gallbladder.

Answers and Explanations

1. The correct answer is (**B**). Cystic fibrosis (CF) is an autosomal recessive disorder with a disease incidence in the Caucasian population of about 1:1500 and a corresponding carrier state of about 1:20. Currently, CF represents the most common lethal genetic disease in the Caucasian population. The disease is much less common among African Americans and Asians. (*McMillan, 1490; Rudolph, 1967*)

2. Like Question 1, this question has only one possible correct answer, and you should have been able to come up with that answer before looking at the list of choices. The answer is (**D**), bite of a tick. *Borrelia burgdorferi*, the spirochete that causes Lyme disease, is transmitted to humans by the bite of a tick, most commonly *Ixodes* species, although in some geographic areas, other ticks such as *Ambylomma americanum* (the lone star tick) have been incriminated. (*AAP:Red Book, 428–433*)

3. The correct answer is (**A**). This question is simple in that it deals with well-known and important clinical features of a common disease—minimal-change nephrotic syndrome (MCNS). It is straightforward in that not only is one of the listed choices (**A**) clearly the best, but the other four choices all are incorrect. Minimal-change disease is the most common cause of nephrotic syndrome in childhood, and accounts for more than all other causes combined. The peak incidence is between 2 and 5 years of age. The prognosis is very favorable, and the process rarely progresses to end-stage renal disease. Serum lipids and cholesterol are elevated, as they are with other causes of nephrotic syndrome. Finally, the disease characteristically responds well to treatment with corticosteroids, with only a small minority of patients failing to remit. (*Rudolph, 1691–1693; McMillan, 1796–1797*)

4. The correct answer is (**D**). Optic atrophy is not a recognized complication of phenytoin therapy. Acute hepatic failure, a lymphoma-like syndrome, and Raynaud phenomenon all have been noted *rarely* with this drug. Gingival hyperplasia is a *common* and troublesome side effect, which often can be minimized by scrupulous dental hygiene. If the examinee knew that a lymphoma-like syndrome has been reported with phenytoin and focused in on that without carefully considering all subsequent choices, he or she might have selected (A). You can avoid such errors by carefully reading the question and asking yourself, "What are the common side effects of this drug?" even before looking at the choices. Knowing that gingival hypertrophy is a very common side effect of phenytoin would be sufficient knowledge to answer the question correctly. Another way to approach this question would be to ask yourself, "Of the following side effects, which is *most* frequent?" (*Rudolph, 1292; McMillan, 2054*)

5. This is another straightforward, completely factual question. Only one choice is correct. As a matter of fact, two answers are not only incorrect, they are exact opposites of what actually happens with cocaine, so it should be easy to be confident that they are incorrect. Infants born to women using cocaine, especially crack cocaine, have an increased incidence of prematurity (not postmaturity) and low birth weight (not macrosomia). Intrauterine growth retardation with disproportionate decrease in head size is noted

in infants exposed prenatally to cocaine. The correct answer is (**B**). *(Rudolph, 2023)*

6. Although this question also is quite straightforward, it potentially is more difficult than the preceding questions because several of the agents listed can explain many of the features of this adolescent's illness. If you read the instructions carefully, you noted that you were asked to select *the one best answer,* which does not imply that all other choices are totally without merit. Consider which of the above choices best fits the clinical scenario, and therefore, which is most likely responsible for this patient's illness.

    The correct answer is (**D**). The agent most likely responsible for this child's illness is the Epstein-Barr virus (EBV). The clinical picture is strongly suggestive of mononucleosis. Although this patient could be infected with group A streptococcus or adenovirus, several features are much more characteristic of EBV infection than either of these. They include the fact that the child is a college student, the presence of splenomegaly, and the fact that the adenopathy is posterior rather than anterior and is only slightly tender. While these findings also could be explained by toxoplasmosis, this diagnosis is rarely confirmed as a cause of acute exudative tonsillitis and cervical adenitis in the United States. Although it is appropriate to think of diphtheria in patients with acute exudative tonsillitis, there is nothing specific in this case to suggest that diagnosis. Infectious mononucleosis is clearly *the most likely* diagnosis. *(Rudolph, 1035–1038)*

7. (**D**) Fetal distress is the major risk factor for meconium aspiration. The mechanism involves the loss of anal sphincter tone, passage of meconium into the amniotic fluid, and aspiration by the distressed, gasping infant during the process of birth. The thick meconium obstructs the airways, causing tachypnea, retractions, and grunting.

    This is the type of question in which a little knowledge can go a long way. If you knew that meconium aspiration was a relatively *common* problem in the delivery room, you could eliminate (C) cystic fibrosis (a relatively *uncommon* disease) as its cause. (*Meconium ileus,* which is

associated with cystic fibrosis, has nothing to do with meconium aspiration.) If you realized that aspiration of meconium can only occur before or during delivery, you also could eliminate (B) congenital heart disease and (A) neonatal meningitis, as neither of these generally cause distress during delivery. Finally, you should be able to figure out that a tracheoesophageal fistula, with or without associated esophageal atresia, would lead to aspiration of saliva, milk, or gastric contents after birth but would not predispose to aspiration of meconium. *(Rudolph, 203)*

    A severe pneumonia following meconium aspiration occurs as an in utero response to significant hypoxic or ischemic stress. Infants who have fetal distress, thick meconium, and APGAR scores of less than 7 at 1 and 5 minutes are at increased risk for meconium aspiration syndrome. When meconium staining of amniotic fluid is noted, the appropriate approach to care of the infant according to The Neonatal Resuscitation Program (NRP) of the American Academy of Pediatrics and American Heart Association include intubation when the infant is not vigorous (defined as having poor respiratory efforts, poor muscle tone, and a heart rate less than 100 beats/minute). *(Rudolph, 194)*

8. (**E**) The overall incidence of congenital heart disease in the general population is less than 1% but about 40% of children with Down syndrome have heart defects. The most common lesions in children with Down syndrome include atrioventricular septal defects, ventricular septal defects and atrial septal defect, or patent ductus arteriosus. Atrioventricular septal defects (AV canal) is most often seen in these children, making up approximately 60% of the congenital heart disease found in trisomy 21 but accounting for less than 3% of congenital heart defects in the general population. *(Rudolph, 732)*

9. Prior to the initiation of conjugate *H influenzae* type b (Hib) vaccine in 1990, infection caused by this pathogen was a major cause of morbidity and mortality in the young infant. A Hib polysaccharide vaccine, first licensed in 1985 was not effective in infants less than 2 years of age; unfortunately, the greatest incidence of Hib meningitis was in this age group. The conjugate

vaccines used a process of bonding the polysaccharide to a protein carrier which served as a more effective antigen, greatly improving the immunogenecity in the young child. It is estimated that 95% of Hib-immunized children will develop protective antibody after a primary series starting when the child is 2 months of age.

The correct answer to this question, therefore, is (**B**). It is now recommended that all infants be immunized with the conjugated Hib vaccine. Depending on the brand of vaccine used, infants should receive a series of two or three immunizations between 2 and 6 months of age, followed by one booster dose at 12–15 months of age. (*AAP:Red Book, 314–315*)

10. The correct answer is (**C**). Current pertussis vaccines used in the United States are acellular products which contain two or more purified *Bordetella pertussis* immunogens. These vaccines have a lower risk of adverse events when compared to previously used whole cell pertussis vaccines. In terms of immunogenecity, efficacy, and number of doses, they do not differ but they are more expensive than whole cell products. (*Rudolph, 43, 45*)

11. (**E**) While the etiology of sudden infant death syndrome (SIDS) is not completely elucidated, since 1992, The American Academy of Pediatrics has recommended that infants be placed to sleep on their backs. Since that time, the frequency of prone sleeping has decreased from greater than 70% to approximately 20% of US infants, and the SIDS rate has decreased by more than 40%. (*Rudolph, 936*)

12. Cases of botulism predominantly occuring in infants less than 6 months of age, have followed introduction of nonhuman milk sources in breastfed infants. Honey is considered a potential risk for infection. Because honey can contain spores of *Clostridium botulinum*, this product should not be given to infants under 1 year of age. (*AAP:Red Book, 258, 863*)

13. The risk factor for urinary tract infection for the infant in this scenario is the fact that he is an uncirmcised male. Uncircumcised boys in the first year of life have a greater than eightfold higher incidence than girls or circumcised boys.

It is suggested that the presence of the foreskin allows for easier bacterial colonization of the periurethral region. While urinary tract infections can occur in infants with galactosemia or prune belly syndrome, there is no information given to suggest that either diagnosis is present in the infant. Vesicoureteral reflux is present in 25% of infants with urinary tract infection and familial risk is described but is not the likely risk for this infant. Urinary tract infections are caused by *Escherichia coli* in 90% of cases and maternal colonization is a risk for Group B streptococcal infection. (*Rudolph, 306, 1668–1669*)

14. (**E**) Failure to thrive (FTT) is a common pediatric problem characterized by poor growth, especially in regard to weight gain. Today, in the United States, nonorganic causes of FTT account for 30% to more than 50% of the cases in most series and are responsible for more cases than any other etiology. Nonorganic causes encompass a diverse spectrum extending from poverty and lack of food, through poor parenting skills and misguided feeding to frank neglect or abuse. Knowledge of the common reasons for failure to thrive allows one to eliminate the other choices because none of the other choices listed accounts for more than 5% or 10% of cases. If gastrointestinal problems had been a choice, the question would have been more difficult, because gastrointestinal disorders account for up to 25% of cases of FTT in most series. (*McMillan, 1048–1049; Rudolph, 7–8*)

15. (**B**) Retinoblastoma is the most likely cause of this child's strabismus and white pupillary reflex (leukokoria, *cat's eye reflex*). Although rhabdomyosarcoma may involve the orbit, it is extrinsic to the globe and does not cause a white pupillary reflex. Other causes of leukokoria include visceral lava migrans (*Toxocara canis* infection) and retrolental fibroplasia. Although retinoblastoma is rare, the association with leukokoria is a classic and important pediatric entity with which all students, pediatric house officers and practitioners should be familiar. (*Rudolph, 2395–2396*)

16. This format is common on national medical examinations. It makes the question difficult

because it requires recall rather than recognition. The question asks you to identify a disease or condition but does not provide a list of diagnoses from which to choose; instead, it provides a list of associated findings, in this case, treatments. To answer the question correctly you must analyze the clinical findings and recall the disease rather than selecting (recognizing) it from a list.

The sudden onset of neurologic signs or symptoms in a previously well toddler always ought to raise suspicion of a toxin or poisoning. The correct answer is (**B**). This child is a victim of organophosphate poisoning. Organophosphate and carbamate insecticides are widely used throughout the United States and are important causes of poisoning in children. These drugs produce both muscarinic effects (rhinorrhea, wheezing, pulmonary edema, salivation, vomiting, cramps, bradycardia, and pinpoint pupils) as well as nicotinic effects (twitching, weakness and paralysis, convulsions, coma, and respiratory failure). These children often ingest the toxic substance unobserved, and the diagnosis must be suspected on the basis of the clinical picture even when there is no history of ingestion or exposure. Atropine will reverse the muscarinic effects of these agents and is a useful part of treatment. Edrophonium is a short and rapidly acting cholinergic drug used diagnostically to reverse the muscle weakness of myasthenia gravis. Myasthenia, however, would not explain the pinpoint pupils, salivation, wheezing, bradycardia, or convulsions. *(Rudolph, 373–374)*

17. (**E**) The child described probably has congenital adrenal hyperplasia (CAH), an inborn metabolic error of the adrenal cortex. The acidosis (HCO_3^- 12 meq/L) helps to rule out pyloric stenosis as the cause of the emesis, as most infants with pyloric stenosis have a metabolic alkalosis. The enzyme deficiency in CAH results in decreased production of cortisol and other adrenal cortical hormones and secondary hypertrophy of the adrenal gland. Accumulation of androgen-like precursors of cortisol during fetal development leads to masculinization of the female fetus and ambiguous genitalia, which is an important clue in this case. The low serum

sodium and high serum potassium levels are classic findings in this condition, reflecting the lack of mineralocorticoids. In addition to the use of saline, administration of a mineralocorticoid such as cortisone or hydrocortisone is critical. The elevated serum potassium level usually responds rapidly to administration of saline and steroids, and specific therapy with exchange resins or glucose and insulin usually is unnecessary.

As did the preceding question, this question tests the examinee's ability of recall rather than recognition, a more difficult but clinically more relevant skill. Instead of providing a list of diseases or syndromes as possible answers, it provides a list of additional features or findings, one of which is associated with the disorder in question. In this case, as in the preceding question, the feature to be selected is the appropriate therapy. The question tests more than the examinee's ability to recite the treatment of hyperkalemia. It tests his or her ability to analyze the clinical situation, make a correct diagnosis, set priorities, and tailor therapy to the specific pathophysiology involved. *(Rudolph, 2032–2041)*

18. Again, this question requires recall rather than recognition. The stem of the question gives no information except the age and sex of the patient and a description of the skin lesions—tender erythematous nodules on the extensor surfaces of the legs. On the basis of these data you must decide what disease the patient most likely has. Which of the following best fits the skin lesions described: erythema nodosum, rheumatic nodules, subcutaneous fat necrosis, hematomas, septic emboli, or Henoch-Schöenlein purpura?

The correct answer is (**C**). To answer this question you must not only identify the rash as erythema nodosum (an uncommon but not rare disease) but you must also know that group A β-hemolytic streptococcal infection is a common cause. Erythema nodosum is a reactive phenomenon characterized by tender, erythematous nodules 1–2 cm in diameter. The lesions usually are on the extensor surfaces of the extremities and are more common on the legs. This rash is seen in a variety of infections including histoplasmosis, tuberculosis, coccidioidomycosis, and group A streptococcal infection. Today, the most common cause in an otherwise well child in the United States is group A streptococcal infection. *(McMillan, 911; Rudolph, 1237)*

19. The differences between adults and children are frequently emphasized in medical training. The differences between adults and adolescents should also be recognized. The differential diagnosis for many conditions, such as an intrathoracic mass seen in this case, is age dependent. While carcinoma of the lung is a leading cause of intrathoracic mass in adults, it is very rare in adolescents, even those who have a significant smoking history. That eliminates choices (A), (B), and (C). While it is true that Wilms tumor frequently metastasizes to the lung, this malignancy almost always presents in the first few years of age and would be unheard of in an 18-year-old. That leaves lymphoma as the only remaining choice and the most likely diagnosis. (**D**) is the correct answer. Other causes, such as tuberculosis, histoplasmosis, and sarcoid need to be considered but were not listed as choices. *(Rudolph, 1608)*

20. Here again, you are required to make a diagnosis but are not given a list of diseases from which to choose. You should analyze the data, identify the important features, and generate a list of most likely diagnoses. The major problems appear to be fever, a localized rash, and meningeal inflammation (headache and stiff neck). The malaise, fatigue, lethargy, generalized lymphadenopathy, and arthralgia are less specific. Of note is the fact that the child was bitten by a tick a week prior to the onset of the illness. If the tick bite is related to the illness, it would suggest an infectious etiology. The systemic findings, the central clearing of the rash, and the time course permit us to rule out a simple cellulitis. Knowledge of the common infections carried by ticks as well as the epidemiology of such infections is essential to correctly answering the question. Rocky Mountain spotted fever, Lyme disease, tularemia, babesiosis, and Colorado tick fever are all spread by ticks, but only Lyme disease fits with the localized rash described— erythema migrans. This disease is caused by the spirochete *B burgdorferi* and over 90% of cases originate from 10 states in the US (Connecticut,

Delaware, Maryland, Massachusetts, Minnesota, New Jersey, New York, Pennsylvania, Rhode Island, and Wisconsin). The organism is susceptible to a number of antibiotics, including amoxicillin and doxycycline. The correct answer is (**E**). *(McMillan, 1171–1173; Rudolph: Color Plate, 22:1212–1213)*

21. This question also challenges you to identify a disease without providing a list of diagnoses from which to choose. What disease do you believe this child most likely has: juvenile idiopathic arthritis, inflammatory bowel disease, cystic fibrosis, Henoch-Schönlein purpura (HSP), *Salmonella* infection?

    The correct answer is (**D**). This child has anaphylactoid purpura, also known as HSP. This is an important and not rare pediatric entity, well known to pediatricians and pediatric residents but not so well known by students. The question is difficult because the scenario given is infrequent although well recognized in this disorder. The major features of this disease are colicky abdominal pain, nephritis, arthritis, and a characteristic purpuric rash limited to the area below the waist. The purpuric rash listed as a possible answer does not specify location or distribution, but is still the best answer. If you missed this question, was it because you were not familiar with HSP or because you did not recognize it from this presentation? The only atypical feature in this case is that the child was taken to the operating room. When abdominal pain is the first complaint, diagnosis is virtually impossible until other features appear. *(Rudolph:Color Plate, 12:1212–1213)*

22. What disorder do you believe this child probably has: psychomotor seizures, Tourette syndrome, drug abuse, brain tumor, or psychologic disorder?

    The child most likely has Tourette syndrome, a disorder characterized by blinking, twitching, grimacing, and jerking movements that often have a repetitive and semipurposeful character. Like simple habit tics, the movements usually can be voluntarily suppressed momentarily, disappear during sleep, and are made worse by emotional tension. These features could mislead the examinee to assume a psychologic etiology. Ultimately, the muscles of respiration and swallowing become involved so that throat clearing, coughing, snorting, hiccups, and other noises are common. Coprolalia, echolalia, and spitting are classic features but are not always present. The correct answer is (**D**). Haloperidol is the drug of choice for Tourette syndrome, although not all patients require this therapy. Haloperidol relieves symptoms in 80% of patients, clonidine has also been found to be helpful in some patients. Corticosteroids are not appropriate in this patient. Referral to a child psychiatrist may be a useful adjunct but has not been shown to have consistent positive effects. An EEG is helpful to diagnose epilepsy, but in this case, the child can stop the movements when asked, so the movements are clearly not indicative of seizure activity. (*Rudolph, 462*)

23. This question deals with a rare but dramatic pediatric syndrome. What is the significance of the hemangioma on one side of the face? If you can identify the disease, can you then anticipate the findings on CT scan? Do you think this child has congenital toxoplasmosis, holoprosencephaly, Sturge-Weber disease, subdural effusions, porencephalic cyst? Providing a list of diagnoses would have changed the question from one of recall to one of recognition.

    The association of a unilateral facial hemangioma, particularly in the distribution of the trigeminal nerve, and focal seizures suggests Sturge-Weber disease, also referred to as Sturge-Weber-Dmitri syndrome and encephalotrigeminal angiomatosis. Incidentally, national examinations often use eponyms for diseases and syndromes even when other specific names exist. Examples include Down syndrome rather than trisomy 21 and Werdnig-Hoffmann disease for spinomuscular atrophy. Sturge-Weber disease is characterized by a port-wine capillary nevus on the face (classically in the distribution of the first division of the trigeminal nerve), focal seizures on the contralateral side, and intracranial calcifications on the ipsilateral side. Therefore, the correct answer to Question 23 is (**C**), gyriform calcifications. The intracranial pathology is caused by hemangiomatous changes of the meninges. This is a congenital disorder, probably of nongenetic basis. The seizures often are very difficult to control. Other common features include mental deficiency and a contralateral hemiparesis. (*Rudolph, 2347*)

24. This question is exceedingly difficult, so your first task is to establish a probable diagnosis. If you were not able to deduce the diagnosis from the question, how about from the list of answers?

TABLE 1-1.

Urinary Finding	Disease
Dermatan and heparan sulfate	Hurler syndrome
Galactose	Galactosemia
Mannose	Mannosidosis
Odor of maple syrup	Branched-chain
aminoacidemia	
Odor of sweaty feet	Isovaleryl CoA
dehydrogenase deficiency	

The correct answer is (**A**). The child described has Hurler syndrome, a form of mucopolysaccharidosis. This rare, autosomal recessive disorder is characterized by growth retardation that generally starts after the first year of life. Classically, facial features become coarse and eventually appear gargoyle-like. Hepatosplenomegaly results from the accumulation of mucopolysaccharide and often is striking. Bone and joint involvement with kyphosis and joint contractures are frequent. Corneal clouding results from the deposition of mucopolysaccharide in that organ. The accumulation of mucopolysaccharide within the brain leads to mental retardation.

If you were not familiar with Hurler syndrome and did not know that it is characterized by dermatan and heparan sulfate in the urine, you would not be able to answer the question. On the other hand, you might know that information and still not be able to answer the question if you could not successfully recall the disease and match the features to the patient in the question. Exploring each potential answer and trying to recall the conditions with which it is associated could help. (*Rudolph, 2329*)

25. (**D**) In a matching question with six or fewer choices, it is practical to read and briefly think about each lettered choice before attempting to answer the numbered questions.

    The lesions of molluscum contagiosum are typically quite small, from pinhead size to

5 or 10 mm in diameter. Larger lesions do occur but are infrequent. The lesions usually have an easily recognized appearance: round, dome-shaped papules with a translucent top and a waxy, whitish material inside. Umbilication is common, especially of larger lesions. The condition is caused by a DNA pox virus and is spread by direct contact with an infected individual. Lesions may occur anywhere but are most common on the arms and trunk. *(McMillan, 831; Rudolph, 1056, 1220)*

26. **(C)** Condyloma acuminatum are soft, fleshy, papular, or pedunculated lesions occurring around the genitalia and/or rectum. Although these lesions are caused by the human papillomavirus and are sexually transmitted in adolescents and older children, it is now believed that most cases in infants and very young children are not sexually acquired but are rather acquired during passage through the birth canal. *(Rudolph, 267)*

27. **(E)** The typical lesion of pityriasis rosea is an ovoid, pink papule or plaque with fine scales. Lesions typically follow tension lines on the skin, giving the appearance of the branches of a pine tree or a Christmas tree on the patient's back. A single lesion appearing a week or two before other lesions is a common occurrence and is referred to as a herald patch. *(Rudolph, 1181)*

28. In this type of matching question, up to 26 options are presented for each item. The choices represent a long differential diagnosis for the infant with hyperbilirubinemia. When the list of options is long (more than six), it becomes inefficient and time consuming to evaluate each possible lettered choice for each numbered item. However, it is helpful to scan or preview the list of options. Then, for each numbered item, decide what the best answer would be and look for it in the list of possible choices.

    It is clear that the 3-day-old term infant in this question has unconjugated hyperbilirubinemia but is otherwise well and has no evidence of hemolysis. The most likely cause of these findings would be physiologic jaundice, a generally benign condition of neonates associated with hepatic immaturity and a peak bilirubin level of less than 13 mg/dL on day of life 3 or 4 for a term infant and 15 mg/dL or less on day 5–7 for a preterm infant. Since physiologic jaundice is one of the options listed **(Q)**, the examinee need look no further. However, if time permits, scanning the list for other potential answers would be a wise safety measure. Although it is true that some of the other conditions listed, such as breast milk jaundice or Crigler-Najjar syndrome, could cause similar findings, we are not told that the infant is being breast-fed, and Crigler-Najjar syndrome is exceedingly rare. Physiologic jaundice is clearly the most likely cause and therefore the best choice. *(McMillan, 199–200)*

29. **(C)** This 5-week-old infant has persistent mixed hyperbilirubinemia, suggesting a hepatic disorder. The normal liver enzymes indicate an obstructive rather than an inflammatory condition. Finally, the inability to visualize a gallbladder on ultrasound examination makes biliary atresia the only plausible diagnosis. Prolonged jaundice in the otherwise healthy neonate can signal a potentially lethal hepatic disorder and in the case of biliary atresia, it is essential to understand that timely diagnosis is key in improving the prognosis for affected infants. Intervention with hepatic portoenterostomy which can prevent the progression to liver failure is associated with poorer outcomes in infants whose diagnosis is made beyond 2 months of age. *(Rudolph, 1506–1507; McMillan, 199–200)*

30. **(H)** This infant has had severe, persistent unconjugated hyperbilirubinemia for 4 weeks but is otherwise well. The normal serum levels of conjugated bilirubin and hepatic enzymes rule out most forms of liver disease (obstructive or inflammatory), and there is no evidence of hemolysis. The Coombs test was negative, and the hyperbilirubinemia is too severe and prolonged for either a blood group incompatibility or breast milk jaundice. Such a course for neonatal jaundice is very rare, and therefore one must consider rare causes. Crigler-Najjar syndrome, a congenital deficiency of hepatic enzymes involved in conjugation of bilirubin, is the only disorder that could explain this patient's findings. *(Rudolph, 166, 1489)*

SELECTED READINGS

AAP. Circumcision policy statement. *Pediatrics* 1999;103: 686–693.

Craig JC, Knight JF, et al. Effect of circumcision of urinary tract infection in preschool boys. *J Pediatr.* 1996;128:23–27.

CHAPTER 2

General Pediatrics

Catalina Kersten, MD

This chapter is designed to include topics not covered in other chapters, and to reinforce important concepts that may be discussed elsewhere in the book.

Questions

DIRECTIONS (Questions 1 through 88): Each of the numbered items or incomplete statements in this section is followed by answers or by completions of the statement. Select the one lettered answer or completion that is best in each case.

1. A 6-year-old girl presents with unilateral non-painful, nonsuppurative conjunctivitis and preauricular lymphadenitis. What is the most likely causative organism?

    (A) Mycobacterium avium
    (B) *Bartonella henselae*
    (C) Adenovirus
    (D) *Staphylococcus aureus*
    (E) *Chlamydia trachomatis*

2. You suspect the diagnosis of Werdnig-Hoffman disease in an infant with severe hypotonia. Which other finding will support this diagnosis?

    (A) normal deep tendon reflexes
    (B) seizures
    (C) fasciculations of the tongue
    (D) recurrent fevers
    (E) atrophy of the optic nerve

3. A 16-month-old girl presents with acute onset of truncal ataxia with vomiting, nystagmus, and dysarthria. She is afebrile and has no nuchal rigidity. Which of the following historical items would help you to identify a cause for these symptoms?

    (A) elevated lead level at the age of one year
    (B) febrile seizure episode at the age of 13 months

    (C) sore throat with blisters on palate 3 weeks ago
    (D) febrile illness with rash 2 months ago
    (E) first MMR vaccination 1 month ago

4. You follow a patient with craniosynostosis and congenital malformations of the head and face in your clinic. What other congenital malformations will you most likely find in this patient?

    (A) trachea and esophagus malformations
    (B) heart malformations
    (C) genitourinary tract malformations
    (D) extremity malformations
    (E) spine malformations

5. A 12-year-old boy has migratory arthritis with red, warm, and swollen joints. He has serologic evidence of recent group A streptococcal infection. Arthritis in this condition is characterized by which of the following?

    (A) usually nonpainful
    (B) heals without deformity
    (C) appears after the fever subsides
    (D) seen only in patients with concurrent carditis
    (E) involves large and small joints equally

6. A 2-month-old infant has severe dyspnea and cyanosis. Chest roentgenogram reveals minimal cardiomegaly and a diffuse reticular pattern of the lung fields. Which of the following best explains these findings?

    (A) acute viral myocarditis
    (B) hypoplastic left heart syndrome

(C) pulmonary artery atresia

(D) total anomalous pulmonary drainage with venous obstruction

(E) transposition of the great arteries

7. You suspect the diagnosis of a brain tumor in a 2-year-old girl with a recent history of ataxia, slurred speech, and early morning vomiting. Which statement about childhood brain tumors is true?

(A) Most are located in the midline and/or below the tentorium cerebri.

(B) Brain tumors are a rare type of cancer in childhood.

(C) Signs of increased intracranial pressure are rare on presentation.

(D) Seizures are the presenting complaint in most cases.

(E) Most cases occur in the first year of life.

8. An 8-month-old child has vomiting and screaming episodes for 12 hours. Physical examination reveals a sausage-shaped mass in the right upper quadrant. Which of the following would be most useful?

(A) passage of nasogastric tube

(B) examination of a stool specimen for ova and parasites

(C) blood culture

(D) abdominal ultrasound

(E) barium enema study

9. A 4-year-old boy has failed to grow and has evidence of exocrine pancreatic insufficiency. What is the most likely cause for this?

(A) acute pancreatitis

(B) biliary atresia

(C) Swachman-Diamond syndrome

(D) congenital absence of the pancreas

(E) cystic fibrosis

10. A 5-year-old girl presents with fever and headache. Imaging of the brain reveals a ring-enhancing lesion. Which of the following is the most likely underlying condition in this child?

(A) chronic renal failure

(B) idiopathic or familial epilepsy

(C) congenital cyanotic heart disease

(D) chronic or recurrent tonsillitis

(E) Langerhans cell histiocytosis

11. A 5-year-old girl diagnosed with pauciarticular juvenile idiopathic arthritis has a positive anti-nuclear antibody test. Which of the following would most likely be found in this patient?

(A) pericarditis

(B) nephritis

(C) uveitis

(D) splenomegaly

(E) lymphadenopathy

12. A 2-year-old African-American child presents with painful swelling of the hands and feet. Laboratory evaluation reveals hemoglobin of 9 g/dL with white blood cell count of 11,500 and platelet count of 250,000. Which additional laboratory test will support your diagnosis?

(A) skeletal survey

(B) VDRL testing

(C) bone marrow aspiration

(D) hemoglobin electrophoresis

(E) serum calcium measurement

13. A 2-week-old infant presents with apnea. The infant was born at term after an uncomplicated pregnancy. The mother of this baby had rhinorrhea and cough that started 3 weeks ago and now she has a severe persistent cough with post-tussive emesis. Which treatment should be initiated?

(A) ceftriaxone

(B) amoxicillin

(C) azithromycin

(D) vancomycin

(E) amantidine

14. An 18-month-old toddler has microcytic anemia. Which dietary history finding best explains this?

   (A) pica
   (B) lack of fresh vegetables in the diet
   (C) intake of inadequate amounts of fruit juice
   (D) intake of excessive amounts of vitamin C
   (E) intake of large amounts of unmodified cow's milk

15. A 2-year-old toddler has a large abdominal mass and pancytopenia. Which of the following diagnoses would most likely be established by bone marrow aspiration?

   (A) hepatoblastoma
   (B) neuroblastoma
   (C) renal cell carcinoma
   (D) rhabdomyosarcoma
   (E) Wilms tumor

16. A 14-month-old boy has a 4-month history of intermittent diarrhea. He frequently has explosive bowel movements containing food particles. He is growing well, is otherwise healthy, and has a normal physical examination. What should be the next step?

   (A) reassurance of parents
   (B) stool culture
   (C) total serum qualitative immunoglobulin measurement
   (D) qualitative fecal fat
   (E) prescribe oral antidiarrheal agent

17. A child with polyosteotic fibrous dysplasia of the bones and abnormal skin pigmentation is diagnosed with McCune-Albright syndrome. What other problem is this patient most likely to develop?

   (A) anemia
   (B) deafness
   (C) precocious puberty
   (D) multiple neurofibromas
   (E) chronic glomerulonephritis

18. A normal 6-month-old infant has a continuous cardiac murmur and bounding peripheral pulses. What step should be taken next?

   (A) karyotype evaluation
   (B) surgical or catheter correction of the defect
   (C) life-long endocarditis prophylaxis for at-risk procedures
   (D) repeating examination at the age of 12 months
   (E) reassuring of the parents

19. A newborn has delayed passage of meconium stools and barium enema radiograph shows dilated proximal colon and small obstructed distal colon. What should be the next diagnostic test?

   (A) abdominal CT-scan
   (B) stool studies
   (C) rectal suction biopsies
   (D) sweat chloride testing
   (E) chromosome analysis

20. An 8-year-old boy is referred for new-onset seizures. Which of the following would mostly support a diagnosis of complex partial (psychomotor) seizures?

   (A) normal mental state, consciousness, and responsiveness during seizure
   (B) a brief tonic-clonic phase
   (C) automatisms
   (D) three-per-second spike-and-wave pattern on EEG
   (E) normal mental state, consciousness, and responsiveness after seizure

21. A 14-year-old female has progressive headaches. Examination shows bilateral papillary edema. CT-scan of the brain is normal. What should be the next diagnostic test?

   (A) lumbar puncture with opening pressure
   (B) MRI of the brain
   (C) orbital CT-scan
   (D) urine toxicology screen
   (E) serum beta HCG measurement

22. An infant is born to a mother who is HBsAg positive. What should be the next step?

(A) Check hepatitis B serology on infant and give hepatits B immune globulin if indicated.

(B) Give infant hepatitis B immune globulin.

(C) Vaccinate infant with hepatitis B vaccine.

(D) Give infant hepatitis B immune globulin and hepatitis B vaccine.

(E) Start infant on formula and discourage breastfeeding.

23. A 38-week infant is born to a mother with gestational diabetes. Birth weight is 4255 g. What would you expect to see most commonly in this infant?

(A) neural tube defect

(B) small left colon syndrome

(C) cardiomegaly

(D) hydronephrosis

(E) renal dysplasia

24. A newborn has been diagnosed with aniridia. Which of the following tests should be performed on this patient?

(A) chest radiograph

(B) alpha-fetoprotein measurement

(C) renal function testing

(D) testicular examination

(E) renal ultrasound

25. A 12-year-old girl develops jaundice, progressive tremors, and emotional lability. You are most likely to find which of the following during physical examination?

(A) head circumference greater than 95th percentile

(B) brown discoloration of the limbic region of the cornea

(C) bilateral conductive hearing loss

(D) generalized lymphadenopathy

(E) sacral hair tuft and dimple

26. A 12-month-old infant is unable to sit by herself and parents have noticed an exaggerated startle response. What are you most likely to find on physical examination?

(A) holosystolic murmur

(B) absent knee-jerk reflex

(C) syndactyly

(D) cherry red macular spot

(E) bilateral inguinal hernias

27. An infant has been diagnosed with congenital hypoparathyroidism. What are you most likely to find on evaluation?

(A) microcephaly

(B) hyponatremia

(C) hyperkalemia

(D) goiter

(E) candidiasis

28. A 14-month-old boy has severe eczema, recurrent sinus and ear infections, and thrombocytopenia. What is the inheritance pattern of this disorder?

(A) X-linked

(B) autosomal dominant

(C) autosomal recessive

(D) random mutation

(E) multifactorial

29. A 12-year-old girl has had progressive muscle weakness over the past weeks. She has also developed an erythematous, scaly rash on the face, arms and thighs, and a lacy rash on her upper eyelids. What is the next best laboratory study?

(A) rheumatoid factor

(B) erythrocyte sedimentation rate (ESR)

(C) urine analysis

(D) serum creatinine kinase

(E) antinuclear antibody (ANA) panel

30. A 12-month-old girl has been diagnosed with transient erythroblastopenia of childhood (TEC). Which statement about this disorder is correct?

   (A) Corticosteroid treatment is usually beneficial.
   (B) Red blood cell transfusions may be necessary.
   (C) Hepatosplenomegaly is usually present.
   (D) Spontaneous recovery is uncommon.
   (E) Parvovirus infection has been associated with this disease.

31. A 2-year-old girl is listless and pale. You obtain a complete blood count and find that the patient has severe megaloblastic anemia. What additional history explains this?

   (A) eats only organically grown products
   (B) drinks exclusively goat milk
   (C) has required phototherapy in neonatal period
   (D) has required multiple antibiotics for middle ear infections
   (E) is an infant of a diabetic mother

32. A 12-month-old child has had poor weight gain. The child started to have loose stools at the age of 8 months and has a very poor appetite. On examination, you see a clingy, irritable child with very little subcutaneous fat and a protuberant abdomen. What is the next best test?

   (A) IgA-endomysial antibody
   (B) urine analysis
   (C) sweat chloride
   (D) quantitative immunoglobulins
   (E) fecal blood

33. A 7-year-old girl develops secondary nocturnal enuresis. What is the next best study?

   (A) renal ultrasound
   (B) voiding cystourethrogram
   (C) abdominal radiograph
   (D) urine analysis
   (E) creatinine clearance

34. A 5-year-old girl suffers from a second episode with meningococcal meningitis. What is the best next laboratory study?

   (A) quantitative immunoglobulin levels
   (B) T-cell subset analysis
   (C) CH_{50}
   (D) quantitative nitroblue tetrazolium test
   (E) delayed hypersensitivity skin testing

35. A 2-year-old child is referred to you for evaluation of child abuse. On physical examination, you find a pale child with diffuse petechiae and bilateral proptosis with periorbital ecchymoses. Which of the following statements is true about this condition?

   (A) Age at presentation correlates directly with survival.
   (B) A full skeletal survey should be obtained next.
   (C) Hematuria is a common finding.
   (D) It usually presents between 4 and 8 years of age.
   (E) Spontaneous regression has occurred in some children.

36. Which study is the most important to obtain in a 2-year-old child with Beckwith-Wiedemann syndrome and an abdominal mass?

   (A) hepatobiliary scintigraphy
   (B) upper gastrointestinal endoscopy
   (C) urine catecholamine levels
   (D) serum alpha-fetoprotein level
   (E) voiding cystourethrogram

37. A 9-year-old African-American child presents with anemia and stroke. What is the most likely finding with hemoglobin electrophoresis?

   (A) HbS 45%
   (B) HbA 65%
   (C) HbA_2 15%
   (D) HbF 15%
   (E) HbC 45%

38. A 2-year-old boy from Sudan has failure to thrive, chronic diarrhea, and severe candidiasis. You suspect HIV infection. Which of the following organisms would most likely be found on stool examination?

    (A) rotavirus
    (B) *Salmonella*
    (C) *Cryptosporidium* species
    (D) *Giardia*
    (E) *Yersinia enterocolitica*

39. A 5-year-old boy has severe pharyngitis and culture is positive for group A streptococci. Of the following suppurative and nonsuppurative complications of group A streptococcal pharyngitis and skin infections, which is associated only with pharyngeal infections?

    (A) scarlatina
    (B) toxic shock syndrome
    (C) rheumatic fever
    (D) necrotizing fasciitis
    (E) glomerulonephritis

40. A 7-year-old boy has abdominal pain and a rash that started several days ago. On examination, you notice a palpable purpuric rash over his calves and buttocks with swelling of both ankles. Abdominal examination is unremarkable. What is the most likely laboratory finding?

    (A) decreased platelet count
    (B) hypochromic microcytic anemia
    (C) elevated blood urea nitrogen and creatinine
    (D) low C3 complement levels
    (E) normal clotting parameters

41. A mother with mild mental retardation has a 10-year-old son with severe mental retardation. The boy is tall, has a long face with prominent jaw and large ears. Which statement about his condition is true?

    (A) Premutation carriers generally have phenotypic manifestations.
    (B) Inheritance is autosomal dominant.
    (C) It is the most common form of inherited mental retardation.

    (D) Affected males typically have microorchidism.
    (E) A single gene point mutation is the cause of this syndrome.

42. A 4-month-old female infant has generalized hypotonia, small ears, inner epicanthal folds, clinodactyly, and wide-spaced first and second toes. For which of the following problems is she most at risk?

    (A) leukemia
    (B) patent ductus arteriosus
    (C) seizure disorder
    (D) hearing loss
    (E) gastrointestinal tract anomalies

43. What is the most important test to obtain a diagnosis in a 14-year-old girl with primary amenorrhea, and short stature, who has a history of repaired coarctation of the aorta in infancy?

    (A) sweat chloride testing
    (B) karyotyping
    (C) fluorescent in situ hybridization (FISH) of chromosome 22q11
    (D) pelvic ultrasonography
    (E) lymphocyte subset analysis

44. What are the blood requirements for transfusion of a patient with hypocalcemia, heart defect, and recurrent infections?

    (A) leukocyte depleted
    (B) HLA matched
    (C) CMV negative
    (D) O negative
    (E) irradiated

45. What hematologic abnormality should you suspect in a newborn with bilateral absence of radii?

    (A) thrombocytopenia
    (B) anemia
    (C) neutropenia
    (D) pancytopenia
    (E) lymphopenia

46. What laboratory abnormality do you expect to find in a 3-year-old child with severe mental retardation, coarse facies, hazy corneas, hepatosplenomegaly, and multiple skeletal x-ray abnormalities?

    (A) increased serum homocystine
    (B) deficiency of leucocyte hexosaminidase A
    (C) urinary excretion of dermatan sulfate and heparan sulfate
    (D) deficiency of liver glucose-6-phosphatase activity
    (E) increased serum uric acid

47. A 3-month-old infant is brought to the hospital because of altered mental status changes. Examination shows a sleepy baby who is difficult to arouse. Fundoscopic examination shows retinal hemorrhages. Examination otherwise is unremarkable. What is the best next diagnostic test?

    (A) spinal tap
    (B) hematology profile with smear review
    (C) CT-scan of the head
    (D) skull radiographs
    (E) EEG

48. A previously healthy 5-year-old girl has acute onset of edema and oliguria. Laboratory studies reveal hypoalbuminemia and hypercholesterolemia. Which of the following is the major cause for mortality with this condition?

    (A) bacterial peritonitis
    (B) acute renal failure
    (C) hyperlipidemia
    (D) congestive heart failure
    (E) hypertension

49. A previously healthy 9-year-old boy has had diarrhea for 6 weeks that started after he returned from camp. He has had anorexia, abdominal cramps with abdominal distension, and a 4 pound weight loss. His stools are large, foul-smelling but do not contain blood. What is the best treatment?

    (A) avoidance of lactose in diet
    (B) gluten-free diet
    (C) oral prednisone

    (D) trimethroprim-sulfamethoxazole
    (E) metronidazole

50. A 16-year-old adolescent has morbid obesity. Which of the following conditions is the most common cause for pulmonary insufficiency in obese adolescents?

    (A) pneumothorax
    (B) gastric esophageal reflux disease
    (C) congestive heart failure
    (D) asthma
    (E) sleep apnea

51. The parents of an 8-year-old boy are concerned about their son's short stature. What should be the most important next step?

    (A) measurement of body mass index
    (B) determination of genital maturation stage
    (C) bone age measurement
    (D) determination of height velocity
    (E) determination of weight/height ratio

52. A 7-year-old boy has chronic fecal soiling but only rarely has a voluntary bowel movement. What is the most common explanation for his problem?

    (A) Hirschsprung disease
    (B) functional fecal retention
    (C) hypothyroidism
    (D) lead poisoning
    (E) iron therapy

53. A 6-month-old boy is found to have very low levels of IgG, IgM, and IgA. Which of the following organisms is most likely to cause problems in this patient?

    (A) enterovirus
    (B) herpesvirus
    (C) *Shigella*
    (D) *Escherichia coli*
    (E) *Mycobacterium tuberculosis*

54. An infant is born to a mother who acquired primary CMV infection during pregnancy. What will be the most likely finding in this infant?

(A) hepatosplenomegaly and jaundice

(B) subclinical infection

(C) microcephaly and intrauterine growth retardation

(D) sensorineural hearing loss

(E) thrombocytopenia and purpura

55. A healthy adolescent is found to have elevated blood pressure on several occasions. Which statement is correct?

(A) Obesity is rarely associated with hypertension among adolescents.

(B) Essential hypertension is the most common cause of hypertension among adolescents.

(C) The incidence in Caucasian adolescents is twice that of African-American adolescents.

(D) Most pediatric patients with hypertension are symptomatic.

(E) An adolescent with hypertension should not participate in sports.

56. A 14-year-old girl has irregular menstrual bleeding since menarche 1 year ago. What is the most common cause for this?

(A) immature hypothalamic-pituitary-ovarian axis

(B) polycystic ovarian syndrome

(C) blood dyscrasia

(D) systemic illness

(E) sexually transmitted disease

57. A 3-year-old girl has a mild febrile illness with mild URI symptoms. She has an erythematous rash on both cheeks. Her pregnant mother had arthralgias of the hands wrists, knees, and ankles a week ago. What should be the next action?

(A) Closely monitor the child's sibling who has spherocytosis.

(B) Exclude the child from daycare until rash has resolved.

(C) Exclude the pregnant daycare providers until no further cases are diagnosed for 2 weeks.

(D) Give the mother IVIG.

(E) Give the sibling with spherocytosis IVIG.

58. A 14-year-old boy has an acutely painful and swollen scrotum. What should be the next step?

(A) fine needle aspiration

(B) bone marrow aspiration

(C) surgical exploration

(D) oral antibiotics

(E) bed rest and analgesia

59. A 16-year-old boy presents with fever, fatique, and sore throat. Examination reveals exudative pharyngitis, generalized lymphadenopathy, and mild splenomegaly. Laboratory studies show elevated WBC count with presence of atypical lymphocytes. What is the best action?

(A) no participation in contact sports for next 2–4 weeks

(B) 2-week treatment with oral prednisone

(C) 2-week treatment with oral acyclovir and prednisone

(D) 10 days of oral penicillin

(E) strict bed rest

60. A 4-year-old girl had bloody diarrhea for several days. One week later she develops periorbital edema and fatique. What is the most likely laboratory finding?

(A) elevated PT and PTT

(B) positive ANA

(C) decreased C3 and C4

(D) hypoalbuminemia

(E) anemia and thrombocytopenia

61. An infant with failure to thrive has rectal prolapse. What test will most likely provide the diagnosis?

(A) abdominal CT-scan

(B) rectal biopsies

(C) liver function testing

(D) barium enema study

(E) sweat chloride test

62. A 16-month-old toddler has painless rectal bleeding. His stools have currant jelly consistency. Physical examination of the patient, including rectal examination, is completely normal. A routine barium study is normal. Which of the following is true for this condition?

    (A) Plain abdominal radiographs are usually diagnostic.
    (B) It is the most common congenital gastrointestinal anomaly.
    (C) The abnormality typically is located within 1 cm of the ileocecal valve.
    (D) Most common presentation is partial or complete bowel obstruction.
    (E) It usually becomes clinically apparent after 2 years of age.

63. A 5-day-old infant boy is jaundiced. The total bilirubin level is 14 mg/dL and the direct bilirubin is 4 mg/dL. Which of the following tests is the most appropriate?

    (A) blood type and direct antibody test on the infant's blood
    (B) blood type and direct antibody test on the mother's blood
    (C) urine analysis and culture
    (D) hepatitis serology
    (E) examination of infant's blood smear

64. An 18-year-old boy presents with acute severe chest pain. EKG and enzyme studies confirm an acute myocardial infarction. Cardiac catherization reveals a coronary artery aneurysm with thrombosis. Which constellation of symptoms in his past could explain this finding?

    (A) conjunctivitis, fever, cervical lymphadenopathy
    (B) meningitis, conjunctivitis, pallor
    (C) cervical lymphadenopathy, hepatitis, rash
    (D) fever, irritability, pancreatitis
    (E) hepatosplenomegaly, rash, conjunctivitis

65. A 2-year-old girl has persistent seborrheic dermatitis in the diaper area. In addition she has chronically draining infected ears. In which location do bony lesions most often occur in patients with this disorder?

    (A) ribs
    (B) femur
    (C) sternum
    (D) skull
    (E) humerus

66. A 3-year-boy with severe hypotonia and mild mental retardation is severely obese. He is obsessed with eating and does not have a sense of satiation. What abnormality will you most likely find?

    (A) macrocephaly
    (B) height greater than 95%
    (C) large hands and feet
    (D) thyromegaly
    (E) micropenis and cryptorchidism

67. A 3-year-old girl develops petechiae and bruises on her extremities while she is recovering from a cold. She is brought to medical attention after she has a transient nosebleed. Physical examination shows a toddler with widespread petechiae and bruising who otherwise looks healthy. What is the best treatment for this patient?

    (A) plasmapheresis
    (B) intravenous gammaglobulin
    (C) vincristine and methotrexate
    (D) intravenous antibiotics
    (E) platelet transfusion

68. A 3-month-old infant has persistent stridor. What is the most likely cause?

    (A) vascular ring
    (B) laryngomalacia
    (C) tracheomalacia
    (D) laryngeal cleft
    (E) subglottic stenosis

69. A newborn girl with ambiguous genitalia has severe vomiting with weight loss. What will be the most likely finding?

(A) decreased urinary excretion of 17-ketosteroids

(B) decreased plasma dehydroepiandrosterone sulfate level

(C) increased plasma cortisol

(D) hyponatremia and hyperkalemia

(E) decreased serum ACTH

70. A 9-year-old has hematuria and an increased serologic titer to antistreptolysin O (ASO). What will be the most likely finding?

(A) decreased serum C3

(B) IgA deposits in kidney biopsy

(C) decreased serum albumin

(D) decreased urinary protein/creatine ratio

(E) hypercalciuria

71. A 6-year-old girl with short stature has webbing of the neck, a low posterior hairline, a broad chest, and cubitus valgus. Which organ is affected most frequently in patients with this syndrome?

(A) heart

(B) kidneys

(C) ovaries

(D) thyroid

(E) intestines

72. A 15-year-old female has a 1 year history of secondary amenorrhea. She is an avid gymnast and has an intese fear of becoming fat. Her weight is at 80% of ideal body weight. For what long-term irreversible complication is this patient at greatest risk?

(A) cardiac arrythmias

(B) hypothyroidism

(C) visual impairment

(D) infertility

(E) osteoporosis

73. A newborn boy was diagnosed prenatally with bilateral hydronephrosis, distended bladder, and oligohydramnios. What will be the most likely diagnosis?

(A) urethral strictures

(B) anterior urethral valves

(C) prune-belly syndrome

(D) posterior urethral valves

(E) meatal stenosis

74. A healthy 2-day-old infant has multiple, firm, yellow-white papules on an erythematous base that are widely dispersed over much of the skin. What will be the most likely microscopic finding?

(A) multinucleated giant cells

(B) eosinophilic infiltrate

(C) cytoplasmic inclusion bodies

(D) gram-positive cocci in clusters

(E) IgA deposits

75. A 13-month-old toddler has a tibia fracture after an insignificant fall. Other family members have blue sclerae and recurrent fractures in childhood. For what other problem is this toddler at increased risk?

(A) presenile hearing loss

(B) mental retardation

(C) seizures

(D) recurrent pneumonia

(E) hydrocephalus

76. A 4-week-old male infant has vomiting and a hypochloremic metabolic alkalosis. What is the next best study?

(A) urine organic acids

(B) urine 17-hydroxy progesterone

(C) stool-culture

(D) abdominal ultrasound

(E) head ultrasound

77. A newborn boy has deficiency of the abdominal muscles and urinary tract abnormalities. What other anomaly will you most likely find?

(A) imperforate anus

(B) undescended testes

(C) mental retardation

(D) congenital heart disease

(E) congenital aganglionic megacolon

78. A 15-month-old boy has strabismus and a white pupillary reflex. Ophthalmologic examination reveals a white retinal mass. This patient is at increased risk for development of which other tumor?

    (A) leukemia
    (B) lymphoma
    (C) osteosarcoma
    (D) Ewing sarcoma
    (E) rhabdomyosarcoma

79. A previously healthy 3-month-old infant develops generalized weakness with difficulty in sucking, swallowing, and crying, and labored breathing. No fever is present. Which study will most likely provide the diagnosis?

    (A) stool culture
    (B) blood culture
    (C) head CT-scan
    (D) nerve conduction velocity testing
    (E) cerebrospinal fluid analysis

80. A 3-year-old boy presents with acute right leg pain and a limp. There is no history of trauma. He holds his right hip in external rotation and flexion and he has mild restriction of range of motion. He appears otherwise well and is afebrile. His WBC is normal and ESR is 25 mm/h. What is the best treatment option at this time?

    (A) intravenous antibiotics
    (B) surgical drainage of the right hip joint
    (C) anti-inflammatory drugs and bed rest
    (D) oral antibiotics
    (E) intra-articular corticosteroids

81. You have followed a 7-month-old infant who has failed to gain weight. Birth weight was 3250 g; the child currently weighs 5.5 kg. In your office, the baby takes an 8-oz bottle with ease and does not vomit. What is the next best step?

    (A) placement of nasogastric feeding tube
    (B) hospitalization of the child with unlimited feedings
    (C) contact child protective services for placement in foster care

    (D) a barium swallowing study
    (E) scheduled return visit in 1 month

82. A patient with streptococcal pharyngitis develops tender red bumps along her entire tibia. What is the most likely diagnosis?

    (A) sarcoidosis
    (B) cellulitis
    (C) thrombophlebitis
    (D) insect bites
    (E) erythema nodosum

83. A 2-year-old child develops apnea, cyanosis, and loss of consciousness with repeated generalized clonic jerks after being scolded by his mother. On examination, the child appears completely normal. What is the best treatment option?

    (A) tegretol
    (B) valproic acid
    (C) antiarrhythmics
    (D) cardiac pacemaker
    (E) counseling of parents

84. A 16-year-old high school soccer player complains of chronic knee pain that has not been associated with an injury. The pain is worse upon going upstairs and after sitting for prolonged periods. The only abnormal finding on examination is peripatellar tenderness. What is the best next action?

    (A) arthroscopy
    (B) thigh strengthening exercise
    (C) knee brace
    (D) immobilization with cast
    (E) anti-inflammatory drugs

85. You evaluate an 8-year-old girl with hyperactivity and inattentiveness. Which of the following manifestations is required to make a diagnosis of attention-deficit hyperactivity disorder?

    (A) occurrence before the age of 10 years
    (B) concurrent learning disability
    (C) impulsivity
    (D) history of birth trauma
    (E) a sibling with the diagnosis of ADHD

86. You counsel the new parents of a baby boy with hypospadias about circumcision. Which information will you most likely share with the parents?

(A) There is clearly an increased risk for penile cancer in uncircumcised males.

(B) Urinary tract infections are 10–15 times more common in uncircumcised infants.

(C) Circumcision reduces the risk of sexually transmitted diseases.

(D) Complications following circumcision are very rare.

(E) Circumcision can be safely done in infants with hypospadias.

87. A 14-year-old boy has had several measurements of blood pressure. His systolic blood pressure has been above 99th percentile for age and diastolic blood pressure has ranged between 90th to 94th percentile. What should you advise this young man?

(A) Complete restriction of exercise is necessary.

(B) Patient can participate in competitive sports if there are no signs of target organ damage.

(C) Participation in competitive sports need to be restricted until hypertension is under adequate control.

(D) Complete restriction of exercise with exception of isometric activities is necessary.

(E) Full participation in all sports without restrictions.

DIRECTIONS (Questions 88 through 112): Each set of matching questions in this section consists of a list of five to eight lettered options followed by several numbered items. For each numbered item select the one lettered option with which it is most closely associated. Each lettered option may be selected once, more than once, or not at all.

Questions 88 through 93

(A) Ventricular septal defect
(B) Atrial septal defect
(C) Bicuspid aortic valves
(D) Coronary aneurysm
(E) Third-degree heart block
(F) Aortic aneurysm
(G) Supravalvular aortic stenosis
(H) Pulmonary stenosis

88. Williams syndrome

89. Neonatal lupus

90. Noonan syndrome

91. Kawasaki disease

92. Turner syndrome

93. Marfan syndrome

Questions 94 through 98

(A) 6 weeks of age
(B) 8 weeks of age
(C) 12 weeks of age
(D) 16 weeks of age
(E) 6 months of age
(F) 8 months of age
(G) 12 months of age

94. Sits without support

95. Hands together in midline

96. Bangs two cubes

97. Thumb–finger grasp

98. Disappearance of Moro reflex

Questions 99 through 104

(A) Hb 12 g/dL; WBC 11,500/mm^3; platelets 160,000/mm^3; reticulocytes 1%

(B) Hb 12 g/dL; WBC 11,500/mm^3; platelets 25,000/mm^3; reticulocytes 1%

(C) Hb 5.5 g/dL; WBC 3000/mm^3; platelets 35,000/mm^3; reticulocytes 0.5%

(D) Hb 5.5 g/dL; WBD 8000/mm^3; platelets 400,000/mm^3; reticulocytes 0.5%

(E) Hb 8 g/dL; WBC 19,500/mm^3; platelets 170,000/mm^3; reticulocytes 14%

99. Idiopathic thrombocytopenic purpura

100. Normal 2-year-old child

101. Sickle cell disease, not in crisis

102. Iron deficiency anemia

103. Acute lymphoblastic leukemia

104. Acquired aplastic pancytopenia

Questions 105 through 107

(A) Congenital aganglionic megacolon
(B) Duodenal atresia
(C) Jejunoileal atresia
(D) Intestinal malrotation
(E) Meconium ileus

105. Cystic fibrosis

106. Midgut volvulus

107. Enterocolitis

Questions 108 through 112

(A) Sensorineural deafness
(B) Limb abnormalities
(C) Short stature
(D) Glaucoma
(E) Hydrocephalus
(F) Tram-track calcifications
(G) Saddle nose
(H) Skin, eye, mouth infection

108. Neonatal herpes virus infection

109. Congenital cytomegalovirus infection

110. Congenital toxoplasmosis

111. Congenital syphilis

112. Congenital varicella

Answers and Explanations

1. **(B)** This patient presents with Parinaud oculoglandular syndrome. This syndrome is the most common atypical presentation of cat scratch disease (CSD) but can also occur with tularemia, tuberculosis, and syphilis. CSD is one of the most common causes of subacute lymphadenitis in children. *Bartonella henselae* is the organism that has been associated with the clinical syndrome of CSD. *Bartonella henselae* is transmitted among cats by fleas and bacteremic cats transmit the disease to humans through saliva. Human-to-human transmission does not occur. The conjunctiva is the site of inoculation in oculoglandular syndrome and the conjunctivitis is typically painless and nonsuppurative. A conjunctival granuloma may be present at the inoculation site. Lymphadenopathy most often occurs in the preauricular nodes and less commonly submandibular. *(English, 27:123–127, 2006)*

2. **(C)** Werdnig-Hoffmann disease is an autosomal recessive disorder affecting the anterior horn cells and the motor nuclei of the brainstem. Loss of motor function begins in infancy and progresses fairly rapidly, leading in most cases to ventilatory failure within the first 2 years of life. Clinical features include hypotonia, weakness or paralysis, hyporeflexia, and muscle fasciculations, which are most readily noted in the tongue. Seizures, optic atrophy, and fever are not features of this disorder. There also is a rare, late-onset, more slowly progressive degenerative disorder of the anterior horn cells referred to as Kugelberg-Welander disease. *(Behrman, 2075–2076)*

3. **(C)** This patient most likely has acute cerebellar ataxia. This occurs primarily in children between the age of 1–3 years and is a diagnosis of exclusion. It is often preceded by a viral illness 2–3 weeks prior to onset of symptoms and is thought to represent an autoimmune response to the viral agent affecting the cerebellum. Recognized viral etiologies include varicella, coxsackievirus, or echovirus infection. Other infectious causes of acute ataxia that must be excluded are cerebellar abscess and acute labyrinthitis which is associated with middle ear infection. Toxic causes of acute ataxia such as alcohol, thallium, and phenytoin must be ruled out as well. Brain tumors of the frontal lobe and cerebellum as well as neuroblastoma may all present with ataxia. *(Behrman, 2020)*

4. **(D)** Craniosynostosis is the condition of premature fusion of one or more of the cranial sutures and occurs both as an isolated abnormality and in association with a wide variety of congenital malformations, syndromes, and chromosomal abnormalities. Excluding abnormalities of the head and face, the extremities are the organs most frequently involved with associated defects. The most common and best known such syndrome is the autosomal dominant Apert syndrome. Craniosynostosis plus extensive syndactyly of the fingers and toes occur with this syndrome. *(Behrman, 1992–1993)*

5. **(B)** The arthritis of acute rheumatic fever is a painful acute migratory polyarthritis. Although any joint can be involved, it is primarily the large joints of the extremities that are affected in most cases. Pain and swelling in one joint subsides as another joint becomes symptomatic. Eventually, all joints heal without deformity or other permanent sequelae. Fever and arthritis usually occur concomitantly but may occur in the presence or absence of carditis. *(Behrman, 876)*

6. **(D)** The clinical findings described are classic for the entity of total anomalous pulmonary venous return with obstruction of the veins. In this condition, the pulmonary veins drain to the right rather than the left atrium. After mixing with systemic venous return in the right atrium, some of the oxygenated pulmonary venous blood shunts across the foramen ovale (which is kept open by the increased right atrial pressure), providing a right-to-left shunt of partially oxygenated blood into the systemic circulation. In many cases, the pulmonary venous return is not directly into the right atrium but rather takes a devious route, often coursing below the diaphragm before reaching the right atrium. In such instances, venous obstruction is the rule, and cyanosis results both from the right-to-left shunt and from wet, congested lungs. A diffuse reticular pattern to the lung fields is characteristically seen on radiograph. Although the heart may be considerably enlarged in patients without venous obstruction, it is characteristically normal or only minimally enlarged in those with obstruction. *(Behrman, 1538–1539)*

7. **(A)** Brain tumors, although rare in the first year of life, are the second most common type of cancer in childhood, exceeded only by leukemia. More than half of the tumors in children are located below the tentorium, and about three-quarters are in the midline. For this reason, increased intracranial pressure from obstruction of the third or fourth ventricle is a common finding. Seizures can be the presenting complaint but are not in the majority of cases. *(Behrman, 1702–1703)*

8. **(E)** The infant described most likely has an intussusception of the intestine. This condition is most frequent in the second half of the first year of life and involves the telescoping of one segment of bowel into another, most frequently the ileum into the colon (ileocolic intussusception). Intermittent abdominal pain and vomiting are common features. Mild fever and leukocytosis are frequent. Very often the intussusceptum can be palpated as a sausage-shaped mass. Circulation to the intussuscepted bowel can be impaired, resulting in discharge of a bloody, mucous stool—the so-called "currant jelly" stool. Barium enema is the procedure of choice because it can be therapeutic as well as diagnostic. Under fluoroscopic visualization, the radiologist usually is able to employ the hydrostatic pressure of the enema to reduce the intussuscepted bowel. *(Behrman, 1242–1243)*

9. **(E)** Cystic fibrosis is the most common cause of pancreatic insufficiency in childhood, accounting for almost all cases. Biliary atresia is not associated with pancreatic insufficiency. Congenital hypoplasia or absence of the pancreas is recognized but rare. Schwachman syndrome is a rare condition of unknown cause characterized by pancreatic insufficiency and neutropenia. Acute pancreatitis usually does not lead to pancreatic insufficiency. *(Behrman, 1299–1300)*

10. **(C)** Brain abscess is an infrequent but not rare disorder of childhood. Most childhood brain abscesses occur between age 4 and 8 years. Recognized predisposing conditions include penetrating head injury, brain surgery, immunodeficiency, cystic fibrosis, right-to-left intracardiac shunts, and infection of the middle ear, mastoid, or facial sinuses. Right-to-left intracardiac shunts in children with cyanotic congenital heart disease bypass the macrophage-filtering mechanism of the lungs and increase the access of bacteria to the brain. In these children, cerebral hypoxia and focal encephalomalacia also may predispose to infection. *(Behrman, 2047–2048)*

11. **(C)** There are three classic clinical presentations of juvenile idiopathic arthritis (JIA)—acute systemic, pauciarticular, and polyarticular. The figure demonstrates the typical knee arthritis seen in a girl with pauciarticular disease (see Figure 2-1). The frequency of ANA seropositivity is highest in girls with younger age at onset of disease. Among children who have oligoarthritis and uveitis there is highest prevalence of positive ANAs. Determination of ANA seropositivity is therefore helpful in identifying children most at risk for chronic uveitis. *(Cassidy, 224)*

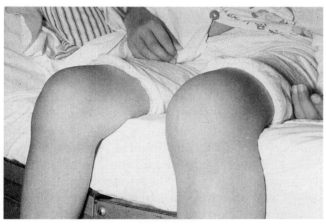

Figure 2-1
(Courtesy of Mary Anne Jackson, MD)

12. **(D)** The child described has the classic hand-foot syndrome seen in infants and toddlers with sickle cell disease. Dactylitis, presumably secondary to infarction of the small bones, causes painful swelling of the hands and feet. Hemoglobin electrophoresis would show presence of high levels of HbS. *(Behrman, 1624–1625)*

13. **(C)** There are many causes of apnea in infants. The extent of the diagnostic workup depends on many factors such as history and physical examination findings. In this case, the symptoms of the mother should raise significant concern for presence of pertussis, a well-recognized cause for apnea in young infants. Pertussis, caused by *B pertussis*, is endemic and the annual incidence has risen in the past year. Coughing adolescents and adults currently are the major reservoir for *B pertussis*. Erythromycin for 14 days in the past has been the standard treatment but current recommendations suggest azithromycin is effective and a shorter duration of therapy is needed. It should be instituted when pertussis is suspected or confirmed to limit the spread of infection; the clinical benefit to the patient who has been coughing for longer than 2 weeks is neglible. New vaccines recently have been licensed for booster immunizations of adolescents and adults (Tdap) and will hopefully serve to reduce the risk of exposure of young infants to the pool of susceptible older patients. *(Behrman, 908–912)*

14. **(E)** Inadequate dietary iron is the leading cause of iron deficiency anemia in children. Milk has low iron content, and the iron in cow's milk is not well absorbed. If a large percentage of dietary calories come from milk, the diet is apt to be low in iron. Additionally, microscopic gastrointestinal blood loss associated with the intake of unmodified cow's milk can contribute to iron deficiency. *(Behrman, 1614–1615)*

15. **(B)** Although rhabdomyosarcoma and infrequently hepatoblastoma, can metastasize to bone, few solid cancers of childhood spread to bone as regularly as neuroblastoma. Additionally, whereas bone metastases of other tumors tend to be focal, involvement by neuroblastoma frequently is diffuse. In some series of neuroblastoma, bone marrow involvement has exceeded 50% of cases. Thus, bone marrow aspiration, even in the absence of radiographic evidence of osseous involvement, is more likely to be diagnostic in neuroblastoma than in any other solid cancer of childhood. *(Behrman, 1709–1710)*

16. **(A)** The patient described most likely has chronic nonspecific diarrhea (CNSD) also called toddler's diarrhea. The diagnosis of this common condition is based on history and physical examination. The presence of normal growth and normal physical examination in the absence of other signs or symptoms despite 4 months of diarrhea makes this the most likely diagnosis. Therefore, reassurance of the parents should occur and no further workup is necessary. It is important that in the process of this office visit, the physician reviews the diet normal for this age including amounts of fruit juices. Antidiarrheal agents are rarely appropriate for infants and children. *(Keating, 25:5–13, 2005)*

17. **(C)** The McCune-Albright syndrome consists of fibrous dysplasia of bone, multiple, large pigmented nevi (generally on only one side of the trunk), and precocious puberty, which is more common in females than in males. Other endocrine disorders occur less frequently and include hyperthyroidism and hyperadrenalism (Cushing syndrome). *(Behrman, 1867)*

18. **(B)** The combination of the continous murmur combined with the wide pulse pressure is typical for a patent ductus arteriosus (PDA). The increased left ventricular output, coupled with runoff from the aorta through the ductus, produces a widened pulse pressure and a bounding or collapsing pulse. The increased flow to the lungs and back to the left ventricle causes hypertrophy of that chamber rather than of the right ventricle. Other more rare conditions such as coronary arteriovenous fistulas, aberrant left coronary artery with massive right coronary collaterals, and truncus arteriosus with torrential pulmonary flow may display similar dynamics as PDA. Spontaneous clusure of the ductus after infancy is extremely rare and patients require surgical or catheter closure. These patients do not need life-long SBE prophylaxis. *(Behrman, 1510–1512, 1569)*

19. **(C)** Congenital megacolon (Hirschsprung disease) is the result of congenital absence of ganglion cells in a segment of large bowel. Absent or deficient peristalsis in the affected segment results in functional obstruction. This causes constipation and distention of bowel proximal to the aganglionic area. It is this chronically distended bowel that has led to the name megacolon. Severe cases present as neonatal intestinal obstruction. Practically all normal, full-term born neonates pass meconium in the first 48 hours of life. Hirschprung disease should be considered in any full-term infant with delayed passage of stool. Rectal manometry and rectal suction biosy are the easiest and most reliable indicators of Hirschprung disease. *(Behrman, 1239–1240)*

20. **(C)** Complex partial seizures is the current name for what previously was termed temporal lobe or psychomotor seizures. Complex partial seizures are characterized by alterations of mental status, consciousness, or responsiveness. During the seizure, there may be confusion, emotional reactions, feelings of detachment, and hallucinations. Automatisms (semipurposeful but inappropriate motor acts) are frequent. There is no tonic or clonic component. Postictal confusion is common. The usual EEG finding is spike-wave activity over one or both temporal lobe regions. A three-per-second spike-and-wave pattern on EEG is characteristic of absence seizures. *(Behrman,1995–1996)*

21. **(A)** This patient has pseudotumor cerebri which is a clinical syndrome that mimics brain tumors. It is characterized by increased intracranial pressure with normal size, position, and anatomy of the ventricles. It is caused by impaired reabsorption of cerebrospinal fluid with or without increased intracerebral blood volume. The causes of pseudotumor cerebri are numerous and involve metabolic, toxic, infectious, hematologic, and anatomic etiologies. A cause is not always identified. The most common symptom is headache. Optic atrophy and blindness are the most serious complications. Treatment options include serial spinal taps to relieve the pressure, acetazolomide, and steroids. *(Behrman, 2048–2049)*

22. **(D)** Hepatitis B vaccines are highly efficacious in preventing perinatal transmission of HBV. Infants born to HBsAg-positive mothers should receive the first dose within 12–24 hours after birth. These infants also should receive hepatitis B immune globulin (HBIG) in the first day of life. Although HBV is found in breast milk, breastfeeding has not been shown to raise the risk of HBV transmission. *(Stellwagen, 27:89–97, 2006)*

23. **(C)** Infants of diabetic mothers tend to be large as a result of increased body fat and enlarged viscera. They may have any of the diverse manifestations of hypoglycemia. A greater incidence of respiratory distress syndrome appears in infants of diabetic mothers. Approximately 30% of these infants have cardiomegaly and heart failure occurs in 5% to 10% of diabetic mothers. Infants of diabetic mothers have a threefold increased incidence of congenital

anomalies. Cardiac malformations and lumbosacral agenesis are among the most common. Neural tube defects, renal anomalies, duodenal or anorectal atresia, holoprosencephaly, and small left colon syndrome also may occur. The incidence of Down syndrome may also be increased. *(Behrman, 613–614)*

24. **(E)** Aniridia involves the whole eye and should not be thought of as an isolated iris defect. Iris tissue usually is present but is hypoplastic. It usually occurs bilaterally and vision is severely impaired. Aniridia can either be a sporadic occurrence or can have an autosomal dominant inheritance pattern. One-fifth of the patients with sporadic anirida will develop Wilms tumor. These patients will need surveillance with renal ultrasound every 4–6 months. There is also an association between Wilms tumor, aniridia, genitourinary anomalies, and mental retardation (WAGR acronym). *(Behrman, 2089)*

25. **(B)** The patient most likely has Wilson disease. Wilson disease or hepatolenticular degeneration is an autosomal recessive disorder of copper metabolism. Copper accumulates in the brain, liver, and cornea where deposits are visible as brown rings (Kayser-Fleischer). Untreated, this disorder ultimately leads to death secondary to hepatic, neurologic, renal, or hematologic complications. Chelation therapy with oral penicillamine should start as early as possible. *(Behrman, 1321–1322)*

26. **(D)** The patient most likely has the infantile form of Tay-Sachs disease. Tay-Sachs is a member of the family of lipid storage diseases. These diseases have a deficiency of a lysosomal hydrolase enzyme, leading to the lysosomal accumulation of specific sphingolipids. Common features of these disorders are neurodegeneration and organomegaly. Tay-Sachs disease is caused by deficiency of hexosaminidase A and is inherited as an autosomal trait with a carrier frequency of 1/25 in the Ashkenazi Jewish population. The infantile form of this disease will often become manifest in early childhood with loss of milestones, increased startle reaction (hyperacusis), and cherry-red spot on retinoscopy. *(Behrman, 462–463)*

27. **(E)** The 22q11 deletion syndrome is characterized by aplasia or hypoplasia of the thymus and parathyroid glands: this results from dysmorphogenesis of the third and fourth pharyngeal pouches during early embryogensis. Other organs that are formed during the same time period are frequently affected as well. Facial abnormalities, esophageal atresia, bifid uvula, and congenital heart disease are some of the anomalies associated with this syndrome. Patients with complete 22q11 deletion syndrome have problems early in life with increased susceptibility to infectious agents such as viruses and fungi. Microcephaly, hyponatremia, hyperkalemia, and goiter are not associated with this syndrome. *(Behrman, 694)*

28. **(B)** The patient described most likely has Wiskott-Aldrich syndrome. This syndrome is characterized by thrombocytopenia, atopic dermatitis, and severe immunodeficiency. The inheritance pattern is X-linked and affects only boys. Severe atopic dermatitis and recurrent infections usually become manifest during the first year of life. These children are susceptible to infections with encapsulated bacteria such as pneumococci, resulting in frequent otitis media, sinusitis, pneumonia, and sepsis. Infections with Pneumocystis carinii, herpes virus, and cytomegalovirus can also become a problem. The only curable treatment is bone marrow transplantation. *(Behrman, 699)*

29. **(D)** The patient has the classical symptoms of juvenile dermatomyositis (JDM). Patients with this disorder usually present with a combination of malaise, fever, fatigue, muscle weakness, and rash. Determination of serum levels of muscle enzymes is important for diagnosis and monitoring the disease course once therapy has been instituted. Rheumatoid factor tests in children with JDM are almost always negative. Antinuclear antibodies (ANAs) can be positive in JDM, however, this would not be the first test of choice. Erythrocyte sedimentation rate is a nonspecific indicator of inflammation and of little help in making a diagnosis of JDM. Renal abnormalities are rare in JDM. *(Cassidy, 407, 424)*

30. **(B)** Corticosteroid therapy is frequently beneficial in the treatment of Diamond-Blackfan syndrome (congenital pure red cell aplasia), but does not appear to have any value in the treatment of TEC. TEC is a transient disorder and usually resolves spontaneously by 1–2 months. Diamond-Blackfan syndrome can become a chronic disease if there is no response to prednisone. Hepatosplenomegaly is not a feature of TEC. Red blood cell transfusions may be necessary for TEC. However, parvovirus infection has been associated with conditions resulting in low hemoglobin concentrations. These include, among others, transient aplastic crisis in children with homolytic anemias and chronic erythroid hypoplasia in immunodeficient patients. Parvovirus infection has not been associated with TEC. *(Behrman, 1606–1608)*

31. **(B)** Megaloblastic anemia in children almost always results from a deficiency of folic acid, vitamin B_{12}, or both. In the peripheral blood, red blood cells are large and frequently hypersegmented neutrophils appear. Folic acid is abundant in many foods, including green vegetables, fruits, and animal organs. Human and cow milk provide adequate amounts of folic acid, but goat milk is clearly deficient in folic acid. Vitamin B_{12} is present in many foods and dietary deficiency is therefore rare. It can be seen in vegans who do not consume any animal products. *(Behrman, 1611)*

32. **(A)** The child described most likely has celiac disease or gluten-sensitive enteropathy. This disorder is the result of small bowel mucosal damage caused by sensitivity to dietary gluten and has an incidence in the United States of approximately 1:10,000. The incidence appears higher in Europe. Symptoms typically start after gluten is introduced in the diet. The clinical spectrum of this disease is wide but failure to thrive, diarrhea, irritability, vomiting, and anorexia are common. The sensitivity and specificity of serum IgA-endomysial antibody testing is very high, but histologic findings on small bowel biopsy remain the standard for making the diagnosis. *(Behrman, 1264–1266)*

33. **(D)** Secondary nocturnal enuresis is defined by the occurrence of nighttime bedwetting after being dry for a minimum of 6 months. An organic cause can only be found in 2% to 3% of patients with nocturnal enuresis. Any organic factors or disease should be ruled out during the office visit. Every child with enuresis should have a urine analysis. Diabetes mellitus, diabetes insipidus, or urinary tract infections can be quickly diagnosed or ruled out. *(Schmitt 18:183–190, 1997)*

34. **(C)** A defect in complement function should be suspected in any patient with recurrent pyogenic infections or recurrent Neisseria meningitidis or N gonorrhea infections. Testing for total hemolytic complement activity (CH_{50}) is a good screening tool for complement abnormalities. *(Behrman, 728–729)*

35. **(E)** The child presented most likely has metastatic neuroblastoma. The median age at diagnosis is 2 years. Age, stage of disease at diagnosis, and biology of the tumor are prognostic factors in neuroblastoma. Children under the age of 1 year with limited disease and without mycn gene amplification have a 95% survival. Imaging with CT scan or MRI, bone scans, and bone marrow biopsy are part of the staging for this disease. Bone radiographs may be abnormal but are not used for staging purposes. Hematuria is not a common feature of this tumor. There are a number of well-documented cases in infants who had complete regression of their tumor without medical intervention. *(Behrman, 1709–1710)*

36. **(D)** Beckwith-Wiedemann syndrome is characterized by neonatal overgrowth. Infants are large for gestational age, have macroglossia, hepatosplenomegaly, and often difficult to control hypoglycemia. Children with this disorder are at increased risk for development of Wilms tumor, hepatoblastoma, and adrenocortical carcinoma. Serum alpha-fetoprotein is elevated in about 90% of patients with hepatoblastoma. *(Behrman, 1712, 1725)*

37. **(D)** The presented patient most likely has sickle cell disease. As many as 10% of patients with sickle cell anemia will exhibit sequelae of

strokes. The diagnosis of sickle cell disease can be made by hemoglobin electrophoresis. A patient who is homozygous for the sickle cell gene has no normal hemoglobin (HbA$_1$), will have a high amount of sickle hemoglobin (HbS), and an increased amount of fetal hemoglobin (HbF). A carrier of the sickle cell gene will have about 50% HbA$_1$ and less than 50% HbS. (*Behrman, 1624–1627*)

38. **(C)** The detection of *Cryptosporidium* in the stool of a patient with chronic diarrhea and malnutrition in the setting of human immunodeficiency virus (HIV) infection would be most likely. This water borne protozoa can been seen in otherwise healthy children but diarrhea is usually self-limited in such cases. Rotavirus, Giardia, Salmonella, and Yersinia have all been associated with gastroenteritis in healthy children and recovery of these organisms would not support a diagnosis of HIV infection. (*Red Book, 271*)

39. **(C)** The incidence of group A streptococcal disease depends on the age group, the season, the climate, and degree of contact with infected individuals. Suppurative and nonsuppurative complications from group A streptococcal disease have increased. Streptococcal skin infections can cause impetigo, cellulitis, erysipelas, and necrotizing fasciitis. Nonsuppurative complications from streptococcal skin infections include scarlatina, poststreptococcal glomerulonephritis, and toxic shock syndrome. Acute rheumatic fever is a nonsuppurative complication from streptococcal pharyngitis but is not associated with streptococcal skin infections. (*Behrman, 873–874*)

40. **(E)** The child described most likely has Henoch-Schönlein purpura (HSP). HSP typically develops in a previously healthy child with a distinctive rash that often involves the extensor surfaces of the lower extremities. Arthritis or arthralgia develops in 75% of cases and most patients have some gastrointestinal symptoms. Intussusception can be a serious complication occurring in about 5% of patients. Renal involvement is detected in about half of the patients and can range from mild to very severe. One percent of patients will develop end-stage renal disease. The diagnosis can be difficult to make when gastrointestinal symptoms or arthritis precede the rash. Laboratory studies are typically not helpful in making the diagnosis. Clotting functions are generally normal and platelet counts in these patients are normal or elevated. Remember, HSP is associated with nonthrombocytopenic purpura (see Figure 2-2). (*Behrman, 826–828; Zitelli, 248–250*)

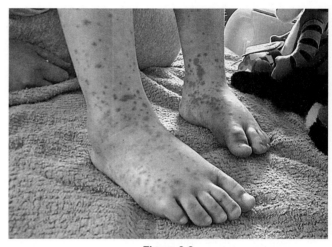

Figure 2-2
(*Courtesy of Mary Anne Jackson, MD*)

41. **(C)** The patient described has signs and symptoms that are very suggestive of fragile X syndrome. Fragile X syndrome is the most frequent cause of hereditary mental retardation. This syndrome is caused by amplification of CGC triplets on the X chromosome. Both male and female premutation carriers of this syndrome typically have no phenotypic manifestations. Premutations can expand to full mutations only in female meiotic transmission. Affected males typically develop testicular enlargement after puberty. (*Behrman, 388; Jones, 160–162*)

42. **(D)** The described patient has classical signs and symptoms of trisomy 21. The occurrence of trisomy 21 or Down syndrome increases with advancing maternal age. There is no single physical finding that makes a diagnosis of Down syndrome; rather, the combination of minor and major anomalies often leads to a diagnosis. All the listed anomalies are more

common in Down syndrome, however, hearing loss affecting more than 60% of patients is the most common. About 40% of patients have cardiac abnormalities with endocardial cushion defect being the most common. *(Jones, 7–11)*

43. **(B)** The patient has classical findings of Turner syndrome. Patients with this syndrome have an XO karyotype. Short stature is the cardinal finding in all girls with Turner syndrome. Ovarian dysgenesis is present and sexual maturation usually fails to occur, although a small percentage of girls may have spontaneous breast development and menstrual periods. Other clinical features that may be present are webbed neck, low hairline, and wide-spaced nipples. Cardiac defects occur in about half of the patients and bicuspid aortic valves are the most commonly found abnormality. Renal abnormalities, such as horseshoe kidney, occur in a majority of patients. *(Behrman, 1931–1934; Jones, 76–81)*

44. **(E)** The patient described most likely has 22q11 deletion syndrome. Dysmorphogenesis of the third and fourth pharyngeal pouches during early embryogenesis leads to thymic and hypoparathyroid aplasia in varying degrees of severity. When absence of the thymus is complete, patients suffer from a severe combined immunodeficiency (SCID) with abnormalities of both B-lymphocyte and T-lymphocyte functions. These infants are at risk for graft versus host disease (GVHD) from nonirradiated blood products and may actually develop GVHD from maternal derived cells in their circulation. 22q11 deletion syndrome can be part of the CATCH 22 syndrome (cardiac, abnormal facies, thymic hypoplasia, cleft palate, hypocalcemia), which includes the broad clinical spectrum of conditions with chromosome 22q11.2 deletions. *(Behrman, 694)*

45. **(A)** Thrombocytopenia absent radius (TAR) syndrome is one of the congenital thrombocytopenia syndromes. The thrombocytopenia severity usually lessens with advancing age. Patients may occasionally have other congenital abnormalities. Wiskott-Aldrich syndrome (WAS) is another congenital thrombocytopenia syndrome in which boys are affected with

thrombocytopenia, eczema, and severe immunodeficiencies. Congenital amegakaryocytic thrombocytopenia usually presents in the first weeks of life with petechiae and purpura. *(Jones, 364–365; Behrman, 1672)*

46. **(C)** The patient described has all the features of mucopolysaccharidosis I (MPS I) or Hurler syndrome. The MPS are inherited disorders characterized by deficiency of lysosomal enzymes needed to break down glycosaminoglycans, the intralysosomal accumulation of glycosaminoglycans, and excessive urinary excretion of glycosaminoglycans such as dermatan sulfate, heparan sulfate, or keratan sulfate. The MPS disorders share many clinical features although in varying degrees of severity. The course is often chronic and progressive, many organs are involved, and typically organomegaly and abnormal facial features and dysostosis multiplex on skeletal radiographs are present. Hurler syndrome is the most severe in this group of disorders and is due to a deficiency of alpha-l-iduronidase. *(Behrman, 483–486; Jones, 524–527)*

47. **(C)** Approximately 85% of shaken babies have retinal hemorrhages. Other findings that are highly suggestive of shaking injury are posterior rib fractures, methaphysial fractures (bucket-handle fractures), and subdural hematomas. These patients may present with coma, convulsions, apnea, and increased intracranial pressure. Often there are no external marks. All children under the age of 2 years in whom physical abuse is suspected should have an initial roentgenologic bone survey done and a repeat study in 7–10 days to reveal healing of fractures that may have been missed on initial film. *(Behrman, 123–124, American Academy of Pediatrics Section on Radiology, 105:1345–1348, 2000)*

48. **(A)** About 75% of nephrotic syndrome in children 1–12 years of age is due to minimal-change disease. The mortality in minimal-change nephrotic syndrome is about 1%–2%. Most of the mortality is related to an increased susceptibility for infections, with bacterial peritonitis being the most serious one. The majority of the remainder of deaths is due to thromboembolic events. Hyperlipidemia is associated with

nephrotic syndrome, but is generally not associated with clinical complications. Acute renal failure can occur with intravascular volume depletion and decreased renal perfusion but is easily treatable. *(Roth, 23:237–247, 2002)*

49. **(E)** The patient most likely has *Giardia intestinalis* infection. Giardiasis occurs worldwide and is endemic in developing countries where sanitation is poor. It is also the most common parasite identified in stool specimens in the United States. Transmission generally occurs through ingestion of cysts from unwashed hands that were in contact with infected feces. Outbreaks can occur from contaminated drinking water and recreational pools. It causes significant morbidity in child-care centers and chronic residential institutions. The clinical manifestations of giardiasis can range from asymptomatic colonization to acute or chronic diarrhea and malabsorption. The current treatment is oral metronidazole for 10 days. *(Behrman, 1125–1127)*

50. **(E)** Obesity in children is on the rise and is reaching epidemic proportions in the United States. Current estimates indicate that 20%–25% of children between the age of 6–19 years are obese. Obesity is a significant risk factor for many serious medical problems. These patients are at risk for psychologic problems, pulmonary insufficiency, skeletal abnormalities, metabolic diseases, cardiovascular diseases, and malignancies. Sleep apnea resulting from upper airway obstruction can be a dangerous complication and is the most common cause for pulmonary insufficiency in obese patients. *(Klish, 19:312–315, 1998)*

51. **(D)** Following and graphing a child's growth is an important tool to assess the general health of the child. Standard growth curves from growth data of different ethnic groups are available. However, the distinction between normal and abnormal growth is not always easy to make. The single most critical factor to determine whether the growth of a child is normal is to determine the height velocity. An easy way to decide if the height velocity is normal is by observing whether the height is crossing percentiles on the linear growth curve. *(Rose, 26: 404–413, 2005)*

52. **(B)** Constipation is a source of frustration for patients, families, and health-care workers. Hard stools, pain with defecation, or failure to pass three stools per week are usually labeled as constipation. There are functional and nonfunctional etiologies of constipation. Functional fecal retention is the most common explanation for childhood constipation. This can first start around potty training time or as a normal avoidance technique in the context of painful anal inflammation. It may be accompanied by early satiety, increasing irritability, and abdominal pain. Unabated functional fecal retention eventually leads to encopresis. *(Abi-Hanna 19:23–31, 1998)*

53. **(A)** The patient most likely has X-linked agammaglobulinemia. Patients with this immunodeficiency typically have no symptoms during the first 6–9 months of life because of passive transfer of maternal antibodies. Thereafter, they are susceptible for severe infections with extracellular pyogenic organisms such as *Streptococcus pneumoniae* and *Haemophilus influenzae*. Fungal infections typically do not occur and viral infections are generally handled well with the exception of hepatitis viruses and enteroviruses. *(Behrman, 689–690)*

54. **(B)** Apprixmately 1%–4% of pregnant women in the United States acquire primary CMV infection during pregnancy. A fetus may become infected as a result of primary and recurrent maternal infection, but risk for fetal infection is greatest with maternal primary CMV infection. Only 5% of all infected infants show the full spectrum of congenital CMV disease with intrauterine growth retardation, prematurity, hepatosplenomegaly, jaundice, thrombocytopenia, purpura, microcephaly, and intracranial calcifications. Another 5% of congenitally infected infants have mild infection. About 90% of congenitally infected infants have subclinical but chronic CMV infection. Sensorineural hearing loss occurs in approximately 7% of infected infants and can even occur in infants who were asymptomatic at birth. *(Behrman, 1066–1069)*

55. **(B)** Hypertension is classified as primary (essential) or secondary. Essential hypertension is a diagnosis of exclusion. Essential hypertension is

the most common cause of hypertension in adults but is a significant pediatric diagnosis only in the adolescent age group. The younger the patient and the more severe the hypertension, the more likely a secondary cause will be found. Coarctation of the aorta is responsible for about a third of the cases of neonatal hypertension. As in adults, hypertension in African-American adolescents is about twice as common as in Caucasian adolescents. Most pediatric patients with hypertension are asymptomatic. Sports participation should not be limited on the basis of hypertension alone. Regular exercise should be part of lifestyle recommendations, especially if the hypertension is associated with obesity. *(Norwood, 23:197–208, 2002)*

56. **(A)** Dysfunctional uterine bleeding (DUB) is most common in the first 2 years after menarche. Almost all cases of DUB during adolescence are due to anovulatory cycles. The most common reason for anovulatory cycles at this age group is immaturity of the hypothalamic-pituitary-ovarian axis. There are other causes for anovulation that must be ruled out. Polycystic ovarian syndrome (PCOS) affects about 5%–10% of women and is associated with irregular menses and physical signs of hyperandrogenism. Systemic illness, especially if associated with significant weight loss, can lead to anovulation. The most common endocrine disorder associated with anovulation is hypothyroidism but hyperprolactinemia and Cushing syndrome are also associated. Abnormal uterine bleeding can sometimes be the first presenting symptom of a blood dyscrasia. These disorders most often present as regular but heavy menses. Sexually transmitted diseases as well as complications of pregnancy can present with irregular and/or painful menses. *(Rimsza 23:227–232, 2002)*

57. **(A)** The child and mother exhibit classical symptoms of human parvovirus B19 infection also called fifth disease or erythema infectiosum. Prodromal symptoms are usually mild and diagnosis is often made when the characteristic rash appears. Initally the rash starts on the face and children have what is often described as a "slapped-cheek" appearance. The rash spreads readily to the rest of the body with a diffuse macular erythema. Central clearing of the macules then occurs rapidly and gives the rash a lacy, reticulated appearance. Joint symptoms are very common in adults and may be the only clinical manifestation of parvovirus B19 infection. The primary target of parvovirus B19 is the erythroid cell line. Children with erythema infectiosum are most infectious prior to the onset of the rash, therefore, exclusion from school or day care after the rash develops is not indicated. Pregnant caregives in day care or schools need not be excluded. Parvovirus B19 has also been associated with hydrops fetalis in pregnant women. It also can cause a more serious transient aplastic crisis in patients with chronic hemolytic diseases. Postexposure prophylaxis with IVIG for pregnant women or patients with chronic hematologic disorders is not indicated. *(Behrman, 1048–1050)*

58. **(C)** Testicular torsion is the most common cause of testicular pain and swelling in adolescent boys. It rarely occurs under the age of 10 years. It is caused by excessive mobility of the testis because of inadequate fixation within the scrotum. After several hours, ischemia to the testis will occur and spermatogenesis is lost. Rapid surgical exploration is indicated when there is suspicion of testicular torsion to preserve function. *(Behrman, 1818–1819)*

59. **(A)** Signs and symptoms in this patient are consistent with infectious mononucleosis most likely caused by Epstein-Barr virus (EBV). A presumptive diagnosis can be made with typical clincal presentation and presence of atypical lymphocytosis. Serologic testing can confirm the diagnosis. Very few healthy adolescents with infectious mononucleosis experience severe complications. The most feared complication is splenic rupture which has a reported occurrence rate of 0.2% in adults and is usually associated with blunt trauma to the abdomen. Participation in contact sports should therefore be avoided for several weeks or until splenomegaly has resolved. Corticosteroids are indicated only if there is severe airway obstruction because of tonsillar enlargement. Acyclovir does not alter the course of the disease. *(Behrman, 1064–1066)*

60. **(E)** The patient exhibits signs and symptoms of hemolytic uremic syndrome (HUS) after an episode of gasteroenteritis most likely caused by enterohemorrhagic strain of E coli. This syndrome is characterized by microangiopathic hemolysis, thrombocytopenia, and acute renal failure. The typical history, clinical picture, and laboratory findings confirm the diagnosis in most patients. Treatment is mainly supportive, frequent peritoneal dialysis needs to be initiated. Mortality is less than 10% with aggressive management of the acute renal failure. Most of the patients will recover normal renal function. *(Behrman, 1746–1747)*

61. **(E)** Rectal prolapse can occur with many disorders such as acute diarrhea, Ehlers-Danlos syndrome, chronic constipation, ulcerative colitis, and cystic fibrosis. For an infant with failure to thrive, the most common diagnosis is cystic fibrosis. However, most cases of rectal prolapse are idiopathic. Usually the protruding rectal mucosa can be reduced by gentle pressure. Controlling the pancreatic steatorrhea with pancreatic enzyme replacement provides adequate treatment in cystic fibrosis. Surgical intervention is occasionally required. Sweat chloride testing remains the fastest and easiest way to diagnose cystic fibrosis. The test may be difficult in the first few weeks of life because of low sweat volumes. The procedure requires care and accuracy and is therefore best done in a laboratory with significant experience. *(Behrman, 1289; 1448–1449)*

62. **(B)** The presented patient has signs and symptoms of Meckel diverticulum, a remnant of the omphalomesenteric duct or the vitelline duct. In the fetus this duct connects the gut to the yolk sac. Meckel diverticulum is the most common congenital gastrointestinal anomaly and occurs in 2%–3% of all infants. They are located within 100 cm of the ileocecal valve. Most of the symptomatic Meckel diverticula are lined with acid-secreting mucosa. The most common symptom is painless rectal bleeding caused by ulceration of the adjacent normal ileal mucosa. Symptoms usually arise in the first 2 years of life, but can occur throughout the first decade. Confirmation of a Meckel diverticulum can be difficult. Plain abdominal radiographs and routine barium studies are usually not helpful. The most sensitive study is a scan with technetium-99m pertechnetate, which is taken up by the mucus-secreting cells of the ectopic gastric mucosa. Surgical excision is the treatment for symptomatic Meckel diverticula. *(Behrman, 1236–1237)*

63. **(C)** The differential diagnosis of jaundice is extensive, but may be divided by elevation of unconjugated (indirect) or conjugated (direct) bilirubin. Elevation of conjugated bilirubin is always pathologic. Causes of direct hyperbilirubinemia generally are infectious or metabolic in nature or otherwise related to intra- or extra-hepatic pathology. Isoimmune hemolysis is a cause of unconjugated hyperbilirubinemia. *(Behrman, 1309–1311; American Academy of Pediatrics Subcommittee on Hyperbilirubinemia, 114, 297–316, 2004)*

64. **(A)** Kawasaki disease, also known as mucocutaneous lymph node syndrome, is the most common cause of acquired heart disease in pediatrics. Criteria for diagnosis are fever for greater than 5 days plus four of the following five features: conjunctivitis, cervical adenitis, mucous membrane changes, a polymorphous rash of the trunk and extremities, and distal extremity changes. The illness can be divided into three phases. The acute phase is characterized by fever, conjunctivitis, cervical adenopathy, rash, mucous membrane changes, extremity swelling, and erythema which are seen in the first 10 days. A subacute phase occurs over the next 7-14 days and is manifested by a decrease in fever, development of thrombocytosis, and distal extremity skin desquamation. Coronary artery aneurysms, which occur in approximately 25% of untreated patients develop 10-40 days into the course. Early treatment with intravenous immunoglobulin and salicylates reduces the risk of developing coronary artery aneurysms. *(Behrman, 823–826)*

65. **(D)** This patient most likely has Langerhans cell histiocytosis (LCH). Three classes of childhood histiocytosis are recognized. They all have in common a prominent accumulation of cells of the monocyte-macrophage lineage. Accumulation can occur in different organs. Eosinophilic

granuloma, Hand-Schüller-Christian disease, and Letterer-Siwe disease are all included in the Class I histiocytoses and are commonly described as LCH. LCH can present as localized or generalized disease. The skeleton is involved in 80% of the patients and bony lesions are most commonly seen in the skull. Chronically draining infected ears can occur with destruction in the mastoid area. About 50% of patients have skin involvement during their course, which is often a seborrheic dermatitis of the scalp or diaper region. *(Behrman 1727–1730)*

66. **(E)** Prader-Willi syndrome is characterized by hypotonia, hypogonadism, obesity, short stature, mental retardation, and undescended testis in males. Although there may be feeding difficulties in infancy, these children eventually develop excessive appetites and obesity. The obesity accentuates the appearance of a micropenis. Hypotonia becomes less marked with time. Hands and feet are generally very small. Microcephaly can be an occasional abnormality. Approximately 70% of affected individuals have a microdeletion of the long arm of the paternal derived chromosome 15. The majority of the remainder are due to two maternal copies of the long arm of chromosome 15 and no paternal copy. *(Jones, 223–227)*

67. **(B)** This patient most likely has idiopathic thrombocytopenic purpura (ITP). ITP is the most common cause of isolated thrombocytopenia in otherwise healthy children. At least half of the cases are preceded by a viral infection. There are no other abnormal physical findings besides the bleeding manifestations. For acute ITP the three most common used therapeutics are prednisone, IVIG, and anti-d immunoglobulin. Platelet transfusions are only indicated in the rare instance of life-threatening bleeding. *(Buchanan, 26:395–402, 2005)*

68. **(B)** Stridor is a musical inspiratory sound of a single pitch produced by narrowing of the extrathoracic airway. Laryngomalacia is the most common cause of persistent stridor in infants, and is usually present by 6 weeks of age. Laryngomalacia is caused by underdevelopment of the cartilaginous support of the supraglottic airway structures. It generally is a benign disorder, which resolves as the cartilaginous support develops, usually by the age of 2 years. Diagnosis is confirmed by direct visualization of the larynx during an endoscopic procedure. *(Behrman, 1409–1410)*

69. **(D)** Congenital adrenal hyperplasia (CAH) with salt-losing disease should be considered in any infant with failure to thrive and ambiguous external genitals. CAH is a family of autosomal recessive disorders of adrenal steroidogenesis that lead to cortisol deficiency. Because of the cortisol deficiency, ACTH levels are increased with resulting adrenocortical hyperplasia and overproduction of intermediary steroid metabolites. Deficiency of 21-hydroxylase accounts for 90% of CAH cases. CAH can lead to a salt-losing disease such as should be suspected in this patient. Laboratory studies would show hyponatremia and hyperkalemia. The diagnosis can be confirmed by increased urinary secretion of 17-ketosteroids and increased plasma levels of dehydroepiandrosterone sulfate (DHEAS). Glucocorticoids should be administered to inhibit the excessive production of androgens and patients with salt-losing disease may also require a mineralocorticoid. *(Behrman, 1909–1914)*

70. **(A)** The differential diagnosis of hematuria in children includes glomerular diseases, extraglomerular renal diseases, and various nonrenal diseases. The glomerular diseases include acute or chronic glomerulonephritis, IgA nephropathy, benign familial hematuria, Alport syndrome, systemic vasculitis, and hemolytic uremic syndrome. Hypercalciuria can also cause hematuria. Serum complement, both total and C3, is decreased in conditions such as poststreptococcal glomerulonephritis, systemic lupus erythematosus, and bacterial endocarditis. Hematuria with a positive ASO and decreased C3 levels confirms a diagnosis of poststreptococcal glomerulonephritis. *(Behrman, 1740–1741)*

71. (C) The patient described has typical findings of Turner syndrome. Half of the patients with Turner syndrome only have one X chromosome (45,X). The other half of patients have a varying amount of mosaicism. At birth these infants are often small with low birth weight and have characteristic edema of the dorsa of the hands and feet and loose skin folds at the nape of the neck. If the diagnosis is not made during childhood, these girls will come to medical attention at puberty because sexual maturation fails to occur. In the absence of one X chromosome, the death of oocytes occurs much more rapidly and nearly all oocytes will be gone by the age of 2 years. The ovaries eventually are described as "streaks" and consist mostly of connective tissue. Associated defects with Turner syndrome are common. About 30% of patients have cardiac anomolies, most often bicusped aortic valves. Renal malformations and autoimmune thyroid disease are also commonly found. Increased incidence of inflammatory bowel disease and gastrointestinal bleeding have been described as well. *(Behrman, 1931–1934)*

72. (E) The patient has key diagnostic criteria of anorexia nervosa as pulished in the DSM-IV. These criteria include fear of becoming obese, disturbance in body image perception, body weight greater than or equal to 15% below expected, and in females the absence of at least three consecutive menstrual cycles. An estimated 0.5% of adolescents and young adults have anorexia nervosa based on DSM-IV criteria. Disturbances in almost any organ can be seen. Congestive heart failure, electrolyte disturbances, and cardiac arrhythmias contribute to the acute mortality, which is about 10%. All these complications are reversible with appropriate management. Amenorrhea can play a major role in the development of osteopenia and osteoporosis and this is the one complication that can have long-term irreversible implications. *(Fisher, 27:5–14, 2006)*

73. (D) Posterior urethral valves are the most common cause of severe obstructive uropathy in newborns. They only occur in boys and in about 30% of patients will lead to end-stage renal disease or chronic renal insufficiency. If the obstruction is very severe, the diagnosis is sometimes made in utero and these infants carry the worst prognosis because they often have associated oligohydramnios and pulmonary hypoplasia. Urethral strictures in males are usually the result of trauma and they are exceptional in females. Anterior urethral valves are very rare. Meatal stenosis is an acquired condition that can occur after circumcision and almost never leads to obstructive uropathy. *(Behrman, 1802–1803)*

74. (B) The neonate most likely has erythema toxicum which is a very common, benign, self-limited eruption. It occurs in approximately 50% of full-term infants and preterm infants are affected less frequently. Lesions may be sparse or numerous and can involve the entire skin but palms and soles are usually spared. The peak incidence occurs on the second day of life, but new lesions may erupt during the first several days of life. The cause of erythema toxicum is unknown. The course is brief and no treatment is necessary. The pustules represent collections of eosinophils in the stratum corneum or deeper in the epidermis. Cultures of the pustules are sterile. *(Behrman, 2162)*

75. (A) This patient most likely has osteogenesis imperfecta (OI) type I. OI is the most common genetic cause of osteoporosis and is caused by defects in type I collagen. There are four recognized forms of OI. Type I is the mildest and can be found in large pedigrees such as in this clinical scenario. Blue sclerae, recurrent fractures in childhood, and presenile hearing loss (30%–60%) may occur in multiple family members. Seizures, mental retardation, and hydrocephalus are not part of this disorder. These patients have mild short stature compared to nonaffected family members. Type II is much more severe and most infants are stillborn or die in the first year of life. Type III is the most severe, nonlethal form and results in significant physical disability. These patients have extreme short stature. Type IV is moderately severe and may present at birth with in utero fractures. Type IV patients have moderate short stature. Patients with Type II OI often die in early life and have a reduced life span because of cardiopulmonary complications. Patients with Type I and Type IV OI have a normal life span. *(Behrman, 2336–2338)*

76. **(D)** The infant presented most likely has pyloric stenosis. Pyloric stenosis is four times as common in boys as in girls. There is a genetic predisposition; infants of mothers with pyloric stenosis have a much higher incidence of pyloric stenosis than the general population. It often presents as nonbilious vomiting in the first weeks of life. The vomiting may become projectile and classically a hypochloremic metabolic alkalosis will develop. The infants generally appear hungry and experienced examiners can feel the thickened pyloric muscle (olive) in most of the cases. After the alkalosis has been corrected, pyloromyotomy can be performed. Elevated urine organic acids can be found in certain metabolic disorders such as organic acidemias, but they would not lead to alkalosis. Measurement of serum or urine 17-hydroxy progesterone would be helpful to diagnose adrenal insufficiency. Adrenal insufficiency may cause persistent vomiting but would not cause alkalosis. Children with gastroenteritis typically have diarrhea and are more prone to develop a metabolic acidosis. *(Behrman, 1229–1231)*

77. **(B)** The infant most likely has prune-belly syndrome, also known as Eagle-Barrett triad. This syndrome occurs mostly in males; only 5% of the patients are females. It is characterized by a deficiency in abdominal muscles, undescended testes, and urinary tract abnormalities. Imperforate anus, mental retardation, congenital heart disease, and congenital aganglionic megacolon (Hirschprung disease) are not associated with this syndrome. *(Behrman, 1801–1802)*

78. **(C)** This patient most likely has retinoblastoma. Retinoblastoma is the most common primary malignant intraocular tumor of childhood and is rarely diagnosed beyond the age of 2 years. Bilateral involvement is evident in 20%–30% of patients. Approximately 30% of retinoblastomas are hereditary. Patients with hereditary retinoblastoma have a significantly increased

risk of developing osteosarcoma. This is thought to be related to loss of heterozygosity of the *Rb gene* which is a tumor suppressor gene. *(Behrman, 1722–1723)*

79. **(A)** The infant most likely suffers from botulism. Botulism is an acute flaccid paralysis caused by the neurotoxin produced by *Clostridium botulinum*. Infant botulism is a life-threatening condition that often is misdiagnosed at onset. In the majority of cases, sepsis is the suspected diagnosis at admission. Botulinum toxin is neurotoxic; it binds irreversibly at cholinergic synapses, blocks the release of acetylcholine, and causes impaired neuromuscular and autonomic transmission. Sensory nerves are not affected and bulbar involvement is severe. In infants, inhalation and subsequent swallowing of airborne clostridial spores most likely cause the disease and prevention is therefore difficult. The only avoidable source of botulinum spores is honey. Honey should not be given to children under the age of 1 year. Routine laboratory studies including cerebrospinal fluid analysis are normal. Nerve conduction velocity and sensory nerve function are normal in botulism. The diagnosis is established by demonstrating the presence of *C botulinum* organisms or toxin in stool. *(Behrman 947–950)*

80. **(C)** Transient synovitis is the most common cause for limping in a healthy child at this age. Transient synovitis classically occurs 1–2 weeks after a nonspecific upper respiratory tract infection. Transient synovitis is a diagnosis of exclusion. Osteomyelitis and septic arthritis must be excluded. Patients with transient synovitis are usually afebrile or may have a low-grade fever. Laboratory studies are usually normal, although a mild elevation in the erythrocyte sedimentation rate may be seen. Ultrasound of the hip can demonstrate a hip joint effusion. Treatment of this disorder is symptomatic with nonsteroidal anti-inflammatory medications. *(Behrman, 808–809)*

81. **(B)** This child most likely has nonorganic (no known medical condition) failure to thrive (FTT) which is far more common than organic (marked by an underlying medical condition)

FTT. Nonorganic FTT is due to lack of adequate caloric intake. Typically, there is an abnormality in the infant–mother relationship. The best-offered option for this child with a weight of 5.5 kg (far below the fifth percentile) is to hospitalize the infant. Unlimited amount of calories should be given, weight should be followed closely and the mother–child interaction should be carefully observed. Typically, children with nonorganic FTT who are in a controlled healthy environment will gain more than 2 oz/day for the first week. It is reasonable and practical to avoid laboratory studies as long as the child is showing good weight gain with this approach. None of the other offered choices are valid options at this point in time. *(Behrman, 133–134)*

82. **(E)** The patient most likely has erythema nodosum, which is characterized by pretibial tender erythematous nodules. Common infectious diseases that have been associated with erythema nodosum are streptococcal pharyngitis, tuberculosis, and other infectious diseases due to *Yersinia*, histoplasmosis, and coccidioidomycosis. Other associated noninfectious diseases are inflammatory bowel disease, sarcoidosis, and spondyloarthropathy. *(Behrman, 794)*

83. **(E)** The patient most likely had a breath-holding spell. These are always provoked by upsetting or scolding a child. The peak age for occurrence is 2 years. The child typically has a brief shrill followed by apnea, cyanosis, and loss of consciousness. Posturing and generalized clonic jerks may occur during an episode. The clinical setting and the occurrence of apnea and cyanosis usually differentiate breath-holding spells from seizure disorders. The best approach is to do a thorough examination followed by an explanation to the parents of the mechanism of breath-holding spells. Breath-holding spells can recur and it is important for parents not to reinforce the child's behavior. *(Behrman, 2010)*

84. **(B)** Patellofemoral pain syndrome is the most common cause of chronic anterior knee pain. As in this patient, it typically worsens upon going up the stairs, after sitting for prolonged periods, or after squatting or running. The finding of peripatellar tenderness on examination confirms the diagnosis. Intensity of treatment is based on the severity of the symptoms and is focused on improving strength and flexibility of the vastus medialis muscle. *(Behrman, 2310–2311)*

85. **(C)** Attention-deficit hyperactivity disorder (ADHD) is characterized by problems with task attendance, motoric overactivity, and impulsivity. According to DSM-IV criteria, the symptoms must be evident before the age of 7 years and must be present in at least two different settings, such as school and home. They must also impair the child's functioning. The prevalence of comorbidities is high. Oppositional and aggressive behaviors, anxiety, mood disorders, and concurrent learning difficulties are some of the more common ones. Comorbidities do not have to be present to meet the diagnostic criteria for ADHD. The presence of another child in the family with ADHD or a history of birth trauma are not criteria of the diagnostics. *(Behrman:107–110)*

86. **(B)** There are many controversies around the subject of circumcision in newborn boys. The American Academy of Pediatrics issued a circumcision policy statement in 1999 and reaffirmed the statement in 2005. The only solid evidence regarding the benefit of circumcision is that urinary tract infections (UTI) are much less common in circumcised infants than in uncircumcised infants. The increased risk for UTI in uncircumcised infants is primarily in the first 6 months, although the risk remains increased at least through the age of 5 years. There is no solid evidence that circumcision significantly lowers the risk for sexually transmitted diseases or penile cancer. Boys with hypospadias should not be circumcised. *(Behrman, 1814; American Academy of Pediatrics Task Force on Circumcision, 103:686–693, 1999)*

87. **(C)** This patient has severe hypertension with systolic blood pressure above the 99th percentile for age. Youth with severe hypertension need to be restricted from competitive sports and highly static activities until their hypertension

is under control and they have no evidence of target organ damage. Cardiovascular conditioning is less strenuous than competitive athletics and youth with severe hypertension may participate in cardiovascular conditioning. Youth who have significant hypertension (95th to 98th percentile) but have no target organ damage may participate in competitive athletics. *(American Academy of Pediatrics Committee on Sports Medicine and Fitness, 99:637–638, 1997)*

88. **(G)** Supravalvular aortic stenosis is the least common type of aortic stenosis. It may be sporadic, familial, or associated with Williams syndrome. Other features of Williams syndrome include mental retardation, elfin facies, and idiopathic hypercalcemia of infancy. *(Behrman, 1516)*

89. **(E)** An infant born to a mother with lupus may develop the neonatal lupus syndrome. Associated problems are cutaneous lesions, liver disease, thrombocytopenia, neutropenia, pulmonary disease, neurologic disease, and congenital heart block. Except for the congenital heart block which often requires cardiac pacing, these associated problems usually resolve without intervention. *(Behrman, 813)*

90. **(H)** Noonan syndrome is characterized by short stature, webbing of the neck, pectus excavatum, characteristic facies, and cardiac defects, most commonly pulmonary valvular stenosis. *(Behrman, 1513, 1925, 1935)*

91. **(D)** Kawasaki disease leads to aneurysms of the coronary or systemic arteries in up to 25% of untreated patients. Three to four percent of patients with Kawasaki disease, treated with intravenous gammaglobulin, will develop aneurysms. *(Behrman, 1591)*

92. **(C)** Clinical features of Turner syndrome include edema of the dorsa of the hands and feet, webbing of the neck, low posterior hairline, broad chest, and short stature. Sexual maturation fails to occur at the expected age. About one-third of the girls with Turner syndrome have bicuspid aortic valves. *(Behrman, 1931–1934)*

93. **(F)** Classical features of Marfan syndrome include tall stature, ocular abnormalities, arachnodactyly, and scoliosis. Morbidity of Marfan syndrome is substantial; about 80%–100% of patients will develop aortic root dilatation. *(Behrman, 2338–2340)*

94. **(E)**, 95. **(C)**, 96. **(F)**, 97. **(F)**, 98. **(C)** Sitting without support is on average mastered at 6 months of life. Generally a 3-month-old infant can bring the hands together in the midline. An average 8-month-old child can bang two cubes and will have a thumb–finger grasp. The Moro reflex is typically absent by 12 weeks of life. *(Behrman, 33–34)*

99. **(B)** In idiopathic thrombocytopenic purpura (ITP) the platelet count is decreased, usually below 60,000/mm^3, while the remainder of the blood count is normal unless there has been significant bleeding, in which case the Hb may be decreased and the reticulocyte count increased. Most pediatric cases of ITP occur in the first 5–6 years of life. *(Behrman, 1670–1671)*

100. **(A)** An Hb concentration of 12 g/dL and a WBC count of 11,500/mm^3 are within statistical "normal" limits for a 2-year-old child (mean 12.5; 10th percentile 11.5). *(Behrman, 1605)*

101. **(E)** In children with sickle cell disease the Hb is usually between 7 and 10 g/dL, and the WBC count is between 15,000 and 25,000/mm^3. The reticulocyte count is increased except in the presence of an aplastic crisis, when the Hb will be lower with low reticulocyte count. *(Behrman, 1605)*

102. **(D)** In the presence of iron deficiency anemia, the reticulocyte count typically is low. Hemoglobin values of 5 g/dL are not uncommon, and values as low as 2 g/dL are seen occasionally in very severe cases. Striking increases in platelet counts have been noted in children with iron deficiency anemia. *(Behrman, 1614–1616)*

103. **(C)** Acute lymphoblastic leukemia (ALL) often presents with anemia and thrombocytopenia. The total WBC count may be increased, normal,

or decreased. In about 10% of the cases, the peripheral WBC count is below 3000/mm³ at the time of presentation. A more definitive diagnosis of ALL in the absence of increased WBC count and absence of lymphoblasts can only be made by examination of the bone marrow. *(Behrman, 1694–1696)*

104. **(C)** As the name implies, in pancytopenia, all blood elements are quantitatively diminished. The low reticulocyte count reflects failure of the bone marrow, which is the usual cause of pancytopenia. *(Behrman, 1642–1646)*

105. **(E)** Meconium ileus is intestinal obstruction in the newborn caused by impacted meconium in the small bowel, usually the ileum. The condition is essentially always associated with cystic fibrosis. In this disease, meconium is abnormally thick and sticky, partly because of abnormal glycoproteins and partly because of pancreatic insufficiency, and accumulates in the intestinal lumen producing bowel obstruction even before birth. About 10%–15% of infants with cystic fibrosis have meconium ileus at birth. *(Behrman, 1440)*

106. **(D)** Malrotation of the intestines is an abnormality that results from a failure of counterclockwise rotation of the fetal intestine as it returns to the abdominal cavity at about week 10 of gestation. The condition often is associated with duodenal obstruction secondary to constricting peritoneal bands. However, in a small percentage of cases, obstruction results from a midgut volvulus. This is a potentially devastating complication in which the mobile, malrotated bowel twists about the superior mesenteric artery. Infarction and necrosis of major segments of bowel may occur. Midgut volvulus is a surgical emergency. *(Behrman, 1235)*

107. **(A)** Enterocolitis is a well-recognized complication of congenital aganglionic megacolon (Hirschsprung disease) that occurs primarily in undiagnosed or inadequately managed patients. Severe recurrent diarrhea secondary to enterocolitis may be the presenting complaint

in a young infant with congenital megacolon. Recognition of the underlying abnormality is important, as the mortality of secondary enterocolitis (toxic megacolon) can be quite high. *(Behrman, 1239–1240)*

108. **(H)** Neonatal herpes virus infections are usually acquired at the time of delivery and many of the mothers do not have evidence of genital herpes lesions. Fifty percent of infants born to mothers who have their primary infection and are shedding virus at the time of delivery, will become infected compared to less than 5% of babies born to mothers with recurrent genital herpes infection. The infection usually manifests within the first month of life. Three major categories exist. The localized skin, eye, and mouth infection is present in about 30%–40% of infants at onset. Isolated CNS infection and disseminated infection are the other two categories. The morbidity and mortality are high, especially with the systemic form of infections. A high index of suspicion for herpes should arise when dealing with infants and sepsis unresponsive to antibiotics. *(Behrman, 1053–1054)*

109. **(A)** Cytomegalovirus (CMV) is the most common identified etiologic agent in congenital infections. Only 5% of infants with congenital CMV have the full spectrum of hepatosplenomegaly, jaundice, petechia, purpura, and microcephaly. The majority of patients are born with subclinical but chronic CMV infections. The most common sequel of congenital CMV infection is sensorineural hearing loss. *(Behrman, 1067–1068)*

110. **(E)** Congenital infection with *Toxoplasma gondii* can range from asymptomatic infection to severe neonatal disease. As with the other congenital infections, patients can have hepatosplenomegaly, thrombocytopenia, and CNS involvement. Intracranial calcifications with congenital toxoplasmosis are usually diffuse. A unique problem with congenital toxoplasmosis is the occurrence of hydrocephalus in some infants. *(Behrman, 1147–1150)*

111. **(G)** The early manifestations of congenital syphilis can involve many different organ systems. Late manifestations are the consequence of chronic inflammation of bone, teeth, and central nervous system. Hutchinson teeth and saddle nose are some of the characteristic findings that occur at later age. *(Behrman, 978–981)*

112. **(B)** Most of the stigmata of congenital varicella syndrome can be attributed to viral-induced nervous system injury. Stigmata involve mainly the skin, extremities, eyes, and brain. Extremities may be shortened and malformed, often covered with zigzag scarring (cicatrix). *(Behrman, 1059)*

CHAPTER 3

The Neonate

Eugenia K. Pallotto, MD

The neonatal period is defined as the period of life from birth until 4 weeks (28 days) of age. This is a vulnerable period of time in the life of a human since the transition from fetal to extrauterine life involves many complex biochemical and physiologic processes. The newborn infant must adapt from dependence on the maternal placental circulation to self-sufficient functioning of all physiologic systems.

There are many unique disease processes that present during this time period along with a unique set of normal laboratory and physiologic parameters. Many problems of the newborn infant are a result of abnormalities in the transition to extrauterine life either due to prematurity, the effects of an immature immunological system, congenital anomalies, or adverse effects of the events surrounding delivery. Understanding of the unique physiology and pathophysiology associated with this period of life is imperative for the physician to be able to appropriately diagnose and treat the newborn infant.

Questions

DIRECTIONS (Questions 1 through 88): For each of the multiple choice questions in this section select the one lettered answer that is the best response in each case.

1. An infant is diagnosed with a given disorder below. Which of these poses the greatest recurrence risk for this patient's future siblings?

   (A) Hirschsprung disease
   (B) cystic fibrosis
   (C) ventricular septal defect
   (D) trisomy 21
   (E) trisomy 13

2. A term infant with microcephaly, jaundice, and thrombocytopenia is thought to have congenital CMV infection. Your attending physician notes though that 1.5% of all newborns may have asymptomatic congenital cytomegalovirus infection. Which of the following is the most commonly reported sequelae of such infections?

   (A) chorioretinitis
   (B) sensorineural hearing loss
   (C) thrombocytopenia
   (D) poor growth
   (E) liver failure

3. A 2-year-old infant has acquired sensorineural hearing loss. His mother is asking what the most likely cause could be. What is the least likely etiology of acquired sensorineural hearing loss in a toddler?

   (A) hyperbilirubinemia
   (B) congenital infection
   (C) aminoglycoside therapy
   (D) neuroblastoma
   (E) late-onset group B streptococcal meningitis

4. The pediatric surgeon is requesting an echocardiogram on a hospitalized newborn with a congenital defect of the gastrointestinal tract. Which of the following defects has the highest incidence of associated cardiac defects?

   (A) omphalocele
   (B) congenital volvulus
   (C) Hirschsprung disease
   (D) gastroschisis
   (E) pyloric stenosis

5. You are a practicing pediatrician in a state where cystic fibrosis is not a routine part of newborn screening. Which of the following symptoms in a newborn infant would prompt you to test for cystic fibrosis?

   (A) pneumonia
   (B) intrauterine growth retardation
   (C) meconium ileus
   (D) wheezing
   (E) hypochloremic alkalosis

6. An infant is born precipitously to a mother without prenatal care and you are requested to determine the infant's gestational age. Of the following, which physical finding is most indicative of a full-term infant?

(A) veins and tributaries are seen over the abdomen
(B) long lanugo is present on the back
(C) palpable breast tissue of less than 1 cm
(D) pitting edema over the tibia
(E) soft ear pinnae, easily folded

7. A 1-week-old term newborn is in your office for a well-child assessment, physical examination findings are consistent with oral candidiasis (thrush). Which of the following is a correct statement regarding thrush in a term newborn?

(A) responds well to topical therapy with nystatin
(B) requires systemic therapy with amphotericin B
(C) requires both topical (nystatin) and systemic (amphotericin) therapy
(D) requires investigation to rule out 22q11 deletion syndrome
(E) requires no treatment

8. During the delivery room resuscitation of a vigorous term newborn, which of the following should be performed first?

(A) Verify the airway is clear, dry, and stimulate the infant.
(B) The heart rate should be auscultated.
(C) Breath sounds should be auscultated.
(D) The mouth and trachea should be suctioned.
(E) Assess color and administer oxygen if necessary.

9. A low-risk newborn infant has pathologic unconjugated hyperbilirubinemia, which is appopriately diagnosed within the first few hours of life due to the astute observation of rapid, progressive jaundice by the nurse. She is asking why the infant was not jaundiced immediately after birth. Which of the following best describes the major route for excretion of bilirubin in the fetus in utero?

(A) via the kidney
(B) transplacental passage
(C) degradation to biliverdin

(D) reincorporation into hemoglobin
(E) hepatic secretion and storage in the intestinal lumen

10. You are the attending physician for a newborn infant with hemolytic jaundice. The mother did not receive prenatal care with this pregnancy or her prior pregnancy. The direct Coombs test is positive. The mother's blood type is A- and the baby's blood type is O+. Her first baby did not have hemolytic jaundice. What is the most likely cause of the hemolytic jaundice?

(A) ABO incompatibility
(B) Toxoplasmosis
(C) Rh incompatibility
(D) rubella
(E) hereditary spherocytosis

11. The blood bank has received an order for an intrauterine transfusion. A fetus with which of the following would most likely require transfusion prior to birth?

(A) erythroblastosis fetalis
(B) sickle cell anemia
(C) spherocytosis
(D) fetal distress and bradycardia
(E) congenital heart disease

12. The obstetrician performing the intrauterine transfusion is counseling the mother regarding complications of this procedure. Which of the following is the most common complication of intrauterine transfusion?

(A) a transfusion reaction (mismatch)
(B) graft-versus-host reaction
(C) premature onset of labor
(D) acquired immunodeficiency syndrome (AIDS)
(E) renal failure

13. During a routine prenatal visit a mother states she has been reading about kernicterus. She is very concerned that her infant will develop kernicterus if she provides breast milk for the infant since she has also read that some breast-fed infants have high bilirubin levels. Which of the following is most predictive for the development of kernicterus?

    (A) hyperbilirubinemia within the first 24 hours of life
    (B) peak conjugated bilirubin level
    (C) peak unconjugated bilirubin level
    (D) duration of hyperbilirubinemia
    (E) hemoglobin level immediately after birth

14. A medical student in your office is assessing a 1-week-old term infant. The mother has been exclusively breast-feeding and the student is not sure how to interpret the change in the infant's weight compared to the birth weight. Which of the following is the expected weight flux for an infant in the first week of life?

    (A) gain approximately 30 g/day
    (B) gain approximately 60 g/day
    (C) neither gain nor lose weight
    (D) lose approximately 5%–10% of its birth weight
    (E) lose approximately 15% of its birth weight

15. A 3-day-old infant is requiring phototherapy for hyperbilirubinemia. Which of the following risk factors best predicts the occurrence of ABO isoimmune hemolytic disease in a newborn?

    (A) first pregnancy
    (B) more than four pregnancies
    (C) prior Rh disease
    (D) maternal blood type is O and infant is type A
    (E) preexisting maternal anemia

16. The patient in Question 15 was hospitalized for 2 weeks, treated with phototherapy for 12 days, and required a red cell transfusion during the hospitalization. Which of the following is the most common serious late clinical manifestation of ABO disease?

    (A) kernicterus
    (B) congestive heart failure
    (C) gallstones
    (D) bilirubinuria
    (E) iron deficiency

17. Prevention of bilirubin encephalopathy or kernicterus is one of the goals for the appropriate diagnosis and treatment of hyperbilirubinemia. Which of the following mechanisms has a role in preventing these adverse outcomes?

    (A) Unconjugated bilirubin is not lipid soluble.
    (B) Unconjugated bilirubin is tightly bound to albumin.
    (C) Unconjugated bilirubin is tightly bound to hemoglobin.
    (D) The blood–brain barrier is impermeable to unconjugated bilirubin.
    (E) Unconjugated bilirubin is rapidly metabolized by cerebrospinal fluid.

18. You are formulating a differential diagnosis for a newborn infant with respiratory distress. Which of the following is most closely associated with the development of neonatal respiratory distress syndrome (hyaline membrane disease)?

    (A) gestational age
    (B) birth weight
    (C) cesarean section delivery
    (D) maternal diabetes
    (E) meconium in the amniotic fluid

19. Which of the following statements is true regarding infants of comparable weight and gestational age (> 1500 g) in the United States regarding mortality rate?

    (A) There is no difference in mortality rates between males and females and African Americans and Caucasians.
    (B) Males have a higher mortality rate than females, and African Americans have a higher mortality rate than Caucasians.
    (C) Males have a lower mortality rate than females, and African Americans have a lower mortality rate than Caucasians.

(D) Males have a higher mortality rate than females, and African Americans have a lower mortality rate than Caucasians.

(E) Males have a lower mortality rate than females, and African Americans have a higher mortality rate than Caucasians.

20. A 29-week-gestation infant is being resuscitated in the delivery room. Surfactant is given through the endotracheal tube. Which of the following is the most physiologically active component of surfactant?

(A) surfactant protein A
(B) surfactant protein B
(C) neutral lipid
(D) water
(E) phospholipid

21. A 25-week-gestation infant is born to a 25-year-old primigravida, who has had preeclampsia. Which of the following is a true statement describing the neonatal mortality rate for this infant?

(A) It decreases with increasing gestational age from 30 weeks through 43 completed weeks of gestation.
(B) It is not related to birth weight.
(C) It is not related to race.
(D) It is higher than the mortality rates of adolescents.
(E) It has not changed significantly since 1980.

22. During the resuscitation of a preterm infant, a medical student in the delivery room is asking why surfactant is so important to neonatal lung physiology. Which of the following is true of surfactant production as it relates to respiratory distress syndrome in a premature infant?

(A) Surfactant is synthesized and stored in the type I alveolar cells.
(B) Surfactant is synthesized and stored in the type II alveolar cells.
(C) Surfactant is produced by the pulmonary alveolar macrophages.

(D) Surfactant is stored in the interstitial spaces in the lungs.
(E) Surfactant is not produced until after labor ensues.

23. A mother presents in active labor, she did not receive prenatal care and is unsure when her last menstrual period was. Using ultrasound, the estimated gestational age is 30 weeks. Which of the following best describes the average birth weight of a 30-week gestation infant?

(A) 500 g
(B) 1000 g
(C) 1500 g
(D) 2000 g
(E) 2500 g

24. A mother presents for prenatal care with a complicated medical history as listed in the following choices. Which of the conditions most predisposes her fetus to congenital heart disease?

(A) hypertension
(B) diabetes mellitus
(C) atherosclerotic coronary vascular disease
(D) anemia
(E) rheumatoid arthritis

25. On a discharge examination you hear a heart murmur and consult the cardiologist. An echocardiogram was notable for a small ventricular septal defect and a patent foramen ovale. You are notifying the parents of the results and explain to them the role of the foramen ovale in fetal life. Which of the following statements are true?

(A) Blood flows through the foramen ovale from the right ventricle to the left ventricle.
(B) Blood flows through the foramen ovale from the left ventricle to the right ventricle.
(C) Blood flows through the foramen ovale from the left atrium to the right atrium.
(D) Blood flows through the foramen ovale from the right atrium to the left atrium.
(E) Blood must pass through the foramen ovale for blood to enter the right atrium from the umbilical vein.

26. A full-term newborn has a diffuse rash on the day of anticipated discharge. You diagnose erythema toxicum and must discuss this finding with the parents. Which of the following is true?

   (A) more common among term than premature infants
   (B) usually associated with fever and a general toxic state
   (C) uncommon before the fifth day of life
   (D) usually associated with an elevated peripheral white blood cell count
   (E) manifested in less than 10% of newborns

27. A mother is hospitalized with high blood pressue at 35 weeks gestation. The perinatologist recommends obtaining a lecithin–sphingomyelin ratio of the amniotic fluid to aid in the decision for delivery. For which of the following systems does the lecithin–sphingomeylin ratio indicate maturity?

   (A) central nervous system
   (B) lungs
   (C) liver
   (D) kidneys
   (E) immunologic system

28. A hospitalized neonate is given the diagnosis of bronchopulmonary dysplasia (BPD). Which of the following best describes the pathophysiology of BPD?

   (A) An inflammatory insult to the lungs late in fetal development.
   (B) Failure of development of pulmonary arterioles during early fetal life.
   (C) Failure of development of the bronchial buds during early fetal life.
   (D) Intrauterine viral infection.
   (E) The use of oxygen and positive-pressure breathing in the treatment of respiratory distress syndrome.

29. A 32-week-gestation infant is now 24 hours old and has had progressive respiratory distress. Given the infant's clinical course and the radiographic appearance of the lungs the decision has been made, in consultation with the neonatologist, to give surfactant replacement therapy for respiratory distress syndrome. Which of the following is true?

   (A) is considered experimental
   (B) is only useful in infants with birth weight less than 1500 g
   (C) has no known complications
   (D) has not been shown to reduce mortality in very low birth weight infants
   (E) requires tracheal intubation to administer

30. You are examining the chest x-ray of a 4-hour-old infant born at 30 weeks gestation. The infant is breathing 100 times per minute while breathing 100% oxygen and intubation is imminent. You suspect respiratory distress syndrome. Which of the following is the characteristic roentgenographic findings of the infant with respiratory distress syndrome?

   (A) lobar atelectasis and interstitial edema
   (B) bilateral patchy densities and pneumothorax
   (C) diffuse reticulogranular changes and air bronchograms
   (D) diffuse hyperaeration and cardiomegaly
   (E) cardiomegaly and interstitial edema

31. After surfactant therapy, the infant with respiratory distress syndrome is treated with continuous positive airway pressure. Which of the following is the major goal of continuous positive airway pressure?

   (A) prevent infection
   (B) prevent pneumothorax
   (C) improve cardiac output
   (D) raise arterial Po_2
   (E) raise arterial Pco_2

32. A 30-week-gestation infant with respiratory distress syndrome is weaning from the ventilator. He currently has an oxygen saturation of 100% while breathing 50% oxygen on minimal ventilator settings. In a premature infant with respiratory distress syndrome, which of the following may be an adverse effect of supplemental oxygen therapy?

(A) alveolar proteinosis
(B) atelectasis
(C) fire or explosion
(D) kernicterus
(E) retinopathy of prematurity

33. The father of a 26-week-gestation infant, who required intubation at birth, is asking why the infant's lungs were not mature. Which of the following is the pathophysiology mechanism of respiratory distress syndrome in the premature infant?

(A) increased production of pulmonary surfactant
(B) decreased production of pulmonary surfactant
(C) increased metabolism of pulmonary surfactant
(D) decreased metabolism of pulmonary surfactant
(E) rerouting of pulmonary surfactant to the systemic circulation

34. A healthy term infant is circumcised and experiences excessive blood loss eventually requiring transfusion. The most likely diagnosis is which of the following?

(A) factor IX deficiency
(B) factor VIII deficiency
(C) von Willebrand disease
(D) disseminated intravascular coagulopathy
(E) protein C deficiency

35. An irregular red reflex is noted on the initial examination of an infant. The infant is referred to the opthalmologist for evaluation of a cataract. Which of the following is most likely to be associated with a cataract in the newborn?

(A) maple syrup urine disease
(B) glucose-6-phosphate dehydrogenase deficiency
(C) phenylketonuria
(D) galactosemia
(E) propionic acidemia

36. A mother has brought her infant into your office for the first newborn visit. She is very concerned about a pigmented skin lesion that was not discussed with her in the hospital. Which of the following is true of pigmented lesions known as slate gray spots?

(A) They never occur in white infants.
(B) They are identified in over 40% of African American infants.
(C) They consist of small, well-demarcated lesions approximately 2 mm in diameter.
(D) Malignant degeneration is common.
(E) The most common site of occurrence is the nape of the neck.

37. A newborn infant presents with cyanosis and mild tachypnea at about 6 hours of life. The infant is placed in 95% oxyhood and saturations normalize. Which of the following is the most likely diagnosis in this infant?

(A) cyanotic congenital heart disease
(B) lung disease
(C) central nervous system disease
(D) liver disease
(E) methemoglobinemia

38. A 35-week-gestation infant is delivered weighing 3.9 kg, with an omphalocele and a large tongue. No other abnormalities are detected. Which of the following is the most likely diagnosis?

(A) congenital hypothyroidism
(B) trisomy 18
(C) trisomy 13
(D) fetal alcohol syndrome
(E) Beckwith-Wiedemann syndrome

39. A 3-week-old infant is noted to have micro-cephaly, cerebral calcifications on skull x-ray, and blindness. Which of the following is the most likely cause of these findings?

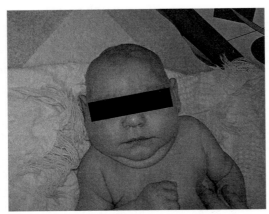

Figure 3-1
(*Courtesy of Angela Myers, MD*)

(A) bilateral subdural hemorrhages
(B) cerebral agenesis
(C) cytomegalovirus infection
(D) erythroblastosis
(E) primary microcephaly

40. A 7-day-old infant develops white, cheesy patches on the tongue and buccal mucosa with mild inflammation of the mucosa. Which of the following organisms is most likely the cause of these oral lesions?

(A) *Candida albicans*
(B) *Listeria monocytogenes*
(C) *Escherichia coli*
(D) group A streptococcus
(E) group B streptococcus

41. You are interviewing a family with a newborn infant. They are new to your practice and you elicit a family history of seizures in both the mother and maternal grandfather. During examination of the infant you note a skin finding that may be associated with the family history of seizures. Which of the following is the most likely skin finding in this infant?

(A) hypopigmented patch
(B) harlequin color change
(C) salmon patch on the nasal glabella
(D) hemangioma of the thigh
(E) pustular melanosis

42. A term, otherwise healthy, neonate has isolated premature synostosis of the sagittal suture. Which of the following is the most likely asso-ciated condition?

(A) scaphocephaly
(B) increased intracranial pressure
(C) microcephaly
(D) hydrocephalus
(E) subdural effusions

43. A healthy newborn is noted to have numerous 3 mm vesicles on the chest and neck, along with several similar-sized hyperpigmented macules in the same distribution. Which of the following is the most likely diagnosis?

(A) mucocutaneous herpes simplex infection
(B) acne neonatorum
(C) erythema toxicum
(D) incontinentia pigmenti
(E) transient neonatal pustular melanosis

44. A newborn infant gags and chokes with feed-ings. He has just had an apneic spell during a feed resulting in significant cyanosis. Which of the following is the most likely diagnosis?

(A) proximal esophageal atresia
(B) hypoplastic left heart syndrome
(C) group B streptococcal sepsis
(D) neonatal herpes simplex infection
(E) pyloric stenosis

45. As a medical student in the newborn nursery, you correctly identify a scalp swelling as a cephalohemtoma. Your attending physician then asks you to describe how you would differenti-ate this from caput succedaneum. Which of the following best describes the way to differentiate a cephalohematoma from caput succedaneum?

(A) absence of a history of prolonged or difficult labor
(B) limitation of swelling to the area over one bone
(C) a normal neurologic examination
(D) a prolonged prothrombin time
(E) a normal lumbar puncture

46. A 40-year-old couple is in your office for genetic counseling prior to having their first child. They are very concerned about advancing maternal age and the possible genetic problems it could cause for their child. Which of the following is the most likely disorder associated with advancing maternal age?

(A) autosomal recessive disorders
(B) nondisjunction chromosome disorders
(C) autosomal dominant disorders
(D) X-linked disorders
(E) inborn errors of metabolism

47. The same couple in Question 46 also is inquiring about the genetic affects of the father's age. Which of the following is the most important disorder associated with advancing paternal age?

(A) autosomal recessive disorders
(B) nondisjunction chromosome disorders
(C) autosomal dominant disorders
(D) X-linked disorders
(E) inborn errors of metabolism

48. A normal newborn is screened for hypoglycemia after birth as per the normal nursery protocol at your hospital. In the asymptomatic term neonate, evaluation and treatment of hypoglycemia should be initiated when the glucose level is at or below which of the following levels?

(A) 10 mg/dL
(B) 20 mg/dL
(C) 40 mg/dL
(D) 60 mg/dL
(E) 80 mg/dL

49. A nurse working in the newborn nursery calls your office because she is concerned about the appearance of the feet of a newborn infant just delivered. Based on her description, the infant has congenital clubfoot. Which of the following systems is most commonly also involved with this disorder?

(A) the central nervous system
(B) the hematopoietic system
(C) the gastrointestinal system
(D) the cardiovascular system
(E) the respiratory system

50. A newborn infant has micrognathia, glossoptosis, and cleft soft palate. These findings are consistent with Pierre Robin sequence. Which of the following life-threatening events is associated with these findings?

(A) heart failure
(B) seizures
(C) intestinal obstruction
(D) metabolic acidosis
(E) upper airway obstruction

51. A consultant in the neonatal intensive care unit is recommending a trial of pyridoxine for a patient. Which of the following problems in a newborn infant might respond to a pharmacologic dose of pyridoxine?

(A) blindness
(B) seizures
(C) jaundice
(D) rash
(E) urinary retention

52. The geneticist is evaluating a patient in the newborn intensive care unit. The possibility of a disorder with a mitochondrial inheritance pattern has been discussed with the family. Which of the following is true of mitochondrial inheritance?

    (A) These disorders commonly follow a paternal line of inheritance.
    (B) These disorders have not been identified in humans thus far.
    (C) Only females are affected.
    (D) Organ systems with low energy demands are the most affected.
    (E) These disorders commonly follow a maternal line of inheritance.

53. A family with an infant in the neonatal intensive care unit is very concerned that their child will have long-term neurologic abnormalities. Of the following, which correlates best with subsequent neurologic abnormalities?

    (A) fetal bradycardia
    (B) failure to breathe at birth
    (C) a low 1-minute Apgar score
    (D) a low 5-minute Apgar score
    (E) seizures in the first 36 hours of life

54. An 8-day-old infant develops inflammatory papules and pustules on the forehead, nose, and malar areas of the face. The child is otherwise well, and the remainder of the physical examination is normal. Which of the following is the most likely diagnosis?

    (A) congenital syphilis
    (B) impetigo
    (C) neonatal acne
    (D) staphylococcal pustulosis
    (E) tuberous sclerosis

55. You are counseling a mother with an abnormal serum alpha-fetoprotein test during a follow-up prenatal visit. The maternal serum alpha-fetoprotein test is most useful in diagnosing which of the following?

    (A) duodenal atresia
    (B) clubfoot
    (C) cleft lip and palate
    (D) myelomeningocele
    (E) alveolar proteinosis

56. A newborn with trisomy 21 develops bilious emesis on the first day of life. An abdominal x-ray reveals a "double bubble sign." Which of the following is the most likely diagnosis?

    (A) annular pancreas
    (B) duodenal atresia
    (C) gastric volvulus
    (D) pyloric stenosis
    (E) Hirschsprung disease

57. A 1700-g infant was asphyxiated at birth, after a successful resuscitation, the infant had numerous apneic episodes. On the third day of life, the infant began to vomit. Abdominal distention and bloody stools were noted. Which of the following is the most likely diagnosis?

    (A) congenital aganglionic megacolon
    (B) intussusception
    (C) necrotizing enterocolitis
    (D) Shigella enteritis
    (E) volvulus

58. A 2-month-old infant is in your office for a well-child examination. The mother is asking you about a red macule on the infant's cheek. She describes it as getting larger over the past few weeks. You suspect this is a capillary hemagioma. The natural history of an elevated capillary or cavernous hemangioma is best described by which of the following statements?

    (A) no significant change in size after birth.
    (B) an increase in size during the first few years after birth and then regression.
    (C) an increase in size during the first decade of life and then no further change.
    (D) a slow but progressive increase in size throughout life.
    (E) a slow but progressive decrease in size starting shortly after birth.

(C) respiratory acidosis and hypoxemia

(D) respiratory and metabolic alkalosis

(E) metabolic acidosis and respiratory alkalosis

100. A college student delivers an infant in the campus housing area after denying her pregnancy and experiencing 6 hours of abdominal pain. Paramedics arrive and find an infant they estimate to be 4–5 lb in weight, crying but slightly dusky. They administer oxygen. The newborn's temperature is 94°F. Hypothermia in this infant would produce which of the following?

(A) decreased oxygen consumption

(B) hypertriglyceridemia

(C) hypercalcemia

(D) hypoglycemia

(E) metabolic alkalosis

101. A 30-day-old, former 24-weeks gestation, 600 g neonate had a difficult initial respiratory course complicated by a tension pneumothorax. She had serial head ultrasound evaluations during the first weeks of life. All previous studies revealed a normal immature brain. Now, the head ultrasound reveals an abnormality. Among the following, which is most likely?

(A) grade II intraventricular hemorrhage

(B) grade IV intraventricular hemorrhage

(C) aqueductal stenosis

(D) periventricular leukomalacia

(E) vein of Galen aneurysm

102. A newborn infant has signs of congestive heart failure. Physical examination does not reveal a significant cardiac murmur. Auscultation of the head reveals a loud cranial bruit. Which of the following is the most likely diagnosis?

(A) polycythemia

(B) hyperthyroidism

(C) ruptured cerebral aneurysm

(D) transposition of the great vessels

(E) arteriovenous malformation of the great vein of Galen

103. A term 4.3-kg infant is delivered vaginally to a 33-year-old woman with juvenile-onset diabetes. The delivery was complicated by severe shoulder dystocia and the infant experienced a brachial plexus injury with limited movement of the right arm. At 72 hours of age, the infant is noted to be tachypneic but he is pink and well perfused. Which of the following is the most likely explanation for his tachypnea?

(A) respiratory distress syndrome (RDS)

(B) diaphragmatic paralysis

(C) pulmonary hemorrhage

(D) pneumothorax

(E) cystic adenomatoid malformation of the lung

104. A term infant is delivered vaginally to an 18-year-old primagravida after an uncomplicated pregnancy. Mother presented with rupture of membranes and a low-grade fever. Labor and delivery proceeded rapidly, maternal antibiotics were not administered prior to delivery of the infant. Maternal screening during pregnancy for group B streptococcus was negative. At 30 hours of age the infant is mottled, not feeding well, and cries when handled. A lumbar puncture is performed and the spinal fluid reveals 660 WBC/mm^3 and a CSF protein of 290 mg/dL. Which of the following is the most likely agent causing this infant's infection?

(A) group B streptococcus

(B) *Escherichia coli*

(C) *Listeria monocytogenes*

(D) *Haemophilus influenzae*

(E) *Streptococcus pneumoniae*

Answers and Explanations

1. **(B)** Cystic fibrosis (CF) is inherited in an autosomal recessive fashion, creating a 25% recurrence risk for subsequent pregnancies. Hirschsprung disease usually is sporadic with a risk of about 3%–5% to siblings of an affected case. There are rare families with Hirschsprung disease transmitted as an autosomal dominant or recessive pattern of inheritance. Ventricular septal defects are also multifactorial in inheritance, the recurrent risk for siblings of a patient with congenital heart disease is 3%–4%. Trisomies are most typically sporadic events and recurrence varies depending on the mother's age. A small proportion of trisomies are transmitted by a parent as part of a balanced translocation with higher recurrence risks in those families. *(Behrman 1239; Brodsky, 165)*

2. **(B)** The majority (90%–95%) of newborn infants infected with cytomegalovirus are asymptomatic at birth. Asymptomatic congenital cytomegalovirus infection is a leading cause of sensorineural hearing loss, which can occur in approximately 7% of infants. Hearing loss is often progressive and may not be detected until the patient is older. Sudden loss of residual hearing at age 4–5 years has been associated with congenital cytomegalovirus. *(Behrman, 1067, 2129)*

3. **(D)** Congenital infections with cytomegalovirus, toxoplasmosis, or syphilis may present with delayed onset of sensorineural hearing loss. Hyperbilirubinemia at levels requiring exchange transfusion is also associated with sensorineural hearing loss. Aminoglycosides put an infant at increased risk for hearing loss particularly when used in combination with other ototoxic drugs or when levels are not appropriately monitored with adequate dosing adjustments in response to these levels. Bacterial meningitis also has a strong association with hearing impairment. Although some cheomotherapeutic agents are associated with hearing loss, neuroblastoma does not have a primary association with sensorineural hearing loss. *(Behrman, 2130)*

4. **(A)** Omphaloceles are among the most common of the abdominal wall defects noted in the newborn and pediatricians must know how to diagnose and provide additional care. In addition, they need to understand the association with other defects. Cardiovascular anomalies occur in 25%–30% of infants with omphaloceles. Omphaloceles also are frequently associated with chromosomal anomalies (50%) and other

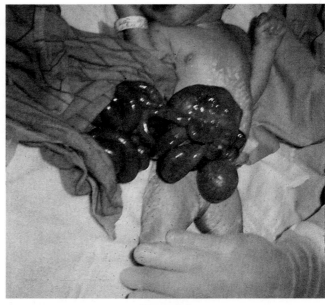

Figure 3-4
(Courtesy of Emily A. Thorell, MD)

syndromes including the Beckwith-Wiedemann syndrome (omphalocele, severe hypoglycemia, macrosomia, and macroglossia). Gastroschisis is a defect of the abdominal wall which is often confused with omphalocele. It is characterized by a defect where the intestines are located outside of the abdomen, and exposed to the air. Unlike omphalocele, there is no sac over the intestines (see Figure 3-4).

The other lesions listed are not typically associated with chromosomal, syndromic, or other nongastrointestinal anomalies. *(Brodsky, 273)*

5. **(C)** The newborn with cystic fibrosis generally is asymptomatic. The most common manifestation, meconium ileus, occurs in 15%–20% of CF patients. The ileum is completely obstructed with meconium, which results in intestinal obstruction. The meconium plug syndrome also is seen with an increased frequency in infants with cystic fibrosis, but it is less specific than meconium ileus. Sweat chloride testing in suspected cases of cystic fibrosis has always been troublesome in the newborn period but DNA testing is now available and is 90%–95% sensitive. In the United States, some states have instituted routine newborn screening for cystic fibrosis. *(Behrman, 1437)*

6. **(C)** Breast hypertrophy is common in full-term infants. The less mature the infant, the smaller the amount of breast tissue. Long lanugo, translucent skin, and a soft ear pinna that does not readily recoil are indicative of prematurity. The Ballard scoring system uses physical findings such as these to determine the gestational age of the newborn. Veins and tributaries over the abdomen and pitting edema over the tibia are associated with pathological conditions and are not used in gestational age assessment. *(Ballard, 1991)*

7. **(A)** Oral candidiasis (thrush) is a common problem and typically does not indicate a serious underlying problem. It is seen frequently in the first few weeks of life. The primary means of infection in healthy newborns is vertical transmission from maternal vaginal moniliasis. It typically requires no immunologic investigation and usually responds rapidly to treatment with oral nystatin suspension. Treating possible sources such as the thumb, the breast, bottle nipples, or pacifier is important to avoid recurrence. If thrush occurs after infancy, or if it is atypically recurrent and/or resistent, investigation of the immune system may be warranted. Immunodeficiency diseases that are associated with T-cell disorders, such as 22q11 deletion syndrome or HIV infection, should be considered. In the sick, premature infant, especially those with central lines or other invasive devices, oral thrush is more serious and may herald systemic infection. *(Burg, 150; Behrman, 588)*

8. **(A)** Resuscitation of the newborn is a systematic procedure with a logical progression of events, which best ensures a successful outcome. The infant should be placed on a warmer, left uncovered, and positioned in the "sniffing" position. If no meconium is present, secretions should be removed from the mouth and then nose with a bulb syringe in order to clear the airway. Once the airway is clear, drying the infant thoroughly will provide stimulation for the infant and will prevent heat loss. Removal of the wet linen is an important step to prevent further heat loss. Assessment of heart rate, respirations, and color should not be completed until these important first steps have been carried out. Suction of the mouth and trachea may be indicated as a first step if meconium is present and the baby is not vigorous. *(Kattwinkel, Lesson 2)*

9. **(B)** Unconjugated bilirubin passes easily across the placenta. This is the major mechanism for fetal elimination of bilirubin. Bilverdin reductase converts biliverdin to bilirubin. The placenta does not eliminate biliverdin, thus there is a fetal advantage to make bilirubin. During fetal life, normal bowel function is not established and the hepatic conjugating system is somewhat dormant so these sytems do not play a prominent role in bilirubin removal. Unconjugated bilirubin (more fat soluble and less water soluble than conjugated bilirubin) easily crosses the placenta to the maternal circulation for disposal by the maternal liver. *(Fanaroff, 1425; Brodsky, 301)*

10. **(C)** Rh hemolytic disease rarely occurs in the first pregnancy, but transfusion of Rh+ blood into an Rh– mother sensitizes the mother resulting initially in production of IgM antibodies, followed by IgG antibody production. Once a mother is sensitized, the following pregnancies result in hemolytic disease. Sensitization is prevented by injection of anti-D gamma globulin (RhoGAM) at 28 weeks' gestation and immediately after delivery. The incidence of Rh incompatibility is 11/10,000 total births. Prior to RhoGAM, it developed in 1% of pregnancies. Hereditary spherocytosis and congenital infections, causing hemolytic disease, are distinguished by negative Coombs testing as well as other clinical characteristic exam findings or peripheral smear findings. ABO incompatibility may occur in the first pregnancy. Subsequent pregnancies are not more severely affected. It would not occur when the fetus is blood type O. *(Brodsky, 289; Behrman, 601)*

11. **(A)** Erythroblastosis fetalis is caused by transplacental passage of maternal antibody active against RBC (red blood cell) antigens. It is characterized by an increased rate of RBC destruction and is an important cause of newborn anemia and jaundice. The severe form is usually a result of Rh incompatibility. If severe anemia develops in utero this can result in fetal hydrops, fetal distress, and possibly fetal death. In severe cases, diagnosed before birth, intrauterine transfusion can improve survival. The transfusion is accomplished by injection of donor blood (packed red cells) into the fetal umbilical vein under ultrasound guidance. Although spherocytosis can cause neonatal jaundice, neither spherocytosis nor sickle cell disease causes serious intrauterine problems. Intrauterine transfusion is not the treatment for fetal distress and bradycardia or congenital heart disease. *(Behrman, 601)*

12. **(C)** Current technology, including the use of ultrasound monitoring during the procedure, has made intrauterine transfusion relatively safe. Premature onset of labor is the major complication but fetal death, fetal bleeding, fetal bradycardia, premature rupture of membranes, and chorioamniotis are all risks of the procedure.

Graft-versus-host reaction has been reported but is rare, irradiation of the blood to kill the lymphocytes prior to transfusion should avoid this. Testing of donor blood for human immunodeficiency virus (HIV) antibody is routine and usually will prevent transfusion transmission of AIDS. Transfusion reactions have not been reported to be a problem, blood should be cross-matched against mother's blood to select the most compatible blood for transfusion. *(Behrman, 601)*

13. **(C)** Kernicterus is a condition of neurologic damage that is the direct result of the toxic effects of bilirubin on the central nervous system. Since unconjugated bilirubin crosses the blood–brain barrier, whereas conjugated bilirubin does not, the risk of kernicterus is most closely related to the serum level of unconjugated bilirubin. The basal ganglia are particularly susceptible to damage with high levels of unconjugated bilirubin. Although kernicterus is more frequently reported when other complicating conditions exist (eg, prematurity, sepsis, isoimmunization), it has also been reported in healthy babies born at or near term. *(Burg, 298)*

14. **(D)** Infants are born in a state of relative extravascular fluid expansion. Through the first week of life, dilute urine and relatively low intake of fluid result in a loss of 5%–10% of their total body mass (up to 10%–15% in premature infants). This weight loss is a normal physiologic loss of fluid from the interstitial fluid space and is not a catabolism of body tissues. *(Merenstein, 351)*

15. **(D)** In most cases of ABO isoimmune hemolytic disease of the newborn, the mother is type O and the infant is type A or B. Mothers with A or B blood types produce mostly IgM antibodies which do not cross the placenta, whereas mothers with blood type O produce mostly IgG antibodies which cross the placenta. Since the IgG antibodies are "naturally" occurring, disease may occur in the first pregnancy. Hemolysis with ABO incompatibility is more mild than Rh disease because A and B antigens are expressed in all tissues of the body, including

the placenta, therefore maternal antibody is diluted and neutralized. Subsequent pregnancies with ABO incompatibility are not more severely affected. This differs from Rh disease where IgG antibodies are made more swiftly with repeat exposure and thus more severe hemolysis is noted with repeat pregnancies. Late anemia can occur with ABO disease. *(Brodsky, 289)*

16. **(B)** Late-onset chronic anemia in ABO isoimmune hemolytic disease is the most common late complication and usually presents as high-output congestive heart failure (CHF). The symptoms of CHF in neonates are usually tachypnea and failure to feed. The hemoglobin will reach its nadir at the sixth to twelfth week of life. Postdischarge montoring of hemoglobin and hematocrit is essential and late transfusion may be needed. Kernicterus and gallstones are uncommon. Bilirubinuria is benign. *(Behrman, 605)*

17. **(B)** Unconjugated bilirubin in the serum is tightly bound to albumin. The unconjugated bilirubin molecule is lipid soluble, and that which is not bound to albumin enters the brain readily. Once the albumin binding sites are saturated, there is an increase in the potentially toxic, free unconjugated bilirubin. A bilirubin/albumin molar ratio of 1 corresponds to approximately 8.5 mg bilirubin per gram of albumin. Factors that are associated with low serum albumin levels (eg, prematurity) and factors that impair bilirubin binding to albumin (eg, acidosis or drugs such as sulfa compounds) can result in kernicterus at lower serum bilirubin levels. *(Merenstein, 548)*

18. **(A)** Prematurity is the strongest predisposing factor to surfactant deficiency disease or respiratory distress syndrome (RDS). While low birth weight infants are also at risk, the risk is more related to the gestational age of the infant. Maternal diabetes does predispose newborns to RDS by causing delayed surfactant release compared to infants of comparable gestational age, but is not as strong of a risk as prematurity itself. Cesarean delivery predisposes more to a condition known as transient tachypnea of the newborn, related to excessive fluid retention within the lungs. Meconium in the amniotic fluid may cause respiratory disease if aspirated into the infant's lungs but the pathophysiology of the disease differs from RDS. *(Brodsky, 71)*

19. **(D)** Males have a higher neonatal mortality rate than females, both overall and when corrected for weight and gestational age. African Americans have a higher rate of prematurity and low birth weight and, therefore, have an overall higher neonatal mortality rate than Caucasians. Among infants of comparable weight and gestational age greater than 1500 g, however, African American infants have a lower mortality than do Caucasian infants. *(Behrman, 52)*

20. **(E)** Pulmonary surfactant is a hydrophobic substance composed mostly of phospholipids (approximately 70%). The majority is DPPC or dipalmitoyl phosphatidylcholine (40%), which is the most physiologically active component of surfactant and most responsible for reduction of surface tension. The total protein contribution is about 10% and neutral lipids about 10%. The proteins appear to be important in structural lipid organization and, to some degree, for regulation of surfactant production. *(Brodsky, 47)*

21. **(D)** Neonatal mortality is highest during the first 24 hours of life. Overall, neonatal mortality accounts for 65% of all infant deaths (deaths before 1 year of age) and is higher than any other period in childhood. Neonatal mortality has declined dramatically between 1980 and 2000 to about 4.6 per 1000 live births. Improved obstetric and neonatal management have contributed to this decline in mortality. The major causes of neonatal mortality are related to preterm birth, low birth weight, and lethal congenital anomalies. While mortality decreases as maturity and birth weight increase, infants who are delivered after 42 weeks gestation have an increased mortality rate compared to their term counterparts. African American newborns still have about twice the infant mortality of Caucasians infants, mostly from complications of preterm delivery. *(Behrman, 519, 641)*

22. **(B)** Pulmonary surfactant is produced in a complex set of structuring steps involving the endoplasmic reticulum and Golgi apparatus of the type II alveolar cells of the lung. It is stored within these cells in structures known as lamellar bodies. Surfactant proteins are expressed in the third trimester. Phosphatidylcholine and phosphatidylglycerol, the predominant lipids in surfactant, increase with lung maturity. Typically, after 34–35 weeks gestation, they are at sufficient levels such that respiratory distress syndrome will not be present, although this varies greatly for individual patients. *(Brodsky, 47)*

23. **(C)** The normally grown 30-week gestation infant weighs 1100–1800 g (mean +2 S.D.). *(Merenstein, 391)*

24. **(B)** Maternal diabetes mellitus during cardiogenesis results in an approximately threefold increased risk of congenital anomalies. This includes cardiac malformations and lumbosacral agenesis. The increased risk is associated with poor maternal glucose control during embryogenesis. In late gestation, poor maternal glucose control predisposes the infant to asymetric septal hypertrophy which can lead to aortic outflow obstruction. *(Behrman, 613)*

25. **(D)** Blood returning from the placenta, to the fetus, via the umbilical vein courses through the ductus venosus. This blood with higher oxygen saturation mixes with the dexoygenated blood returning from the fetus' inferior vena cava, enters the right atrium, and preferentially crosses the foramen ovale into the left atrium. It is then pumped into the aorta by the left ventricle. After birth, expansion of the lungs and an increased arterial Po_2 results in a rapid decrease in pulmonary vascular resistance. Simultaneously, there is an increase in systemic vascular resistance with removal of the low-resistance placental circulation. These events result in a physiologic cessation of flow across the foramen ovale. *(Behrman, 1479)*

26. **(A)** Erythema toxicum is a benign condition seen in 30%–70% of normal, term infants. It is much less common among premature infants, particularly those weighing less than 2500 g.

The skin lesions usually appear within the first 3 days of life and are not associated with any systemic signs or symptoms. They typically last less than 7 days. Infants are afebrile, and the peripheral white blood cell counts are normal. The rash presents with one or more of three types of skin lesions including erythematous macules, wheals, and vesiculopustules on an erythematous base. *(Eichenfield, 91)*

27. **(B)** The lecithin–sphingomyelin ratio of amniotic fluid specimens reflects the composition of fetal lung fluid, which is effluxed from the lungs into the amniotic sac. It is a useful indicator of lung maturity and risk of development of respiratory distress syndrome or hyaline membrane disease. *(Brodsky, 49)*

28. **(E)** Some infants with severe respiratory distress syndrome who require mechanical ventilation and high concentrations of oxygen develop chronic pulmonary changes known as bronchopulmonary dysplasia (BPD). *(Behrman, 580)*

29. **(E)** Surfactant replacement therapy is delivered directly into the lungs via an endotracheal tube. Multiple studies have documented the improvement in survival of infants with respiratory distress syndrome, who receive surfactant replacement after delivery. Common complications include transient hypoxemia and bradycardia associated with the dosage procedure and air leak syndromes from undetected rapid improvement in pulmonary compliance. *(Merenstein, 652)*

30. **(C)** The characteristic chest x-ray findings in infants with respiratory distress syndrome include reduced lung volumes, air bronchograms, reticulogranularity, and lung opacification. The x-ray appearance is frequently characterized as having a homogenous ground glass appearance. These changes are presumed to represent diffuse alveolar atelectasis which increases lung density. Air-filled bronchi (ie, air bronchograms) then stand out against the opaque lung tissue. Lobar densities are infrequent. Pneumothorax does occur as a complication of the disease or its treatment, but not in association with patchy densities. *(Merenstein, 650)*

31. **(D)** The purpose of continuous positive airway pressure (CPAP) is to increase the functional residual capacity and improve oxygenation by improving ventilation and perfusion mismatch. Improvement of ventilation (a decreased arterial CO_2) and maintenance of an adequate cardiac output is desired when providing CPAP, but these parameters may be adversely affected if the appropriate pressure is not provided for the individual patient. Pneumothorax is one of the complications of treatment with continuous positive airway pressure. There is no evidence that continuous positive airway pressure prevents infection. To the contrary, the invasive technology (eg, endotracheal tube) often required can predispose to infection. *(Merenstein, 603)*

32. **(E)** Although the pathophysiologic process in the development of retinopathy of prematurity (ROP) is not completely understood, there are several factors that have been associated with this disease. Although hypoxia may increase the risk and severity of ROP, hyperoxia and oxygen radicals also have an association with increased risk for this disease. Arterial oxygenation should be closely monitored in the premature infant. It is clear that oxygen alone is not the only predisposing factor. Acidosis, apnea of prematurity, anemia, nutritional status, and alterations in cerebral perfusion are other factors that have been associated with ROP in some infants. *(Merenstein, 641)*

33. **(B)** A decrease in production of pulmonary surfactant by alveolar cells has been demonstrated in the lungs of infants and experimental animals with respiratory distress syndrome. The biologic function of surfactant is to lower the surface tension of the alveolar lining and thereby stabilize the alveoli. Absence of surfactant leads to alveolar collapse (atelectasis), which in turn causes the pathophysiologic, clinical, and roentgenographic changes characteristic of this disorder. *(Behrman, 575)*

34. **(B)** In the healthy term male infant, hemophilia A (factor VIII deficiency) and hemophilia B (factor IX deficiency) are the most common severe inherited bleeding disorders. Hemophilia occurs in 1:5000 males with factor VIII deficieny being the most common (85%). Disseminated intravascular coagulopathy (DIC) is unlikely in a healthy infant. von Willebrand factor is high just after birth, making symptoms uncommon in the newborn. Protein C deficiency is associated with thrombosis not bleeding. (Note: Verification that there is no family history of bleeding problems should be done prior to any newborn circumcision. Once bleeding has begun after a fresh circumcision in a patient with factor VIII deficiency, it is very difficult to control.) *(Behrman, 1657–1665)*

35. **(D)** Any opacity of the lens is a cataract. The differential diagnosis for cataracts identified in the neonatal period is wide and includes developmental disorders, congenital infections, and metabolic disorders. Galactosemia, a disorder of carbohydrate metabolism, should be a primary consideration in a neonate presenting with cataracts. *(Behrman, 2105)*

36. **(B)** Blue or slate-gray spots (historically referred to as Mongolian spots) are macular lesions. They are most commonly found on the presacral area, have variably defined margins, and can often be quite large. The incidence is low in Caucasian infants (< 10%), but they are present in more than 80% of African-American, Asian, and East Indian infants. They typically fade with time and malignant degeneration does not occur. Their presence and location should be documented as they may be mistaken for bruising later in infancy. They are thought to be produced from melanocytes that have arrested in their migration from neural crest to epidermis. *(Behrman, 2162)*

37. **(B)** Cyanosis in the newborn can be due to many causes, but by far the most common cause is respiratory disease. If cyanosis is present without respiratory symptoms, such as tachypnea, one must classically consider congenital heart disease or the less commonly identified methemoglobinemia. Cyanosis typically will not normalize in the case of congenital heart disease or methemoglobinemia. Central nervous system diease could also cause cyanosis, but this is typically due to hypoventilation. *(Behrman, 560)*

38. **(E)** Beckwith-Wiedemann syndrome encompasses abdominal wall defects (especially omphalocele), macroglossia, and macrosomia. Its recognition is critical in the immediate newborn period as about one-third to one-half of cases have hypoglycemia. Cases are usually sporadic, the gene is located at 11p15. The characteristic phenotype occurs due to a variety of different genetic mechanisms, which all result in a dosage imbalance of a number of genes clustered at 11p15. Patients with this disorder have an increased risk of abdominal tumors (ie, hepatoblastoma and Wilms tumor) during childhood. Regular screening for these tumors during the early part of childhood is warranted. *(Jones, 175–177)*

39. **(C)** The combination of microcephaly, cerebral calcifications, and blindness is typical of the damage caused to neural tissues by intrauterine infection with either cytomegalovirus or toxoplasmosis. Subdural bleeding results in enlargement of the head. Cerebral agenesis is not associated with calcifications, and erythroblastosis would not explain any of the findings listed. Primary microcephaly is not associated with either cerebral calcifications or blindness. *(Brodsky, 199–201)*

40. **(A)** The findings described are typical of thrush (oral infection with *C albicans*), which is common in young infants. Although *E coli*, L monocytogenes, and group B streptococcus all are important pathogens in the neonatal period, they typically are not associated with pharyngeal infection or oral exudate. Group A streptococcus is a common cause of exudative tonsillitis in the older child but is an extremely rare pathogen in the newborn infant likely due to maternally acquired antibody. Additionally, the exudate noted with group A streptococcal infection would be in the area of the tonsils rather than on the buccal mucosa. *(Behrman, 870, 1392; Brodsky, 204)*

41. **(A)** Neurocutaneous syndromes are characterized by both skin and central nervous system abnormalities. They include a heterogenous group of disorders. Hypopigmented patches observed in the newborn period may be a sign of neurofibromatosis or tuberous sclerosis and would raise great suspicion if seen on the body of an infant with a family history of seizures. The skin lesion of tuberous sclerosis has classically been described as an ash leaf. Neurofibromatosis is likely to have pigmented cafe au lait spots develop over time as well. Salmon patches and pustular melanosis are normal, benign findings in newborn infants. A harlequin color change, while striking, typically is harmless. *(Behrman, 215)*

42. **(A)** The cranium of the child grows at right angles to several sutures, primarily the sagittal, coronal, lambdoidal, and temporal. Isolated premature closure (craniosynostosis) of the sagittal suture results in a long and narrow skull (scaphocephaly) with a slightly greater than normal total circumference. With early fusion of a single suture, there usually are no signs of increased intracranial pressure, and the problem is chiefly cosmetic. Craniosynostosis of multiple sutures, however, often is associated with increased intracranial pressure. *(Behrman, 1992)*

43. **(E)** Transient neonatal pustular melanosis is a benign lesion. It initially appears as a pustules without erythema and evolve into ruptured pustules with scale surrounding a hyperpigmented macule. The hyperpigmented macules can last up to 3 months. They typically cluster under the chin, forehead, neck, or lower back. Pustules may have already ruptured at the time of birth. They are somewhat more common in infants with greater amounts of skin pigment. *(Brodsky, 356)*

44. **(A)** The most common congenital defect of the esophagus is atresia of the proximal segment with a fistula between the distal segment and the trachea. This type of esophageal atresia accounts for 80%–90% of all cases. Attempts to feed the infant will result in regurgitation and may precipitate aspiration. Even prior to feeding, aspiration of gastric secretions may occur through the distal fistula and cause a damaging pneumonitis. Hypoplastic left heart syndrome and group B streptococcal sepsis are more likely to present with apnea or cyanosis unrelated to feeding. Disseminated neonatal herpes simplex infection similarly presents with a sepsis-like picture typical after 4–7 days of age.

Pyloric stenosis generally presents after the first month of life with vomiting. *(Behrman, 1219)*

45. **(B)** Both cephalohematoma and caput are associated with prolonged and difficult labor and delivery. They are also associated with a normal neurologic examination, unless there has been concomittant intracranial trauma. Caput, however, is diffuse and poorly demarcated edema of the scalp, whereas a cephalohematoma is a subperiosteal collection of blood. Therefore, a cephalohematoma is sharply demarcated and limited to a single bone. Cephalohematomas may be bilateral, but each is separate and sharply demarcated. *(Brodsky, 143)*

46. **(B)** There is a clear association between advancing maternal age and nondisjunction chromosome disorders (failure of a chromosome pair to separate). The rate of Down syndrome, the most common chromosome abnormality seen in newborns, increases with advancing maternal age from approximately 1/1500 at age 25 to more than 1/100 by age 40. *(Jones, 7–12)*

47. **(C)** While the association of maternal age and chromosome problems is well known, a lesser discussed phenomenon is the clear relationship of autosomal dominant disorders and paternal age at conception. The paternal age in disorders such as achondroplasia and Marfan syndrome, for example, is substantially higher than the general population. It is thought that the accumulation of DNA replicative errors during spermatogenesis is responsible for this phenomenon. *(Fanaroff, 122)*

48. **(C)** There is not always a correlation between blood glucose levels and classic clinical manifestations of hypoglycemia in the neonate. The lack of symptoms does not indicate that the glucose level is adequate for brain metabolism. Although a clear lower limit glucose level in newborn infants has not been determined, many authorites are recommending that any blood glucose value less than 50 mg/dL in the neonate be evaluated and treated. *(Behrman, 505)*

49. **(A)** Congenital clubfoot (talipes equinovarus) is usually an isolated congenital anomaly. When associated with another disorder, the central nervous system is most commonly involved. It is commonly associated with myelomeningocele. Genitourinary disorders resulting in low amniotic fluid volumes may result in clubfoot if the foot has been held in a deformed position in utero. *(Behrman, 1983, 2256)*

50. **(E)** Hypoplasia of the mandibular area in early gestation results in a posteriorly located tongue during development and impaired closure of posterior palate. The posterior displacement of the tongue can cause significant airway obstruction, which is the most urgent problem encountered in these infants with Pierre Robin sequence. While substantial spontaneous growth of the mandible occurs in many of these patients within a few months, temporary tracheostomy may be required in severe cases. Prone or partially prone positioning may relieve the obstruction in less severe cases. *(Jones, 262; Behrman, 120; Tibesar, 27)*

51. **(B)** So-called pyridoxine dependency is a group of rare, inborn metabolic errors that cause severe neonatal seizures that respond to pharmacologic (as opposed to physiologic) doses of pyridoxine. Although the disorder is extremely rare, it has given rise to the practice of sometimes empirically administering an intravenous dose of pyridoxine to infants with unexplained and otherwise uncontrollable seizures. *(Fanaroff, 1617)*

52. **(E)** Mutations in the mitochondrial DNA can produce specific diseases. In most cases, the functional mitochondria of both males and females are acquired from the mother. The mitochondrial complement passed in the egg may not represent the total mitochondrial population of the mother, thus there can be great variability in disease symptoms within a family. As would be anticipated, disorders of energy metabolism are predominant in this group of disorders. A myopathy or neurologic disease coming from the maternal side should alert the clinician to consider a mitochondrial etiology. Paternal inheritance may occcur, but this is uncommon. *(Behrman, 380)*

53. **(E)** Most infants who experience fetal brady-cardia during labor are not severely asphyxi-ated at birth and ultimately have a good neurologic outcome. Likewise, most infants who fail to breathe initially or are cyanotic at birth and have a low 1-minute Apgar score recover promptly and do well neurologically. Although a low 5-minute Apgar score gener-ally indicates more prolonged oxygen prob-lems and correlates somewhat better with outcome than does the 1-minute score, most of these infants also will be normal. In contrast, a substantial population of newborns with low Apgar scores and seizures in the first 36 hours of life will show neurologic abnormalities on long-term follow-up. *(Volpe, 439-442)*

54. **(C)** The lesions described are typical for neona-tal acne (acne neonatorum), a benign skin erup-tion occurring during the first few weeks of life, probably secondary to transplacental pas-sage of maternal hormones. Comedones are not typically present with neonatal acne. Adenoma sebaceum, one of the several cuta-neous manifestations of tuberous sclerosis, typically is not present in the neonatal period. The distribution and decsription of the rash in this patient are not typical of congenital syphilis, impetigo, or pustulosis. *(Eichenfield, 94, 144–151)*

55. **(D)** The maternal serum alpha-fetoprotein (MSAFP) test is used to screen for open neural tube defects. About 90% of affected pregnancies can be identified. High MSAFP levels are also seen in abdominal wall defects (eg, omphalo-cele) and twin gestation. Low MSAFP levels have been associated with trisomy 18 and 21, incorrect gestational age assessment, and intrauterine growth restriction. Maternal serum testing can be used in combination with ultra-sound and amniocentiesis to fine-tune risk assessments for these disorders. *(Behrman, 535)*

56. **(B)** Intestinal atresia accounts for 30%–40% of all neonatal intestinal obstructions of which duodenal atresia is most common. Bilious vom-iting without abdominal distention is the hall-mark of duodenal obstruction. The double bubble appearance on abdominal radiograph is due to a distended gas-filled stomach and prox-imal duodenum. Down syndrome is associated with all diseases listed except volvulus. Athough annular pancreas does result in a duodenal obstruction, it is seen less commonly than duo-denal atresia. Vomiting due to pyloric stenosis and gastric volvulus is nonbilious and radiograph denotes a dilated stomach. Vomiting due to pyloric stenosis often does not start until after 3 weeks of life. Hirschsprung disease is a lower intestinal obstruction and associated with delayed passage of stools. *(Behrman, 1229-1239; Jones, 8)*

57. **(C)** Necrotizing enterocolitis (NEC) occurs fre-quently among low birth weight infants who have had repeated episodes of hypoxia or poor perfusion. The usual signs of NEC are abdom-inal distention, bloody stools, vomiting, hypothermia, and lethargy. Intussusception is rare in the neonatal period. Volvulus and con-genital aganglionic megacolon (Hirschsprung disease) are unrelated to low birth weight or hypoxia and usually are associated with failure to pass stool. Shigella infection is very uncom-mon in the nursery. *(Behrman, 590, 1239)*

58. **(B)** Most capillary or cavernous hemangiomas are small or even invisible at birth. During the first weeks or months of life, they begin to grow and may become very large before finally start-ing to regress after a few years. Spontaneous regression usually (but not invariably) is com-plete or nearly so. Recognition of the natural history of this lesion permits reassurance of parents and avoidance of unnecessary therapy. The best cosmetic results are achieved by nat-ural regression. Active intervention (surgery or laser therapy) should be advised only when a complication such as trapping of platelets (Kassabach-Merritt syndrome), erosion of tissue, or impairment of a life-threatening func-tion (eg, vision, breathing) is a problem. *(Eichenfield, 336–346)*

59. **(D)** The most immediate task when an infant presents with vesicles and bullae at birth is to rule out infection. Although rare in the new-born period, the infections listed can present with severe disease which may be life threatening

if the infant is not adequately treated with appropriate antibacterial or antiviral therapy and supportive therapy for fluid and electrolyte issues. Decreased immune defenses and a fragile fluid and electrolyte balance can make the situation worse in the newborn period. Staphylococcus aureus infection is most likely. Herpes simplex and gram-negative infections do not generally present with bullous lesions. Epidermolysis bullosa is a group of inherited diseases in which the skin cannot withstand friction and thus skin blistering develops, but is very rare. Severe forms of the disease can also be life threatening. Maternal diabetes is not associated with these skin findings at birth. *(Eichenfield, 137–178)*

60. **(B)** Characteristically, the lesions of erythema toxicum (erythematous macules and papules) are loaded with eosinophils. The cause of this transient disorder of term newborns is unknown, and the lesions resolve spontaneously within a few days. Cultures of the lesions are sterile. It is important not to confuse this totally benign condition with the rash of serious disorders such as staphylococcal pustulosis or disseminated viral infection. *(Eichenfield, 91)*

61. **(B)** Infants born to mothers with hyperparathyroidism often develop transient hypoparathyroidism, resulting in hypocalcemia and hyperphosphatemia. The mechanism, presumably, is suppression of the fetal parathyroid glands by excessive transplacental maternal parathyroid hormone. Occasionally, the mother's condition may be undiagnosed, and otherwise unexplained hypocalcemia in an infant can lead to the diagnosis of hyperparathyroidism in the mother. *(Fanaroff, 1511)*

62. **(B)** Hereditary tyrosinemia is disorder of amino acid metabolism. Tyrosine is ingested from protein and synthesized endogenously from phenylalanine. Normally, the body metabolizes excess tyrosine to carbon dixoide and water. Deficiencies along this metabolic pathway will result in buildup of toxic metabolites (most commonly, fumarylacetoacetate) and hepatocellular dysfunction. The hepatic dysfunction frequently presents as conjugated hyperbilirubinemia, also known as direct hyperbilirubinemia. The other problems listed cause indirect (or unconjugated) hyperbilirubinemia. *(Behrman, 402, 1310–1311)*

63. **(A)** The infant described in this scenario most likely has congenital adrenal hyperplasia of which more than 90% of cases are caused by 21-hydroxylase deficiency. Ambiguous genitalia in association with congenital adrenal hyperplasia usually indicates a female pseudohermaphrodite (46 XX karyotype with ambiguous external genitalia due to excess androgens). This disorder is associated with both cortisol and aldosterone deficiency of which the classic signs and symptoms are progressive weight loss and vomiting, hyponatremia, hyperkalemia, and hypoglycemia. Without treatment, shock, cardiac arryhthmias, and death may occur. In many states, the newborn screening programs will test for congenital adrenal hyperplasia (detection of elevated 17-hydroxy progesterone) in order to identify and treat patients prior to the development of symptoms. Although 3-beta-hydroxysteroid dehydrogenase deficiency may present with both salt wasting and ambiguous genitalia, this disorder is very rare. The other disorders listed do not present with salt wasting and hypotension. *(Brodsky, 314; Behrman, 1909–1915)*

64. **(B)** Infants born to women with active and untreated Graves disease may be hyperthyroid at birth, presumably as a result of transplacental passage of thyroid-stimulating antibodies. These antbodies can cause an increase in fetal thyroid hormone production. If the mother is receiving antithyroid medication, this also crosses the placenta, and the infant may be euthyroid or even hypothyroid at birth. Even if the infant is asymptomatic at birth, the antibodies may persist for several weeks so regular screeing of the infant's thryoid function during the first 4–6 weeks of life is indicated. *(Brodsky, 310)*

65. **(C)** Approximately 75% of neonatal disease is due to HSV 2 (typically genital herpes). Transmission most commonly occurs at delivery due to virus in the birth canal (95%). In utero infection from ascending or transplacental passage is also possible (5%). A primary maternal genital infection is the single greatest

risk for disease in the infant due to the presence of a high viral replication load, longer viral excretion, and lack of maternal antibody passage to the infant. The risk for disease in the infant during a primary maternal infection is 10–20 times higher than in the presence of maternal secondary or recurrent lesions. In most neonates with disease, there is no maternal clinical history of HSV. Prolonged rupture of membranes increases the risk of ascending infection. Fetal scalp monitoring may break the infant's skin barrier and thus is contraindictaed in the presence of known maternal HSV infection. Prematurity is also a risk factor likely due to low transplacental IgG antibodies in premature infants. *(Brodsky, 192)*

66. **(B)** After delivery, the infant is cut off from its continuous calcium supply prompting a precipitous fall in serum calcium over the first 1–2 days. In normal circumstances, this stimulates PTH causing a gradual return to higher serum calcium levels. PTH secretion is inhibited in infants of diabetic mothers. Therefore, hypocalcemia is a common problem in infants of diabetic mothers. *(Polin, 87)*

67. **(E)** Passage of meconium usually occurs within the first 12 hours of life. Approximately 15% of term deliveries have meconium in the amniotic fluid, suggesting meconium was passed in utero. Also, 99% of term infants and 95% of preterm infants will have passed their first meconium stool by the age of 48 hours. In a term infant, failure to pass meconium by 24–48 hours should prompt evaluation for an underlying problem such as intestinal obstruction, Hirschsprung disease, or hypothyroidism. *(Polin, 144; Behrman 527)*

68. **(E)** The description and location of the lesion (beneath fading forceps marks) are typical of subcutaneous fat necrosis, which may follow trauma (forceps). Buccal cellulitis caused by *H influenzae* frequently has a violaceous color but is exceedingly rare in the newborn period and infants are likely to appear systemically ill. *(Eichenfield, 184–185, 420–422)*

69. **(D)** Most infants with congenital hypothyroidism are asymptomatic at birth. Thyroid hormone is critical for normal brain development, deficiency of thyroid hormone during the first 2–3 years of life could result in irreversible brain development. Neonatal screening programs assist the clinician in identifying these infants after birth, although errors in screening occur. Awareness of the subtle clinical signs and symptoms is imperative. The infants may be edematous, have a large posterior fontanelle, have difficulty with feeding, and have a history of prolonged jaundice. *(Polin, 102; Brodsky, 308)*

70. **(A)** Low birth weight, a faster rate of growth, and iatrogenic blood loss are factors that put premature infants at an increased risk of early iron deficiency. They have iron stores adequate for less than 3 months postnatally. Iron stores in a term infant are sufficient for the first 4 to 6 months of life. In cases of hemolysis (such as ABO incompatibility) and physiologic hyperbilirubinemia, iron is not lost from the body. Polycythemia is an elevated hemotocrit commonly seen in cases of intrauterine hypoxia or placenta vascular insufficiency or from placental transfusion such as delayed cord clamping. *(Merenstein, 521–534)*.

71. **(D)** Fetal hemoglobin binds poorly to 2,3-DPG. Because 2,3-DPG binding decreases the affinity of hemoglobin for oxygen, fetal hemoglobin, unbound to 2,3-DPG, has an increased affinity for oxygen. Prenatally this works to the advantage of the fetus in obtaining oxygen from the maternal blood (across the placenta), but postnatally it is to the infant's disadvantage in releasing oxygen at the tissue level. *(Fanaroff, 1089)*

72. **(C)** The mass shown is a typical example of an encephalocele. These lesions consist of herniation of the meninges, with or without brain tissue, through a defect in the skull. They occur most commonly in the occipital region (70%–80% of cases). It is a restricted disorder of neuralation that involves anterior neural tube closure. The precise pathogenesis is unknown. The mass is far too large to be an abscess. There

is no such entity as posterior hydrocephalus. Hydroceles are limited to the scrotum. Myelomeningocele is restricted failure of posterior neural tube closure. Approximately 80% of lesions occur in the lumbar area. *(Volpe, 7–9)*

73. **(C)** The roentgenogram reveals absence of the radius and suggests the thrombocytopenia with absent radius (TAR) syndrome. Affected infants have early thrombocytopenia, which may be associated with bleeding. Infants manifest congenital skeletal malformations of the arm and hand. The other disorders listed are causes of bleeding in the neonatal period but are not typically associated with congenital abnormalities of skeletal development. *(Merenstein, 537)*

74. **(A)** Breast milk jaundice results from an increase in unconjugated bilirubin. Prolonged and exaggerated jaundice occurs because of an inhibitor or inhibitory substance in the breast milk that prolongs increased enterohepatic circulation. The hyperbilirubinemia becomes exaggerated by day 5 of life and persists for 4–14 days followed by a gradual decline. Elevation of bilirubin levels within the first 12 hours of life is typically associated with hemolysis. Since breast milk jaundice is not associated with hemolysis, levels do not escalate within the first day of life and there is not an association with anemia or reticulocytosis. It is a common problem in infants of all races. *(Merenstein, 553)*

75. **(D)** Infants of diabetic mothers present with a variety of problems. The most common is hypoglycemia resulting from hyperinsulinism. Hypoglycemia develops in 25%–50% of infants of diabetic mothers. The probability of hypoglycemia after delivery increases when maternal fasting glucose is high. There is a threefold increase in the incidence of congenital anomlies in these infant including sacral agenesis, congenital cardiac malformations, and intestinal atresias. Large birth weights are common among infants of diabetic mothers which predisposes the babies to birth trauma and asphyxia. Cardiomegaly is common in 30% of these infants, asymmetric septal hypertrophy

may occur that manifests similarly to idopathic hypertrophic subaortic stenosis. This septal hypertrophy typically resolves with time. Hypocalcemia and associated hypomagnesemia is seen frequently, but infants do not typically develop hyponatremia beyond what is normally seen in newborn infants. *(Behrman, 614)*

76. **(E)** Infantile glaucoma typically presents in infants less than 6 months of age, and requires surgical treatment. Signs and symptoms include enlargement and clouding of the cornea, tearing, blepharospasm, and photophobia. It is associated with many other conditions including Marfan syndrome, neurofibromatosis 1, and congenital rubella. It can be associated with a number of chromosomal syndromes but there is not a classic association with trisomy 21. Infantile or congenital gluacoma begins within the first 3 years of life. The white pupil sign is suggestive of a congenital cataract. *(Behrman, 2122)*

77. **(D)** Tachypnea, retractions, cyanosis, and grunting are common findings in neonatal respiratory distress syndrome (RDS). Pallor and poor perfusion may also be present but are is not the most common initial manifestation. Wheezing is not a feature of RDS. The clinical findings relate to the pathogenesis of the disease, which primarily is atelectasis due to collapse of the terminal airways caused by surfactant deficiency. *(Merenstein, 650)*

78. **(B)** Uterine contractions can precipitate a fall in fetal PAO$_2$. The fetus has a limited ability to compensate for hypoxemia. Adults increase their heart rate to increase their total cardiac output while the fetus responds by redistribution of their cardiac output. Blood flow is increased to the brain and heart and perfusion to less critical organs is reduced. Acute hypoxemia leads to acidosis and fetal bradycardia. The fetal heart rate is usually 110–160 beats per minute with considerable beat-to-beat variatiability. Accelerations of the heart rate are normal and not usually of concern. A rate less than 100 beats per minute is unusual and worrisome. A fixed heart rate or decreased beat-to-beat variability often indicates fetal hypoxia (fetal distress). Decelerations may be of no

consequence or may be ominous, depending on their temporal relationship to uterine contractions. Early decelerations are usually benign, whereas late or variable decelerations can indicate fetal distress. *(Merenstein, 26)*

79. **(C)** Infants with a symptomatic pneumothorax typically develop tachypnea, cyanosis, and increased work of breathing. Apnea and irritability may also be an early sign. The chest may appear asymetric and breath sounds may be absent. In a tension pneumothorax, signs of shock including hypotension and bradycardia may be noted. The heart apex is shifted away from the affected side. Prompt diagnosis and treatment is needed. *(Behrman, 586)*

80. **(D)** Since the infant in question was more than 38 weeks gestational age, she is not premature. She is, however, of low birth weight (< 2500 g) and is small for gestational age. This can be confirmed by the use of standard intrauterine growth charts. (Note: Answers (A), (C) and (D) are correct, but (D) is the BEST answer.) *(Merenstein, 21, 94)*

81. **(D)** Clinically significant subdural hemorrhage in the neonatal period is typically a traumatic lesion. The majority of the cases have involved full-term infants. Intraventricular hemorrhages occur primarily in premature infants. Hemorrhagic disease of the newborn can occur in either premature or term infants who do not receive vitamin K prophylaxis, but is not more common in term infants. Both congenital infection and neonatal sepsis are more common in premature than term infants. *(Volpe, 485-493)*

82. **(D)** Meconium ileus results from thick, viscid meconium packed into the terminal ileum. The substance fills the lumen of the small bowel causing a mechanical bowel obstruction. The colon has a resultant small caliber (microcolon) because of lack of use. Progressive abdominal distention and bilious vomiting are the hallmarks of the clinical presentation. Nearly all neonates presenting with meconium ileus have cystic fibrosis. Of neonates with cystic fibrosis, 10%–20% will present with meconium ileus. *(Polin, 174)*

83. **(B)** Neither DIC nor dermal erythropoiesis are recognized manifestations of congenital syphilis. There are a variety of highly characteristic skin manifestations including bullous lesions on the palms and soles. Cutaneous findings of syphilis classically involve the palmar / plantar, perioral and anogenital regions. Mucous membrane involvement may manifest as snuffles, a clear nasal discharge that may be mistaken for a viral upper respiratory infection. Pneumonia and hepatitis may occur but also are seen in many other neonatal infections. *(Eichenfeld, 196; Brodsky, 186)*

84. **(A)** Epiphyseal dysgenesis, the development of multiple foci of ossification, occurs in patients with hypothyroidism that are not treated or are inadequately treated. The development of ossification centers is also retarded in hypothyroidism. About 60% of infants with congenital hypothyroidism have x-ray changes, consient with delayed osseous development, present at birth. The ossification center of the hamate is not normally present at birth, thus x-ray examination of the wrist is of no value in the newborn period. Roentgenographic demonstration of absence of the distal femoral epiphyses in a term infant would be suggestive of hypothyroidism. Although cardiomegaly from myxedema of the heart can be seen, there are so many other, much more common causes of cardiomegaly in the newborn that an enlarged heart would not be suggestive of hypothyroidism. *(Behrman, 1876)*

85. **(E)** Hypoplastic left heart syndrome typically presents within the first few days to weeks of life with tachypnea, lethargy, and poor feeding. The condition of the neonate worsens dramatically with closing of the PDA. Cyanosis may not be obvious initially, but patients develop a grayish blue color of the skin which results from a mix of cyanosis and hypoperfusion. As the PDA closes, progressive shock will develop. The other cyanotic heart lesions listed are more likely to present with cyanosis and tachypnea rather than shock. *(Behrman, 1524–1544)*

86. **(D)** The initial lesions of incontinentia pigmenti are inflammatory bullae that eventually evolve

into hyperpigmented lesions. The bullae are typically present at birth or during the first few weeks of life, although neonates may be born with or develop the hyperpigmented lesions without the preceeding bullous lesions. Mental retardation, seizures, and several other organ system anomalies (eg, eye, skeletal system) are often present. *(Eichenfeld, 377)*

87. **(A)** Amnion nodosum (granules on the amnion) suggests oligohydramnios, which, in conjunction with the "Potter facies" described, is characteristic of bilateral renal agenesis. Esophageal atresia often is associated with poly-hydramnios, not oligohydramnios. None of the features of this case are suggestive of congenital heart disease or infection. *(Behrman, 547, 1783)*

88. **(B)** Cats are the definitive host for *Toxoplasma gondii*, an intracellular parasite that can be transmitted from mother to fetus through the placenta (transplacental transmission). Typically, this is the result of a primary infection in the mother. The most severely infected fetuses aquire the infection during the first trimester of pregnancy. (Note: The table of clinical findings of infants with congenital infections found in Brodsky's *Neonatology Review* on page 201 is worth reviewing!) *(Brodsky, 200)*

89. **(B)** Trisomy 18 (Edwards syndrome) is characterized by severe retardation of growth and mental development. Most of the patients die in early infancy, mortality in the first year of life is 90%. Characteristic abnormalities include low-set and malformed ears, nail hypoplasia, abnormal fisting with index finger overlying third finger, and rocker-bottom feet. The abnormalities of the hands and feet are clinically distinctive features. Congenital heart disease is usual, most commonly a ventricular septal defect or a patent ductus arteriosus. *(Brodsky, 167)*

90. **(A)** The cardinal features of trisomy 13 (Patau syndrome) include cleft lip and palate, holo-prosencephaly, and severe mental retardation. Holoprosencephaly is an incomplete development of the forebrain, often associated with absence of the corpus callosum, fusion of the frontal lobes, and a single ventricle. Other features of trisomy 13 include ocular abnormalities, congenital heart disease, and cutaneous defects of the scalp (eg, cutis aplasia). Greater than 90% of infants die within the first year of life. *(Brodsky, 166)*

91. **(D)** Among live births, Down syndrome is the most common chromosomal abnormality. It occurs in about 1 in 800 live births. Fewer than 5% of patients have a translocation rather than an extra (47) chromosome. Hypotonia and hyperextensible joints are characteristic. Mental retardation is present in all patients, but is less severe than in other trisomy syndromes (ie, tri-somies 13 and 18). Clinodactyly, especially of the fifth finger, a single plamar crease, an increased distance between the first and second toes, upward-slanting palpebral fissures, epi-canthal folds, flat nasal bridge, and flat occiput are some of the physical findings associated with this syndrome. Many of these patients have serious congenital malformations such as congenital heart disease or duodenal atresia. Brushfield spots (tiny white spots that form a ring in the midzone of the iris) are frequently present. *(Brodsky, 168)*

92. **(C)** The cri–du-chat (cry of the cat) syndrome is so named because of the characteristic cry, which is reminiscent of a mewing cat. This characteristic cry is present in infancy but dis-appears as the child grows and usually is gone by the age of 1 or 2 years. The cry is high pitched and distinctive and results from abnormal laryngeal development. These patients also have microcephaly, severe mental retardation, epicanthal folds, downward slant of palpebral fissures, hypertelorism, and low-set ears. The syndrome is associated with a dele-tion of the short arm of chromosome 5. (Note: The student who understands French has an obvious advantage in answering this question.) *(Brodsky, 168)*

93. **(E)** Features of Turner syndrome, 45,X or XO, in the older child include short stature, lack of development of sexual characteristics, primary amenorrhea, webbing of the neck, cubitus

valgus (wide-carrying angle of the arms), and short fourth metacarpals. In the newborn period, redundant skin at the nape of the neck, a low posterior hairline, and edema of the dorsum of the feet are characteristic. Cardiac defects (especially coarctation of the aorta) and renal anomalies are common. Intelligence usually is normal, but perceptual difficulties may be present. *(Brodsky, 176)*

94. **(C)** After birth, intubation and tracheal suction decrease the risk of developing meconium aspiration syndrome in infants who are not vigorous at birth. The infant described in this case is not vigorous (depressed respirations, depressed muscle tone, and/or a heart rate < 100 beats per minute), thus endotracheal intubation with suctioning to remove the meconium is indicated after the infant is delivered. *(Kattwinkel, Lesson 2)*

95. **(C)** While most infants with cytomegalovirus (CMV) infection are asymptomatic at delivery, the combination of growth impairment, hepatosplenomegaly, and the "blueberry muffin" rash of extramedullary hematopoiesis (specifically dermal erythropoiesis) are characteristic of CMV infection. *(Brodsky, 199–201)*

96. **(E)** Jaundice in the first day of life nearly always is a pathologic process in term infants. Hereditary spherocytosis has an incidence of approximately 1/5000 in populations of Northern European origin, less in most other ethnic groups. ABO isoimmune hemolytic anemia occurs much more frequently, in about 3% of pregnancies, and is associated with early-onset jaundice and spherocytes on the blood smear. The spherocytes are generated as splenic disruption of the red cell membrane occurs. Glucose-6-phosphate dehydrogenase deficiency (the most frequently inherited RBC enzyme defect) is associated with normal RBC shape. Patients with disseminated intravascular coagulopathy have bleeding, abnormal coagulation studies, and thrombocytopenia. *(Brodsky, 289–297)*

97. **(D)** Varicella infections in the newborn are frequently life threatening. If the mother has had varicella in the past, her IgG antibody to varicella crosses the placenta and protects the infant for weeks after delivery. Certainly, infants who face exposure without maternal antibody protection acquire the infection at a high rate with serious morbidity, mainly from varicella pneumonia. Varicella immune globulin is useful in preventing acquisition of infection in susceptible infants. Infants are considered susceptible if maternal onset of varicella is 5 days or less before delivery. Varicella immune globulin is not indicated if the mother has zoster. *(Pickering, 711–725)*

98. **(A)** Supraventricular tachycardia (SVT) is the most common tachydysrhythmia in the newborn period. Dual AV nodal pathways, rapid conduction through an accessory bundle, or the existence of an ectopic atrial pacemaker are all potential mechanisms for development of SVT. Often predisposing conditions are identified such as Wolff-Parkinson-White syndrome or structural abnormalities of the heart (eg, Ebstein anomaly). Newborns with SVT gradually develop congestive heart failure if it is not identified. Symptoms of congestive heart failure in the newborn include anxiousness, restlessness, tachypnea, and poor feeding. *(Merenstein, 730)*

99. **(C)** Infants with severe respiratory distress syndrome (hyaline membrane disease) commonly develop hypoxemia and acidosis. Acidosis is usually respiratory (elevation of Pco_2 levels to > 50 torr) but a metabolic acidosis component may also be present. Diffuse atelectasis and ventilation/perfusion mismatch are present in this disease. *(Merenstein, 649–651)*

100. **(D)** In the face of acute cold stress, the infant attempts to conserve heat by vasoconstriction thus reducing heat loss and initiating thermogenesis. Glycogen stores are depleted, oxygen consumption increases. Hypoglycemia and in increased oxygen need is likely to result but hypercalcemia and hypertrigliceridemia are not encountered. As hypothermia continues, the infant uses anaerobic metabolism to increase

heat production. This causes an increased lactic acid production with resultant metabolic acidosis (not metabolic alkalosis). Acrocyanosis, initially present, will progress to central cyanosis, apnea, and bradycardia. The large surface area to mass ratio of the newborn predisposes to this problem. *(Merenstein, 133–135)*

101. **(D)** Periventricular leukomalacia (PVL) is characterized by focal necrotic lesions in the periventricular white matter. Cranial ultrasound can detect focal echo denisities and/or cystic lesions surrounding the lateral ventricles that are diagnostic of PVL. Other imaging techniques may be needed to detect more diffuse injury. These lesions are rarely found in infants greater than 32 weeks gestation. Premature infants are predisposed to the development of PVL due to the complex interaction between the cerebral vasculature and regulation of cerebral blood flow that is gestatonal age dependent. Actively differentiating or myelinating periventricular glial cells are also vulnerable to injury. The findings of PVL may not be evident until 1 month of age or later. Congenital anomalies of the brain and intraventricular hemorrhage usually are readily apparent on imaging in the first days of life. *(Brodsky, 140; Behrman, 562)*

102. **(E)** Congestive heart failure is a common complication of large intracranial arteriovenous fistulas. A cranial bruit usually is readily audible in these patients. The great vein of Galen is a frequent location for such arteriovenous malformations. Hyperthyroidism and polycythemia cause congestive heart failure only rarely and are not associated with a cranial bruit; transposition of the great vessels usually is associated with a cardiac murmur and not with a cranial bruit, although a murmer arising from the heart may be transmitted to the cranium. Ruptured cerebral aneurysms are exceedingly rare in the newborn period and present with neurologic findings rather than heart failure or cranial bruits. *(Behrman, 1974, 2036)*

103. **(B)** Brachial plexus injury results from stretching of the plexus and nerve roots. The upper roots (C5 and C6) are most vulnerable to injury. Phrenic nerve injury on the same side of the injury may occur, which results in diaphragmatic paralysis. This risks are highest for brachial plexus injury if the infant is large for gestational age and/or if the labor and delivery is complicated. Respiratory distress syndrome is uncommon in term infants and almost always presents initially in the first 24 hours of life. Pulmonary hemorrhage, pneumothorax, and cystic adenomatoid malformation can cause cyanosis and respiratory distress but have no association with brachial plexus injury. *(Brodsky, 144, 71–81)*

104. **(A)** The most common cause of neonatal meningitis is group B streptococcus (GBS). *Escherichia coli* generally is the second leading cause. Listeria is less frequent but not uncommon. *Haemophilus influenzae* and *S pneumoniae* are uncommon causes of meningitis during the first month of life. GBS is usually vertically transmitted from the mother either at delivery or from ascending transmission after rupture of membranes. The risk for neonatal infection increases in the presence of prematurity, prolonged rupture of membranes, intrapatum fever, chorior aminionitis, and maternal GBS bacteruria. Vaginal colonization of GBS (or absence of colonization) may be transient, so screening cultures are not 100% predictive of status at delivery. *(Brodsky, 184–186)*

SELECTED READINGS

Polin RA, Fox WW. *Fetal and Neonatal Physiology.* 2nd ed.
Philadelphia, PA: W.B. Saunders Co.; 1998.

CHAPTER 4

Growth and Development

Sarah E. Hampl, MD

An understanding of pediatric growth and development is essential for those entering primary care. This is where it all begins, and wise students will do well to recall their own childhoods as they learn the wide array of physical, developmental, and emotional milestones that today's infants, toddlers, children, and teens achieve. If one is already in the role of parent, learning or recalling of these milestones is an exciting, pleasurable task. However, most students have had little prior experience as a caregiver to children, and may find it difficult to comprehend and remember these milestones and their normal and abnormal variations. A variety of easily read resources exists to facilitate this learning. Spending time caring for or observing infants, toddlers, and school-age children is a valuable method of naturally learning their activities and behaviors.

Questions

DIRECTIONS (Questions 1 through 92): For each of the multiple choice questions in this section select the one lettered answer that is the best response in each case.

1. Third-year medical students are rotating in the normal newborn nursery. The students learn that most neonates actually lose weight after birth. One student asks what the average rate of weight gain is following the initial period of weight loss. After 2 weeks of age, a term neonate will gain an average of which of the following increments of weight?

   (A) 15 g/day or 1/2 oz/day
   (B) 30 g/day or 1 oz/day
   (C) 45 g/day or $1^1/_2$ oz/day
   (D) 60 g/day or 2 oz/day
   (E) 120 g/day or 4 oz/day

2. A mother brings her 6-month-old son in for a checkup. She is concerned that when she is playing with him and puts a toy behind her back, he does not try to find it. Object permanence, the understanding that objects continue to exist even when not seen, is a major milestone that occurs closest to which of the following ages?

   (A) 9–12 months
   (B) 15 months
   (C) 18 months
   (D) 24 months
   (E) 30 months

3. A 6-month-old girl, comes in for her checkup with her mother and grandmother. A look in the girl's mouth reveals no teeth. What is the usual age for the eruption of the primary teeth?

   (A) 2–4 months
   (B) 4–6 months
   (C) 6–8 months
   (D) 8–10 months
   (E) 10–12 months

4. The girl's grandmother goes on to report that she is sure that her grandaughter will be left-handed, just like her. Consistent use of a dominant hand is established at which of the following ages?

   (A) 12 months
   (B) 24 months
   (C) 4–6 years
   (D) 7 years
   (E) 9 years

5. A group of nursing students are learning about how vision screening is done in the primary care office. One student asks at what age visual acuity reaches 20/20. Normal visual acuity typically occurs at which of the following ages?

   (A) 1 week
   (B) 6 months
   (C) 1 year
   (D) 4–5 years
   (E) 7–9 years

6. The father of a 3-year-old boy brings him in with a 2-week history of purulent rhinorrhea and an occasional headache in the frontal area. He requests that you perform sinus films to

determine if his son has frontal sinusitis. What is the earliest age at which the frontal sinuses can be visualized radiographically?

(A) 3 years
(B) 4 years
(C) 6 years
(D) 8 years
(E) 10 years

7. A medical student is rotating with a local pediatrician who uses the Parents' Evaluations of Developmental Status (PEDS) questionnaire. Which of the following characteristics best describes this screening test?

(A) Used to evaluate development of children 10–14 years
(B) Screens for development in children less than 8 years
(C) Utilizes a 100-question format
(D) Used to evaluate teen adjustment
(E) Less than 50% sensitivity, but high specificity for diagnosing emotional disorders in children

8. A third-year college student reports that she took a pregnancy test which was positive this morning. She had moderate alcohol use for the last 2 months and was worried that development of the embryo might be affected. Which of the following gestational ages describes the embryonic period?

(A) up to 5 weeks
(B) up to 9 weeks
(C) up to 12 weeks
(D) up to 16 weeks
(E) up to 20 weeks

9. At 4-weeks gestation, she has not experienced fetal movements. Which of the following best describes the occurrence of first fetal movements, or quickening?

(A) 12 weeks
(B) 16 weeks
(C) 20 weeks
(D) 24 weeks
(E) 28 weeks

10. A worried mother brings her 2-year-old to the pediatrician for a well-child check. She is concerned because the child still has only 50 words in his vocabulary. Which of the following best describes the characteristic age of a toddler who speaks 50 words?

(A) 12 months
(B) 15 months
(C) 18 months
(D) 24 months
(E) 36 months

11. The mother of a 3-year-old boy reports that he is "on the go" all the time. Typically, children stop taking daytime naps at which of the following ages?

(A) 18 months
(B) 24 months
(C) 30 months
(D) 36 months
(E) 48 months

12. Pediatric residents are performing camp physicals for Girl Scouts. A 9-year-old girl asks how she will know that she is beginning puberty. In girls, which of the following is the first visible sign of puberty?

(A) development of breast buds
(B) appearance of early pubic hair
(C) menarche
(D) enlargement of the clitoris
(E) appearance of axillary hair

13. While giving a talk about growing up to the parents of 4-H youth, a father asks the pediatrician if it is considered normal for a boy to have signs of puberty at age 8. The median age for entering puberty in boys is at what age?

(A) 8 years
(B) 10 years
(C) 12 years
(D) 13 years
(E) 15 years

14. A 10-year-old female patient, who is at sexual maturity rating (SMR) stage II is the shortest girl in her class and her mother wonders when she will have her next growth spurt. Maximal height gain velocity in girls occurs during which of the following SMR?

    (A) I
    (B) II
    (C) III
    (D) IV
    (E) V

15. The grandmother of an 8-year-old boy presents with him for his preschool checkup and is concerned because he has not grown in height for the last 2 years. Which of the following best approximates the prepubertal annual increase in height?

    (A) 1–2 cm
    (B) 3–4 cm
    (C) 5–7 cm
    (D) 8–10 cm
    (E) 12–14 cm

16. The causes of childhood obesity are being reviewed by a group of pediatric residents. In children, obesity is defined as a body mass index (BMI) above which percentile for age and gender?

    (A) 50%
    (B) 75%
    (C) 95%
    (D) 120%
    (E) 150%

17. A mother concerned about her 10-year-old's weight calls your office to find out how to calculate her child's BMI. Your office nurse tells her the BMI can be calculated only if one knows which of the following values?

    (A) Weight
    (B) Height
    (C) Weight and height
    (D) Weight, height, and age
    (E) Weight, height, gender, and age

18. A pediatric endocrinologist has diagnosed constitutional growth delay in a 14-year-old boy. Which of the following are consistent with this diagnosis?

    (A) bone age is normal compared to chronologic age
    (B) prognosis for a normal adult height is good
    (C) family history for childhood short stature
    (D) undernourished for the first year of life
    (E) infant was small for size at birth

19. A 1-week-old infant male presents to his primary care provider's office for his first visit. His mother is concerned because he sleeps a lot. Which of the following is the average amount of sleep per day experienced by infants in the first month of life?

    (A) 12 hours
    (B) 14 hours
    (C) 16 hours
    (D) 18 hours
    (E) 20 hours

20. A 100 kg, 10-year-old presents for well-child care. Which of the following history items should be included when evaluating this obese child?

    (A) family history of hyperparathyroidism
    (B) vigorous physical activities performed by the child
    (C) parents' occupation
    (D) instances of binge drinking by the parent
    (E) presence of learning disabilities in siblings

21. A preschool teacher is concerned that a 24-month-old boy occasionally repeats words spoken to him. She sends a note with mother to his checkup. The boy's physical and neurologic examinations are entirely normal, and the child's developmental landmarks are within normal limits. Which of the following is the most likely description of this child's symptom?

(A) precocious verbal behavior

(B) subtle neurologic abnormality

(C) poor language development

(D) autism spectrum disorder

(E) normal

22. A neonatologist is performing a physical examination with medical students on an infant greater than 24 hours old. Which of the following findings would be considered normal for the neonate at this age?

(A) has a visual preference for geometric shapes over faces

(B) needs 4–6 hours after birth to suck well at the breast

(C) is farsighted

(D) is unable to hear well

(E) learns to differentiate the voice of her mother from that of other women by 4 weeks of age

23. First-time parents of a 1-month-old are anxious to hear what they can expect in the next few months. Which of the following best describes the usual sequence for attainment of gross motor milestones in a young infant?

(A) head control, rolling over, hands together in midline, sits without support

(B) head control, hands together in midline, rolling over, pulls to stand

(C) rolls over, sits without support, hands together in midline, pulls to stand

(D) sits without support, hands together in midline, pulls to stand, walks along

(E) pulls to stand, walks along table, sits without support, hands together at midline

24. The parents of a 15 month old are concerned that their daughter does not seem to be able to stack cubes into a tower like their son could at the same age. Her pediatrician reviews the child's prior fine motor development with the parents. Which of the following best describes the correct sequence of fine motor development one should see in a healthy infant/toddler?

(A) thumb–finger grasp, grasps rattle, transfers objects from hand to hand

(B) grasps rattle, thumb–finger grasp, reaches for objects, transfers objects from hand to hand

(C) grasps rattle, transfers objects from hand to hand, builds tower of two cubes, thumb–finger grasp

(D) reaches for objects, transfers objects from hand to hand, turns pages of book, builds tower of two cubes

(E) grasps rattle, transfers objects from hand to hand, thumb–finger grasp, builds tower of two cubes

25. A 6-year-old boy is proud to show off the first tooth he lost but his mother is concerned because the tooth was one of his canines and a permanent tooth seems to be erupting in this area. Which of the following best describes the correct sequence for eruption of permanent teeth?

(A) central incisors, first premolars, canines, second molars

(B) first molars, central incisors, canines, first premolars

(C) central incisors, lateral incisors, canines, first molars

(D) first molars, lateral incisors, canines, first premolars

(E) lateral incisors, first molars, canines, first premolars

26. The parents of a 6-month-old boy point out that he has just cut his first tooth, and wonder which teeth will come next. Which of the following is the correct sequence for eruption of primary teeth?

(A) central incisors, first molars, second molars, canines

(B) central incisors, lateral incisors, canines, first molars

(C) central incisors, canines, first molars, second molars

(D) central incisors, lateral incisors, first molars, canines

(E) canines, central incisors, lateral incisors, first molars

27. A term newborn infant has a normal weight but height below the 5th percentile. A large posterior fontanelle is the only other finding. A delayed bone age is noted on skeletal survey based on the appearance of ossification centers and further testing reveals the diagnosis of congenital hypothyroidism. In normal neonates, ossification centers are usually radiographically visible at birth in which of the following sites?

    (A) patella
    (B) lunate (carpal)
    (C) proximal tibia
    (D) head of the femur
    (E) distal tibia

28. The grandfather of a 1-year-old brings him in for a checkup and states that the boy received a tricycle for his first birthday but wonders when he will be able to pedal to ride it. Which of the following sequence best demonstrates the correct attainment of motor milestones?

    (A) runs, rides tricycle, skips, hops
    (B) runs, hops, skips, rides tricycle
    (C) runs, goes upstairs alternating feet, rides tricycle, skips
    (D) hops, skips, rides tricycle, goes upstairs alternating feet
    (E) goes upstairs alternating feet, rides tricycle, runs, skips

29. The mother of a 30-month-old brings the primary care provider a note from his parents as teachers (PAT) (early childhood development) specialist. The PAT specialist is concerned by the child's lack of self-feeding skills. Which of the following social development sequences do toddlers follow?

    (A) feeds self, helps to undress, washes hands, domestic role-playing
    (B) handles spoon well, plays in parallel, dresses and undresses, washes hands
    (C) plays in parallel, feeds self, dresses and undresses, washes hands
    (D) plays in parallel, dresses and undresses, washes hands, feeds self
    (E) washes hands, dresses herself, plays in parallel, handles spoon well

30. A group of student nurses is learning about childrens' language development. Their instructor explains that language is a critical barometer of both cognitive and emotional development. With which of the following is speech delay most closely associated?

    (A) 22q11 deletion syndrome
    (B) spina bifida
    (C) diabetes
    (D) child abuse
    (E) asthma

31. The mother of a 2-year-old girl brings her to her pediatrician's office for a checkup. When asked about discipline concerns, the mother expresses worry because the child gets mad and throws herself on the ground screaming. Which of the following statements regarding temper tantrums is correct?

    (A) most often indicate a serious psychosocial problem
    (B) usually appear at the end of the first year
    (C) peak prevalence is between 4 and 6 years
    (D) routinely occur 8–10 times per day
    (E) usually last between 30 and 45 minutes

32. A group of first-year residents is examining the National Center for Health Statistics growth curves for girls and boys. Typically, infants and children stay within one or two growth chart channels. A normal exception to this rule exists for which of the following?

    (A) female infants
    (B) during preschool years (3–6 years)
    (C) up to age 2 years
    (D) male infants
    (E) during adolescence

33. As part of a routine 18-month check-up, a medical student in the outpatient clinic administers the Denver Developmental Screening Test (DDST) to the child. She reports that the child appeared to function at about a 15–18-month level, but he was noncompliant and difficult to test. Which of the following best explains the testing results for this child?

(A) advanced and was stressed by the test

(B) delayed and psychologically disturbed

(C) delayed and was stressed by the test

(D) normal and noncompliance is common at this age

(E) normal but psychologically disturbed

34. The mother of a 6-year-old in first grade reports that he is not keeping up with the other kids in any subject and wants testing to be performed. Evaluation of academic failure at school typically includes which of the following?

(A) hearing and visual evaluation

(B) personality testing

(C) magnetic resonance imaging (MRI) of head

(D) home visit

(E) computed tomography (CT) scan of head

35. Vision milestones are being discussed with a group of student nurses. One student asks when babies can begin to visually follow people as they walk across the room. Fixation and tracking through the visual field are well developed by which of the following ages?

(A) at 7 months gestation

(B) at birth

(C) at 2 months

(D) at 6 months

(E) at 1 year

36. A tired-appearing mother of a 2-month-old boy states he is feeding and sleeping well but cries for a total of 3 hours each day. The baby's examination is normal. Which of the following statements about crying is correct?

(A) Crying increases through the entire first year of life.

(B) Crying usually is a result of hunger.

(C) Any baby crying 3 hours per day, even in light of a normal examination, warrants a medical workup.

(D) This amount of crying is normal for this age.

(E) This degree of crying warrants an immediate skeletal survey.

37. The mother of 9-month-old, who had a normal sleeping pattern in the past, reports he has started awakening and crying once or twice a night. Her primary care physician suggests that this may be a manifestation of separation anxiety. At which of the following ages does separation anxiety usually first manifest?

(A) 1 week

(B) 3–4 months

(C) 8–9 months

(D) 2–3 years

(E) 5–6 years

38. A medical student is checking out a 2-month well-child visit to the attending pediatrician. She remarks that the infant is sleeping with her parents. Which of the following statements regarding cosleeping is true?

(A) Incidence of sudden infant death syndrome (SIDS) is higher in young infants.

(B) Cosleeping is uncommon in countries outside of the United States.

(C) Cosleeping can facilitate transitioning to a child's own crib or bed.

(D) The primary care provider should refer the child for sleep testing.

(E) The infant's parents typically report feeling well rested.

39. A 7-month-old infant presents for well-child care and the physician notes a well-developed Moro reflex, palmar grasp reflex, and tonic neck reflexes on examination. The persistence of neonatal reflexes is an indicator of developmental delay, he tells the mother of the infant. At which age should the Moro reflex typically disappear?

(A) 3 months

(B) 4 months

(C) 6–8 months

(D) 12–16 months

(E) 17–20 months

40. At what age should the tonic neck reflex disappear?

    (A) 3 months
    (B) 4 months
    (C) 6–8 months
    (D) 12–16 months
    (E) 17–20 months

41. At what age should the palmar grasp reflex disappear?

    (A) 3 months
    (B) 4 months
    (C) 6–8 months
    (D) 12–16 months
    (E) 17–20 months

42. A 1-year-old girl who has been in a motor vehicle accident today is alert, but you note a positive Babinski (upgoing plantar) reflexes. At what age does a Babinski reflex disappear?

    (A) 3 months
    (B) 4 months
    (C) 6–8 months
    (D) 15–18 months
    (E) 20–24 months

43. A mother brings her preteen twins (1 girl, 1 boy) in for a checkup and notes that the girl is 2 in taller than her twin. She asks the pediatric nurse practitioner if this could be a sign of puberty. Pubertal growth spurt in females begins on average at what age?

    (A) 8 years
    (B) 10 years
    (C) 12 years
    (D) 14 years
    (E) 16 years

44. The pubertal growth spurt in males occurs at which of the following ages?

    (A) precedes the growth spurt in females by 2 years
    (B) has its onset at the same age as in females but lasts longer

    (C) follows the growth spurt in females by 2 years
    (D) coincides with attainment of the ability to ejaculate
    (E) begins at Tanner IV stage of sexual maturity

45. The father of a 13-year-old boy asks if his son's adult height can be predicted. The peak velocity of growth during adolescence averages which of the following?

    (A) 1–2 cm/yr
    (B) 3–4 cm/yr
    (C) 5–6 cm/yr
    (D) 7–8 cm/yr
    (E) 9–10 cm/yr

46. An adolescent male wearing a baggy T-shirt comes to his pediatrician's office for evaluation of breast development. He is very worried and embarrassed, and he inquires if there is anything that can be done to treat it. Which of the following statements regarding gynecomastia in males during adolescence is correct?

    (A) is distinctly uncommon
    (B) usually occurs at age 14–15 years
    (C) is synonymous with lipomastia
    (D) is often a continuing problem in adulthood
    (E) necessitates basic laboratory testing

47. Concerns about childrens' TV watching are being discussed with a group of parents. The age at which a child can reliably distinguish fantasy from reality occurs at which of the following ages?

    (A) 4 years
    (B) 6 years
    (C) 7 years
    (D) 8 years
    (E) 10 years

48. A 19-year-old G3P3 reports that she had a period of depression after the birth of her second child. She is concerned this could resurface with the birth of the third child. Which of the following statements is true regarding postpartum depression?

(A) Postpartum "blues" are rare in new mothers.

(B) Other family stress usually lessens in the postpartum period.

(C) Teenage mothers have a high rate of depression.

(D) Psychosis is a common feature.

(E) In the majority of cases of postpartum depression, intervention is necessary for resolution of symptoms.

49. The HEADSS inventory is a useful screening tool for adolescents. Which of the following areas are evaluated?

(A) Risk for decreased intelligence quotient

(B) Risk for early coronary artery disease

(C) Risk for diabetes

(D) Risk for normal growth

(E) Risk for depression

50. The tired parents of an infant girl ask if there are any predictive factors for the development of colic. Which of the following best describes risk factors for colic?

(A) Colic usually is associated with infants who are bottle-fed.

(B) Colic typically begins at 41–42 weeks gestational age regardless of gestational age at birth.

(C) Colic is most prevalent among caucasian neonates.

(D) Colic occurs more commonly among females than males.

(E) There are very predictable long-term temperamental outcomes that emerge from a colicky infancy.

51. The parents of a 21-month-old boy are concerned because he used to say a few words and more recently, he is just babbling with no recognizable words. They are worried these may be features of autism. Which of the following is a feature that characterizes autistic spectrum disorders?

(A) Pointing or waving by 18 months

(B) Use of 2 word phrases by 18 months

(C) Decreased eye contact

(D) Nystagmus

(E) Lack of sensitivity to textures or sounds

52. The mother of a 6-month-old girl presents for a well-child check. The baby's weight and length are at the 5th percentile, and her head circumference is at the 25th percentile. Which of the following is a true statement regarding failure to thrive in infants?

(A) more common among Hispanic children

(B) extremely rare in the United States

(C) most often caused by an organic problem

(D) more common among female infants than male infants

(E) a major risk factor for later developmental and behavioral difficulties

53. The parents of a 6-year-old boy bring him to his pediatrician to discuss his behavior patterns. The child's mother is concerned about his behaviors, but his father reports that his son will "grow out of it." Some behavior patterns are considered appropriate at certain developmental stages, but are obviously pathologic if present later on in life. Other behavior patterns are considered pathologic at all ages. Which of the following is an example of the latter?

(A) temper tantrums

(B) lying

(C) oppositional behavior

(D) truancy

(E) rebellion

54. One of this mother's concerns is that her 6-year-old often physically fights with his siblings. Childhood aggression is most commonly associated with which of the following?

(A) girls compared to boys

(B) children small for their age compared to children large for their age

(C) children from smaller families compared to children from larger families

(D) children diagnosed with attention-deficit hyperactivity disorder

(E) children with borderline personality disorder

55. Primary care office nurses are designing a questionnaire to screen for toxin poisoning in their practice. They wonder how to describe pica so that a parent can understand it. Pica is the ingestion of nonnutrient substances like dirt and chalk. Which of the following statements regarding pica is true?

    (A) The median age of onset is 6 years.
    (B) It is often a symptom of family disorganization, poor supervision, and affectional neglect.
    (C) It is caused by iron poisoning and parasitic infestations.
    (D) It usually persists into adolescence.
    (E) It is caused by viral infections.

56. A father brings his twins (1 boy, 1 girl) in for their kindergarten checkup. He is concerned because both children wet the bed at night, and he wonders how long it will last. Which of the following statements regarding nocturnal enuresis is true?

    (A) Prevalence at age 10 years ranges from 7% to 10%.
    (B) A marked familial pattern is often noted.
    (C) Workup routinely recommended in the management includes renal ultrasound and micturating cystourethrogram to rule out kidney disease and vescicoureteric reflux.
    (D) Bed wetting alarms are rarely useful in the management of some children with enuresis.
    (E) Among 5-year-old children, enuresis is more common in females.

57. A pediatrician has followed a child in foster care since infancy. This child has experienced academic and social success despite difficult environmental stresses. Factors which contribute to resiliency in childhood include which of the following?

    (A) difficulty with adaptability to changes
    (B) low level of energy and persistence
    (C) a desire to investigate and master new situations

    (D) absence of sense of personal autonomy
    (E) family history of academic success

58. The mother of a kindergartner is concerned that her child may have a learning disability. Which of the following would be consistent with a learning disability?

    (A) reverses some letters when writing his name
    (B) had delayed speech as toddler
    (C) diagnosis before age 3 years
    (D) has a discrepancy between intelligence and achievement in one or more areas
    (E) cannot read yet

59. The mother of a 2-year-old girl wonders if her daughter's motor skills are age appropriate. Which of the following is a motor skill that most 2-year-olds have attained?

    (A) stands on one foot for 10 seconds
    (B) climbs stairs using alternating feet
    (C) pedals a tricycle
    (D) copies a circle
    (E) builds a tower of 8–10 cubes

60. The mother of a 2-year-old girl is concerned that her daughter is resisting efforts to be toilet-trained. Which of the following recommendations for toilet training are advisable?

    (A) Begin training before age 2 years
    (B) Continue even if the child is extremely resistant
    (C) "Time out" for "accidents"
    (D) Don't begin if more than five wet diapers in a day
    (E) Sticker charts are a useful tool to track successes

61. The normal cognitive development of toddlers is being discussed with a group of medical students. The developmental thrust of the 2-year-old is best expressed by which of the following phrases?

    (A) "me do it"
    (B) "show me how"

(C) "that can't be right"

(D) "why"

(E) "you do it"

62. The mother of a 9-month-old girl reports that she is now waking up at night, after sleeping all night for several months. Nighttime awakening at this age can be treated by which of the following?

(A) Vary the bedtime routine

(B) Avoid the use of a transitional object such as a teddy bear

(C) Give a bottle of formula or breast milk to the infant in bed

(D) Reassure by rocking the infant to sleep

(E) Put infant to bed while drowsy but still awake

63. In discussing the features of the body mass index (BMI) curve for children to a group of medical students, the pediatrician reports that children experience a period of growth called the adiposity rebound, where their body weight begins increasing to a greater degree than their height is increasing. Adiposity rebound typically occurs at which of the following average ages?

(A) 1 week

(B) 1 year

(C) 5 years

(D) 10–12 years

(E) 13–17 years

64. In coordinating pediatric residents to perform head start (early childhood development) physicals and developmental screenings on a group of preschool children, it is mentioned that a child who can walk downstairs alternating his or her feet, do a broad jump, and throw a ball overhand, also would be expected to do which of the following?

(A) add five and five

(B) identify three or four coins

(C) name two or three colors

(D) multiply three times three

(E) write his or her name

65. The mother of a 3-year-old girl reports that her daughter is afraid to go to bed at night. Which of the following are recommended methods of managing nighttime fears?

(A) Perform an exhaustive "search" for monsters in the child's bedroom

(B) Vary the bedtime schedule

(C) Vary the regular nighttime routine prior to bedtime

(D) Allow the child to watch TV and videos for at least one hour prior to bedtime

(E) Visit the child briefly to provide reassurance when the child awakens with fear

66. The parents of a child who recently turned 5 years old bring him in for a well-child check and assessment of school readiness. Regarding school readiness, which of the following is true?

(A) Any concerns about the child's ability to learn will probably resolve if the child delays kindergarten entry for a year.

(B) Previous daycare experience is irrelevant.

(C) The ability to follow 1–3 step directions is an important skill for kindergarten success.

(D) Private schools usually have more access to specialized services than do public schools.

(E) If the child is short for his age, his parents should delay starting him in kindergarten for a year.

67. The pathophysiology of various causes of neonatal cyanosis is being discussed with a group of pediatric residents doing their nursery rotation. In the term newborn, which of the following statements regarding fetal hemoglobin is correct?

(A) Nearly 100% of a neonate's hemoglobin is fetal hemoglobin.

(B) Fetal hemoglobin binds oxygen less tightly than adult hemoglobin.

(C) Oxygenated fetal hemoglobin is blue rather than red.

(D) Fetal hemoglobin prevents sickling of sickle cells.

(E) Fetal hemoglobin hemolyzes easily and is a major cause of neonatal jaundice.

68. A 12-month-old infant presents to her primary care provider's office with respiratory distress. The normal respiratory rate of a 1-year-old child is which of the following?

    (A) over 80 breaths per minute
    (B) between 60 and 80 breaths per minute
    (C) between 35 and 50 breaths per minute
    (D) between 20 and 30 breaths per minute
    (E) between 10 and 12 breaths per minute

69. A pediatric cardiologist is reviewing the electrocardiogram (ECG) of a term infant with tachycardia with a group of pediatric residents. As compared to older children and adults, the ECG of an infant normally shows which of the following findings?

    (A) a shorter RR and shorter PR interval
    (B) a shorter RR and longer PR interval
    (C) a longer RR and shorter PR interval
    (D) a longer RR and shorter PR interval
    (E) an equal RR and PR interval

70. A 2-year-old boy coming in for a checkup is fascinated while his blood pressure is taken, and he remains quiet. The average blood pressure at 2 years of age is most likely to be which of the following values?

    (A) 50/30 mm Hg
    (B) 60/30 mm Hg
    (C) 75/50 mm Hg
    (D) 95/60 mm Hg
    (E) 120/80 mm Hg

71. A 4 week male with a temperature of 101°F has undergone an evaluation for meningitis. The results of his cerebrospinal fluid (CSF) testing return and while no white blood cells are seen and the glucose is normal, the protein is recorded as high at 90 mg/dL. The concentration of protein in the CSF of infants during the first few weeks of life normally may be as high as which of the following?

    (A) 20 mg/dL
    (B) 45 mg/dL
    (C) 125 mg/dL

    (D) 500 mg/dL
    (E) 1000 mg/dL

72. The parents of a 4-year-old boy are concerned because his speech is still not fully understandable. Which of the following best describes a child's conversation at 4 years of age?

    (A) fully understandable, although mispronunciations and grammatical errors are common
    (B) fully understandable, with few if any mispronunciations and grammatical errors
    (C) fully understandable to the parent but not necessarily to others
    (D) somewhat understandable although garbled and indistinct
    (E) somewhat understandable, with mostly correct use of nouns and mostly incorrect use of verbs

73. A 7-year-old girl comes to her pediatrician's office because her teacher is concerned that she may have attention-deficit hyperactivity disorder (ADHD). Hallmarks of ADHD include which of the following?

    (A) Often quiet demeanor
    (B) History of seizures at birth
    (C) History of recurrent ear infections
    (D) Symptom occurrence in more than one environment
    (E) Does not appear to be easily distracted

74. The father of 2- and 8-year-old siblings calls their pediatrician to discuss how he and the childrens' mother can prepare them for the parents' upcoming divorce. Which of the following statements is true regarding children of divorce?

    (A) The emotional availability of one or both parents is often heightened.
    (B) On average, girls have a more difficult time adjusting initially to divorce than boys.
    (C) As boys reach young adulthood, they may experience anxiety about male-female relationships.

(D) The majority of children have adjusted to the altered family circumstance by the second year following the divorce.

(E) Preschool-aged children may demonstrate regressive behavior.

75. The mother of an otherwise healthy infant noticed recently that she could not identify the soft spot in her infant anymore. Based on this piece of history, this child is most likely to be what age?

(A) 3 months
(B) between 3 and 9 months
(C) between 9 and 18 months
(D) between 18 and 24 months
(E) between 24 and 36 months

76. The parents of a 3-month-old boy who is growing well come to the pediatrician's office for a well-child check. Which of the following guidance items regarding growth and development are appropriate to discuss at this visit?

(A) may leave infant unattended on couch or changing table as long as he is not rolling over yet
(B) caution against leaving small items on the floor because infant could pick them up
(C) infant still needs to be fed every 2 hours at night
(D) expect him to coo, smile and laugh
(E) may place infant on his abdomen to sleep

77. A 16-year-old girl presents to her primary care provider's office requesting a pregnancy test due to a late period. Which of the following factors are associated with an increased risk of teen pregnancy?

(A) poor academic performance
(B) rigid parental support and supervision
(C) living in a middle class community
(D) history of drug or alcohol abuse in parent
(E) late onset of puberty

78. A medical student is describing the growth pattern of a child with growth hormone (GH) deficiency. Children with isolated GH deficiency usually have which of the following?

(A) have a normal bone age
(B) have associated mild hypothyroidism
(C) grow parallel to, but below, the normal growth curve
(D) have an associated (compensating) hyperthyroidism
(E) show deceleration of growth velocity and fall away from the growth normal curve

79. Parents bring a 10-year-old boy in for evaluation of short stature. The patient is worried about his eventual adult height. Children with constitutional growth delay (without endocrine abnormality) generally can expect to ultimately achieve which of the following growth descriptions?

(A) very short and obese
(B) short but of proportionate weight
(C) of normal height and weight
(D) very tall but of proportionate weight
(E) very tall and obese

80. The parents of a 7-year-old girl report that she would rather watch TV than play outside. It is estimated that the average school-age American child watches television for about how many hours a week?

(A) 4–8 h/week
(B) 10–14 h/week
(C) 15–20 h/week
(D) 25–30 h/week
(E) 35–40 h/week

81. The inpatient pediatric team is discussing the causes of failure to thrive (FTT) as they evaluate a 9-month-old infant with weight and length below the 5th percentile. Which of the following should be included in the differential diagnosis of infant who is not thriving?

(A) Small atrial septal defect
(B) Acute bacterial meningitis
(C) Cystic fibrosis
(D) Recurrent otitis media
(E) Mild intermittent asthma

82. High school teachers are listening to a lecture about the features of adolescence. Which of the following best describes the period of adolescence?

    (A) immediately before, during, and after puberty
    (B) of maximal physical growth
    (C) of maximal sexual development
    (D) of physiologic adjustment to maturity
    (E) of psychosocial transition from childhood to adulthood

83. The mother of a 16-year-old girl reports that she has noticed declining scholastic grades, refusal to participate in family activities, and an unwillingness to communicate with either parents or peers. These findings in an adolescent usually indicate which of the following?

    (A) a normal stage of development
    (B) a normal response to peer pressure
    (C) a normal reaction to overprotective parents
    (D) a transient phase of ambivalence
    (E) an emotional or psychiatric problem

84. The parents of a 2-year-old boy report he is about to be thrown out of daycare due to biting other children. For the primary care provider, which of the following facts are important to inquire about regarding biting behavior?

    (A) Age when parents introduced solid food
    (B) Toileting behavior
    (C) Age at which child's first tooth erupted
    (D) History of pica
    (E) Concerns about the child's developmental progress

85. A hemoglobin and hematocrit is obtained from a 12-month-old who came to his pediatrician's office for a checkup. Which of the following best describes the normal (average) hemoglobin concentration at 1 year of age?

    (A) 17 g/dL
    (B) 15 g/dL
    (C) 12 g/dL
    (D) 10 g/dL
    (E) 8 g/dL

86. A group of medical students on the newborn nursery rotation are discussing the sensory and physical abilities of a newborn. Which of these abilities is considered normal?

    (A) inability to sense pain
    (B) preference for geometric shapes over mother's face
    (C) 20/20 vision
    (D) grasping a caregiver's finger
    (E) ability to see objects 2–3 feet away

87. The parents of a 4-year-old with recurrent wheezing are both smokers. They inquire about the child's likelihood of becoming a smoker when he reaches adulthood. The phenomenon of children incorporating habits demonstrated by the adults in their lives is known by which of the following terms?

    (A) time in
    (B) incidental learning
    (C) conditioned reinforcement
    (D) fading
    (E) rapprochement

88. Growth milestones are being discussed with a group of medical students in the newborn nursery. During the first year of life, how much weight would an infant who weighs 7.5 lb (3.4 kg) at birth ordinarily gain?

    (A) 5 lb (2.3 kg)
    (B) 10 lb (4.5 kg)
    (C) 15 lb (6.8 kg)
    (D) 20 lb (9 kg)
    (E) 25 lb (11.4 kg)

89. During the second year of life, the average child grows how many centimeters?

    (A) 12–15 cm
    (B) 20–25 cm
    (C) 30–40 cm
    (D) 40–50 cm
    (E) over 50 cm

90. The father of a 2-month-old boy wonders why his son's head looks so big. Which of the following best describes the head growth during the first month of life?

(A) 0.5 cm

(B) 1.25 cm

(C) 2 cm

(D) 5 cm

(E) 7.5 cm

91. The mother of an 11-year-old girl who comes to her pediatrician's office for a checkup notes that her daughter is beginning to develop breast buds. She asks when her daughter might have her first period. Which of the following is a true statement regarding menarche in the adolescent girl?

(A) precedes the spurt in linear growth

(B) occurs simultaneously with Tanner stage II breast development

(C) generally occurs when Tanner stage III breast and pubic hair development have been achieved

(D) occurs simultaneously with Tanner stages IV to V pubic hair and breast development

(E) generally occurs a year or more after Tanner stage V breast and pubic hair development have been achieved

92. A pediatric psychologist is discussing the concept of temperament with a group of residents. Which of the following best describes the term temperament?

(A) A parent's response to a tantrum.

(B) The emotional bond that a child feels with his parent.

(C) The acts of independence that a child demonstrates as she enters toddlerhood.

(D) A child's emotional clinginess to a parent when faced with an unfamiliar situation.

(E) Stable, individual modes of responding to the environment.

DIRECTIONS (Questions 93 through 100): The following group of questions is preceded by a list of lettered answer options. For each question, match the one lettered option that is most closely associated with the question. Each lettered option may be selected once, multiple times, or not at all.

Questions 93 through 97

(A) Parents' Evaluations of Developmental Status (PEDS)

(B) CAGE questionnaire

(C) NICHQ Vanderbilt Assessment Scale

(D) Pediatric Symptom Checklist

(E) Otoacoustic emission test

93. This test measures development of a 1-year-old. What is it?

94. This test measures externalizing and internalizing behavior in a 10-year-old. What is it?

95. This test detects alcohol misuse in an adolescent. What is it?

96. This screens for deafness in a newborn. What is it?

97. This test evaluates potential ADHD in a 7-year-old. What is it?

Questions 98 through 100

(A) 4–6 months

(B) 6–9 months

(C) 15–18 months

(D) 18–24 months

(E) 24–36 months

98. A toddler has started toilet training. What is the typical age of this child?

99. An infant is experiencing stranger anxiety. What is the typical age when this appears?

100. An infant is able to self-feed. What is the usual age?

Answers and Explanations

1. **(B)** Newborns may lose up to 10% of their birth weight in the first few days of life, but with normal nutrition birth weight is regained in approximately 10 days. The infant subsequently gains approximately 30 g/day for the first several months. *(Dixon, 224, 229)*

2. **(A)** At 9–12 months, infants gradually develop the concept of object permanence, or the understanding that objects exist even when they are not seen. Around the time this milestone is achieved, infants develop frontal activity on the electroencephalogram. Infants first apply this concept of object permanence to the image of their mother because of her emotional importance; this realization is a critical part of attachment behavior. *(Dixon, 312)*

3. **(C)** Primary or milk teeth are the initial dentition of children. The first teeth to erupt are the central incisors, at 6–10 months of age. Typically, the mandibular central incisors erupt before the maxillary. The lateral incisors (typically maxillary, followed by mandibular) come in next at 9–13 months of age. The first molars follow at 13–19 months. The canines erupt at around 16–23 months. The second molars are the last to come in at 23–33 months of age. *(Kliegman, 1529)*

4. **(C)** Handedness frequently is established by the fourth year. Frustration may result from attempts to change children's hand preference once handedness is established. Unusually early appearance of handedness, such as before the second year, should raise suspicion of motor weakness of an upper extremity. *(Dixon, 283)*

5. **(D)** At birth, the retina is well developed, but the lens is rather immobile. Fixation and tracking through the visual field are well developed by 2 months of age. Infants prefer to gaze at a human face rather than geometrical designs and they also prefer curved lines, bright colors, and high contrast. Strabismus is common after birth but usually resolves by 3 months of age. Although visual acuity is poor at birth, approximately 20/400, it improves rapidly in the first 6 months of life to 20/40. However, it does not reach 20/20 until about 4 years of age. *(Dixon, 149-151)*

6. **(C)** Development of the paranasal sinuses continues throughout childhood. The ethmoid and maxillary sinuses are present from birth; the frontal and sphenoid sinuses usually appear radiologically around 6 years of age, and frequently develop asymmetrically. Frontal sinuses are absent in 1%–5% of adults. *(Kliegman, 1749)*

7. **(B)** The Parents' Evaluation of Developmental Status (PEDS) is a useful developmental screening tool for the primary care office. It can be used from birth to 8 years, and screens for various kinds of emotional and developmental problems and delays. The PEDS consists of 10 questions, and can be administered in 2–5 minutes. Its sensitivity in detecting children with difficulties is greater than 75%, and specificity in correctly detecting normal development is 70%–80%. *(Dixon, 729)*

8. **(B)** The fetal period begins at the ninth week of gestation and ends at birth. It is preceded by the embryonic period, during which the

rudiments of all major organ systems develop. *(Kliegman, 38)*

9. **(C)** By 20 weeks gestation, most second-time mothers and many first-time mothers feel their baby's first movements. This sensation is known as "quickening." *(Kliegman, 39)*

10. **(D)** Following the realization that words can stand for things, the child's vocabulary balloons from about 10–15 words at 18 months to 100 or more at 3 years. After 18 months, there is a dramatic increase in expressive and receptive vocabulary and by the end of the second year, a quantum leap occurs in language development, such that most children presenting for their 2-year-old checkup are reported to say at least 50 words. *(Dixon, 392)*

11. **(E)** Even during the neonatal period, up to 10 of an infant's average of 16 hours of sleep per day are concentrated at night. This is reflective of an adaptation process which began in the third trimester of pregnancy. Daytime sleep progressively declines in infancy; the 12-month-old typically takes two 1-hour naps during the day. By the age of 3, most toddlers sleep 1 hour during the day, and the majority of 4-year-olds do not take a daytime nap. *(Kliegman, 45)*

12. **(A)** Teenagers have been entering puberty at increasingly earlier ages during the last century, presumably because of better nutrition and improved socioeconomic conditions. The age of menarche decreased by about 4 months per decade during the last century. In the United States, the average age at menarche is 12 years, the average weight is 48 kg, and the average height is 158.5 cm. Although the first measurable sign of puberty in girls is the beginning of the height spurt, the first conspicuous sign usually is development of breast buds between the ages of 8 and 11 years. *(Dixon, 541)*

13. **(B)** The first sign of puberty in boys, testicular enlargement, begins as early as 9.5 years. The appearance of pubic hair is an early event in puberty, but can occur any time between ages 10 and 15 years. The penis begins to grow significantly a year or so after the onset of testicular and pubic hair development, usually between the ages of 10 and 13.5 years. The median age for entering SMR II or puberty in boys is 10.5 years. However, great variability exists in the timing and onset of puberty and growth, and psychosocial development does not necessarily parallel physical changes. *(Dixon, 537-538)*

14. **(C)** Growth acceleration begins in early adolescence, although peak growth velocity is not reached until SMR III in girls and SMR IV in boys. Girls reach their peak height velocity between 11.5 and 12 years of age. The height spurt usually ends by age 14. Girls who mature early will reach their peak height velocity sooner and attain their final height earlier. Girls who mature late will attain a greater ultimate height because of the longer period of growth before the growth spurt. Final height is related to skeletal age at onset of puberty as well as genetic factors. *(Kliegman, 61)*

15. **(C)** Growth is rapid in the first 2 years of life. Infants increase their length by 50% the first year and 25% the next. They triple their birth weight in the first year. After 2 years of age, the growth velocity curve stabilizes into the rate for mid childhood, which is a weight gain of 2–3 kg or 4.5–6.5 lb/yr and a height gain of 5–7 cm or 2–3 in/yr. *(Kliegman, 72)*

16. **(D)** C Growth charts for children ages 2–20 now include body mass index (BMI) charts. Childhood obesity is the most common form of malnutrition in the United States. Other parameters used to detect and quantify obesity include measurement of skinfold thickness in triceps and subscapular regions and measurement of percent body fat by bioelectrical impedance (BIA) or dual x-ray energy absorptiometry (DEXA). BMI varies with age; it typically increases yearly after a nadir between the ages of 2 and 5. Obesity is defined as a BMI greater than <u>95%</u> for age and gender. *(Kliegman, 73)*

17. **(C)** Body mass index (BMI) is calculated as (weight in kilograms)/(height in meters)^2. Once this value is determined, it must be compared

to others of the child's same gender and age. *(Kliegman, 73)*

18. **(B)** Constitutional growth delay has a characteristic pattern of having a late growth spurt during adolescence, therefore in early adolescence the child will be short as compared to his or her peers. However, he or she will continue to grow later in adolescence and reach a normal adult height. Children with constitutional growth delay will be of normal size at birth. Bone age is delayed and is comparable to the height age. Children with constitutional growth delay must be differentiated from those with undernutrition and endocrinologic short stature who also have delayed bone age. *(Kliegman, 2297)*

19. **(C)** The majority of a newborn's early days are spent sleeping. Total requirements for sleep are 16 hr/24 hr in the first month of life, with most of the sleeping hours concentrated at night. Sleep requirements decline slowly over the first year. By the age of 9 months, the average infant sleeps 14 hr/day and by 3 years of age, most toddlers sleep 12 hr/day. *(Kliegman, 45)*

20. **(B)** The topic of childhood obesity must be approached with sensitivity by the primary care provider. Parents often have much guilt surrounding their child's size, and may be defensive when history questions are presented. Key questions to ask include a family history of children with rapid weight gain, the frequency and types of vigorous physical activities performed by the child, the parents' own commitment to physical activity, and the presence of extreme overeating or binging by the child. Additional pertinent questions regarding the child's and family's nutrition habits and the family's perception of influence that the child's weight has upon them should be presented. *(Parker, 253–260)*

21. **(E)** Some echolalia (echoing spoken words) during toddlerhood is common and usually of no concern. When severe or persistent beyond toddlerhood, echolalia may be a sign of disturbed language development, mental retardation, or neurologic disease. Although echolalia

is common in infantile autism, most toddlers who display word repetition are not autistic. (Note: The question did not ask whether autism should be considered [it should] but whether the child probably has autism [he probably does not].) *(Dixon, 363, 391-393)*

22. **(E)** Normal newborns are endowed with a set of reflexes to facilitate survival, including rooting and sucking reflexes, and remarkable sensory abilities. The newborn is no longer considered a blank slate. Instead, the newborn is seen as having genetic strengths and weaknesses in neurocognitive organization that are reflected in temperament, adaptability, responsiveness, and general interaction with the environment. Hearing is well developed at birth, and speech sounds are preferred. The infant learns to recognize his mother's voice and differentiate it from other female voices within the first 3 weeks of life. At birth infants prefer to gaze at a human face rather than geometric designs, and they also prefer curved lines, bright colors, and high contrast. Infants are myopic at birth. They are able to suckle at the breast immediately after birth. *(Dixon,152)*

23. **(B)** The attainment of gross motor milestones begins at approximately 2 months of age with steady head control. This allows better visual interaction between infants and parents. The child is then able to be pulled to sit without head lag at around 3 months of age. Putting hands together in the midline at around 3 months of age allows the infant to examine objects in the midline and manipulate them with both hands. Once the asymmetric Tonic neck reflex is gone, at around 4 months of age, infants are able to begin to roll over, first from stomach to back and finally around 6 months of age from back to stomach. Infants will sit without support at approximately 6 months of age and will pull to stand and cruise around furniture by 9 months of age. The average age of beginning to walk alone is 12 months. *(Dixon, 248, 264, 289, 323)*

24. **(E)** Around the same time as the infant is able to put hands together in the midline, he is able to grasp objects and examine them. This occurs at an average of 3.5 months of age. He can transfer

objects from hand to hand at approximately 5.5 months of age, allowing him to compare objects. He attains thumb–finger grasp at approximately 8 months of age, at which time he begins to feed himself finger foods. At around 1 year of age he is able to turn pages in a book, and by 13 months of age he has attained sufficient visual-motor coordination to scribble. By 15 months of age he can build a tower of two cubes, using objects in combination, and by 22 months of age he can build his tower up to six cubes, which requires visual, gross, and fine motor coordination. *(Dixon, 264,289,315, 317, 377)*

25. **(C)** Growth of the midface and lower face in children occurs gradually. Loss of the deciduous (baby) teeth is a more dramatic sign of maturation, beginning at around 6 years of age, after eruption of the first molars. Replacement with adult teeth occurs at a rate of about 4 per year. The mandibular, then maxillary central incisors are replaced at the same time or just following the eruption of the first molars at around 6–7 years of age. After this, the lateral incisors erupt, at around 7–8 years of age. The adult canines replace the baby teeth at around 9–11 years of age, and next to erupt are the first premolars and then the second premolars. The second molars erupt at around 12 years of age but the third molars (wisdom teeth) do not erupt until 17–21 years of age. *(Kliegman, 1529)*

26. **(D)** The primary teeth form in dental crypts that arise from a band of epithelial cells incorporated into each developing jaw. Organization of adjacent mesenchyme takes place in each area of epithelial growth, and the two elements together comprise the beginning of a tooth. The first primary or deciduous teeth to erupt are the central incisors at 5–7 months of age, followed by the lateral incisors at around 7–10 months of age, and the first molars at around 10–16 months of age. The canines do not erupt until 16–20 months of age. *(Kliegman, 15 21)*

27. **(C)** Ossification centers usually present at birth include the distal femur and the proximal tibia. Reference standards for bone maturation facilitate estimation of bone age. In constitutional growth delay, endocrinologic short stature, and

undernutrition, the bone age is low and is comparable to the height age. In familial short stature, the bone age is normal (compared to chronological age). The most commonly used standards are those of Gruelich and Pyle, which require radiographs of the left hand and wrist; knee films are sometimes added for younger children. *(Kliegman, 27 71)*

28. **(C)** Most children begin to walk independently around the time of their first birthday; some do not walk until 15 months. At 18 months of age, the infant shows improvements in balance and agility, and the ability to run and climb stairs while holding a parent's hand emerges. By 30 months of age, the child is able to go upstairs by himself, alternating feet. By 3 years of age, the child has attained the motor coordination to ride a tricycle. A child is usually hopping by 4 years of age and skipping by 6 years of age. *(Dixon, 335, 470)*

29. **(A)** At approximately 18 months, several cognitive changes come together to mark the conclusion of the sensorimotor period. At this time, the infant can feed himself, seek help when in trouble, and complain when wet or soiled. From this age forward, the child is increasingly independent. By 24 months of age, he helps to undress himself and is able to handle a spoon well. As a 3-year-old, he helps in dressing and undressing, washes his own hands, and engages in "parallel play." By age 5, he is able to fully dress and undress himself. At this time he is likely to engage in domestic role-playing. *(Dixon, 378,406,430, 468)*

30. **(D)** Child abuse and neglect are correlated with delayed language, particularly the ability to convey emotional states. Such delays may contribute to problems of behavior, socialization, and learning. Mental retardation may first become apparent with delayed speech at approximately 2 years, although earlier signs may have been overlooked. Hearing loss is a common cause of speech delay. Consequently, hearing evaluation should be an integral part of the management of delayed speech. The other choices listed do not have a proclivity for speech delay. *(Dixon, 400–401)*

31. **(B)** As children mature, they learn what behaviors are acceptable and how much power they are able to wield by testing limits. Control is a central issue. Inability to control some aspect of the external world, such as how to make a certain toy work or when to leave, often results in a loss of internal control, that is, a temper tantrum. Fear, overtiredness, or physical discomfort can also evoke tantrums. When they are reinforced by intermittent rewards, as when the parent occasionally gives in to the child's demands, tantrums can also become an entrenched strategy for exerting control by the toddler. Tantrums lasting more than 15 minutes or happening regularly more than three times daily can reflect underlying medical, emotional, or social problems. Tantrums normally appear at the end of the first year of life and peak at 2–4 years. Frequent tantrums after 5 years of age usually persist throughout childhood. Clearly, this is an undesirable outcome which, in nearly all children, is avoidable. *(Dixon, 372–373)*

32. **(C)** A newborn's birth weight correlates with the size, nutritional state, and general health of the mother and represents the influence of uterine constraints on ultimate size. After the first 6 months of life, genetic factors influencing ultimate height begin to exert their effect. The growth percentile, therefore, may shift significantly in the first 4–18 months of life. This shift can be either up or down. An infant who is small for gestational age and has a genetic predisposition to larger stature usually experiences accelerated growth in the first 6 months, and by 18 months a stable growth percentile is established. A downward shift is seen in large infants who have a genetic predisposition to short stature. A stable growth percentile should be established by 18 months of age. *(Dixon, 230–231)*

33. **(D)** About half of normal children during the second year of life are noncompliant when faced with a task such as the DDST. This is itself a developmental phenomenon, reflecting the child's movement toward independence and his newfound ability to resist control and do things himself. The range of normal on-screening tests such as the DDST is broad, and a score in the 15–18-month range for an 18-month-old child is not bothersome. Usually, more formal and complete evaluation is indicated for the child who is functioning more than one-third below his chronologic age. *(Dixon, 366)*

34. **(A)** In evaluation of academic failure at school, neuropsychological and educational testing is completed, as well as audiometry and visual testing by the school or the pediatrician. Evaluation for attention-deficit hyperactivity disorder (ADHD) may form part of the evaluation for academic failure. Neuroimaging typically is not part of this evaluation process. Although a home visit may be particularly helpful, it is not commonly carried out by the school personnel. *(Dixon, 480–485)*

35. **(C)** At birth, the retina is well developed but the lens is rather immobile. Fixation and tracking through the visual field are well developed by 2 months of age. The length of time that an infant fixates on a paired visual stimulus has been interpreted as visual preference, and has also been correlated with later cognitive development. *(Dixon, 247)*

36. **(D)** Crying gradually increases during the first 6–12 weeks of age because it is the main modality by which infants express responses to stimuli, both aversive and nonaversive. Crying can be a response to a variety of stimuli, including hunger, a wet diaper, fear, fatigue, and overstimulation. Crying gradually decreases after 12 weeks of age as the infant develops other responses, such as smiling or reaching, or becomes more adept at self-soothing, such as sucking the fingers or the thumb. In the first weeks of life, however, crying can become a distressing problem for the parents, and crying associated with irritability is often labeled as colic. *(Dixon, 234–237)*

37. **(C)** The advent of object constancy corresponds with qualitative changes in social and communicative development. The infant looks back and forth between an approaching stranger and a parent, as if to contrast known from unknown, and may cling or cry anxiously. This occurs around 8–9 months of age. Separations often become more difficult, and infants who

have been sleeping through the night for months begin to awaken regularly and cry, as though remembering that parents are in the next room. *(Dixon, 294)*

38. **(A)** Cosleeping is an accepted phenomenon in many ethnic groups, including African American, Hispanic, and Southeast Asian. It has been implicated as a risk factor in sudden infant death syndrome (SIDS), especially for infants of a mother who smokes. Prolonged cosleeping may predispose children to more significant sleep problems as they get older. Parents, especially fathers, may report less restful sleep. Nonetheless, this issue must be approached with sensitivity by the primary care provider. *(Kliegman, 1738)*

[handwritten: most of these are wrong! D✓]

39. **(C)**, 40. **(C)**, 41. **(D)**, 42. **(C)** Reflex movement begins in fetal development as early as 9 weeks gestation. However, most of the reflexes associated with the newborn develop between 20 and 38 weeks gestation. The Moro reflex disappears by 7 months of age. *[handwritten: 4-5]* Palmar grasp usually disappears by 6 months of age, facilitating release of objects. The Tonic neck reflex, which is elicited by turning the infant's head, resulting in extension of the arm and leg on the side toward which the head is turned and flexion of the opposite side, disappears by 8 months of age, unless myelinization or brain development is pathologic. The Babinski (upgoing toes) sign, which develops in an infant just prior to term, does not disappear until 16 months of *[handwritten: 12-16 mon.]* age, when adequate myelinization has occurred. *(Dixon, 158)*

43. **(B)** Growth acceleration begins in early adolescence, although peak growth velocities are not reached until SMR III or SMR IV. The pubertal growth spurt begins at about 10 years in females and about 12.5 years in males. Different areas of the skeleton attain their peak growth at different times. This is seen most dramatically in the feet, which first develop a growth spurt. This is followed by a rapid increase in leg length, and subsequently in truncal growth. Facial growth occurs after peak height velocity. This asymmetric growth gives the young adolescent a gawky look. *(Dixon, 539)*

44. **(C)** The first sign of puberty in the male, usually between the ages of 10 and 12, is scrotal and testicular growth. The first ejaculation is a notable event and usually begins 1 year after the beginning of testicular growth, but its timing is highly variable. Ninety percent of boys have this experience between the ages of 11 and 15 years. The pubertal growth spurt begins at about 10 years in females and about 2 years later in males. Boys have just over 2 more years of preadolescent growth than girls do; during this time, leg growth increases more dramatically than trunk growth. Girls have a greater spurt in hip width related to stature than boys do, although boys exceed girls in most other areas of bone growth. The growth spurt begins at SMR II and peaks at SMR IV. *(Dixon, 537-539; Kliegman 60-63)*

45. **(E)** The peak velocity of growth among adolescent girls corresponds with SMR III, and among boys with SMR IV. This growth averages 9–10 cm/yr, although this growth is somewhat lower in girls than in boys. However, the period of pubertal development lasts much longer in boys and may not be completed until the age of 18 years. Thelarche (breast development) in girls occurs much earlier than the period of peak growth velocity; it is the first visible sign of puberty and may begin as early as age 8 years. *(Dixon, 537-54;, Kliegman 62-63)*

46. **(B)** Gynecomastia significant enough to be embarrassing for adolescent males occurs in less than 10% of boys, although some degree of breast tissue enlargement is seen in 40%–65% of adolescent boys in the ages of 14–15. This resolves within 2 years on its own in the majority of cases, and rarely is pathologic. Lipomastia refers to soft subcutaneous fat often seen in obese boys and sometimes confused with gynecomastia. *(Kliegman, 2385-2386)*

47. **(C)** Most children younger than age 7 cannot reliably distinguish fantasy from reality. This is particularly relevant given that today's school-age children spend at least 4 hours in front of the TV per day. These young children believe that all the characters act and feel as they are shown on TV, and that the characters live in the TV setting between shows. *(Dixon, 425)*

48. (C) Postpartum depression is a common occurrence among new mothers, affecting up to 80%. This usually resolves itself with hormonal changes back to normal homeostasis, but in 10% a major depression occurs. Depressed parents tend to bring their children to the pediatrician more often. Teenage mothers are particularly vulnerable to depression, especially if there is poor social structure. Even after treatment of a parent with major depression, the children tend to have ongoing problems of functioning. Though maternal psychosis is uncommon, the adjustment of children is related not only to their exposure to psychiatric symptomatology but also to more common, longer term patterns of dysfunctional parenting behaviors and aberrant social interactions. (*Dixon, 207–210*)

49. (E) The HEADSS inventory assists in the psychosocial evaluation of adolescents. Less "sensitive" questions are followed by more sensitive ones. Examples of home questions may include "Where do you live, how many siblings do you have?" Education questions may include, "What is the best/worst part of school for you?" Activities questions may include, "Do you play any sports or exercise?" as well as "What do you like to do with your friends?" Questions about drugs may include, "Are you/your friends using tobacco, marijuana, alcohol, or other drugs?" Sexuality questions may include, "Are any of your friends dating someone, and are they getting involved physically?" Suicide/depression questions may include, "Are you happy with the way you look and feel?" (*Dixon, 550–552*)

50. (B) Colic typically begins at 41–42 weeks gestational age in both term and preterm infants. There are two patterns of colic, the most common being associated with fussiness beginning in the early evening hours and occurring in paroxysms of crying. The second pattern is characterized by paroxysms of crying throughout the day in a hyperirritable infant. There are no differences in prevalence of colic among race, gender, or method of feeding (breast vs bottle). The presence of colic during infancy gives no predictive value for long-term behavioral, temperamental, or psychologic outcomes. (*Dixon, 233–237*)

51. (C) Autism is a neurodevelopmental disorder characterized by impaired socialization, impaired verbal and nonverbal communication, and restricted, repetitive patterns of behavior. Early recognition of autism, preferably before the second year of life, is critical. Referral criteria in the second year of life include no pointing or waving by 18 months, a preference for solitary play, diminished eye contact, and an oversensitivity to textures and noises. Nystagmus is more likely to be associated with an ocular disorder. Lack of use of two-word phrases is a concern after the age of 2 years. (*Dixon, 363–365*)

52. (E) Failure to thrive is a major risk factor for later behavioral and developmental problems. It is diagnosed by persistent and significant deviation from the growth curves along time. Poverty-stricken children are likely to be affected, at 5%–10% prevalence. Although this could represent an organic disorder, by far the most common cause of failure to thrive is psychosocial: the so called nonorganic failure to thrive. (*Kliegman 184-187*)

53. (D) In children less than 6 years of age, oppositional behavior, rebellion, and lying are common as children are just learning to follow societal rules. Temper tantrums may persist from preschoolers up until 5 years of age, usually without pathologic origin. Truancy, or intentional school avoidance, is pathologic at any age. (*Dixon, 448–449*)

54. (D) Several factors contribute to childhood aggression. Boys almost universally are reported to be more aggressive than girls. Larger children often are more aggressive than smaller ones. Children from larger families often are more aggressive than those from smaller families. Conduct-disorder behavior often is associated with psychopathologic conditions. Both attention-deficit hyperactivity disorder and borderline personality disorder (BPD) correlate with aggression. However, ADHD is much more common than BPD, so (D) is the best answer. Of interest is the correlation in boys between severe reading retardation and the development of aggressive conduct disorder. (*Dixon, 446–447*)

55. **(B)** Pica is a chronic eating disorder which involves the eating of nonnutritive substances such as dirt, clay, and peeling paint. The age of onset usually is 1–2 years but may be earlier. This disorder usually remits by middle childhood. Lack of parental nurturing and mental retardation are predisposing factors. Children with pica are at an increased risk for lead poisoning and parasitic infections. Differential diagnoses for this behavior include autism, schizophrenia, and certain physical disorders such as Kleine-Levin syndrome. *(Kliegman, 113)*

56. **(B)** Enuresis, the repeated involuntary or voluntary discharge of the bladder after the age at which bladder control should be maintained, is among the most common problems brought to the pediatrician. Among 5 year olds, enuresis occurs in 7% of males and 3% of females. Twin studies reveal a marked familial pattern. Enuresis is associated with immigration, socioeconomic disadvantage, and family psychopathology. Organic pathology can be found in only a very small number of cases; physical examination and urine analysis are the only routinely indicated tests in enuresis. *(Kliegman, 113-114, 2249-2250)*

57. **(E)** Contributors to resiliency in childhood originate within the child, the caregiving environment, and the larger sociocultural environment. Child-based contributor include an easy adaptability, ability to sustain high levels of activity and to be persistent in achieving goals, a desire to approach and master new situations, and a sense of personal autonomy. *(Levine, 48)*

58. **(D)** The key criterion to the diagnosis of learning disability is a significant discrepancy between the child's estimated intelligence and his or her achievement in one or more learning areas. Although reversal of letters is common in these children, it is not present in all patients and is not a criterion for diagnosis. Furthermore, some reversal of letters may occur in normal children as they begin to learn to write. Children with learning disabilities are usually of average or above average intelligence, but above average intelligence is not a criterion for diagnosis. Similarly, visual or auditory perceptual defects are frequently seen in these patients but are not

criteria for diagnosis. Many of these patients do have emotional, behavioral, or motivational problems in addition to, or in reaction to, their learning disability. *(Dixon, 488)*

59. **(E)** Major gross motor skill milestones of most 3–year-olds include going upstairs alternating feet, jumping from the bottom step, pedaling a tricycle and standing on 1 foot for greater than 3 seconds. A fine motor skill hallmark is copying a circle. It is not until the child is older than 4 that he or she can stand on one foot for greater than 10 seconds. A 2-year-old should be able to build the tower of cubes. *(Dixon, 470)*

60. **(E)** Toilet training generally begins around 2 years of age. Parents should begin when children start staying dry for at least 2 hours at a time, are having regular bowel movements, are able to follow simple instructions, are uncomfortable with dirty diapers and want them to be changed, are asking to use the potty chair, or are asking to wear regular underwear. Children should not be punished for failures. *(Kliegman, 54)*

61. **(A)** Toddlerhood is the period of developing autonomy, when the child normally is seeking to establish his or her own identity and to prove his or her own ability. Toddlers want to control and do everything by themselves. They are too impatient and immature to seek or accept explanations. The toddler's slogan is "me do it." *(Kliegman, 48)*

62. **(E)** While nighttime awakening by infants of this age can be viewed as a setback by parents, the phenomenon is actually a sign that the infant has acquired an important cognitive skill, that of object permanence. The approach to nighttime awakening is the same as for establishing good sleep hygiene; namely that a consistent bedtime, the use of a transitional object, a brief visit to provide reassurance, and putting the baby to sleep while drowsy but still awake. It is not recommended to feed the infant during these episodes. *(Dixon, 305)*

63. **(C)** Body fat comprises about 16% of body weight at birth, increases to about 22% at about a year of age, and then gradually declines.

Velocity of weight gain slows between the ages of 2 and 5 years, and body mass index (BMI) naturally declines. After approximately age 5, the velocity of weight gain compared to that of height gain increases, and BMI increases. This is the period known as the adiposity rebound. Children who experience early adiposity rebound (before the age of 5) are at higher risk for obesity. *(Kliegman, 234)*

64. **(C)** The gross motor tasks described (walking downstairs with alternate feet, throwing overhand, broad jump) are accomplished at 3–4 years of age. A child of this age also should be able to identify two or three colors. The other abilities listed generally come at, or after, 5 years of age. (Note: This format is common in pediatric examination questions about development. The student should recognize that often, as is the case in this question, the correct answer can be surmised even if the reader cannot identify the age of the child described in the body of the question. Logically, in this case, the correct choice must be the one corresponding to the youngest age. The ability to name colors precedes all the other items listed and therefore must be the correct answer. Knowing the sequence of development without knowing the corresponding ages would be sufficient to answer this question.) *(Dixon, 468-470)*

65. **(E)** Daytime experiences or recall of nightmares may precipitate nighttime fears in young children. Parents must remember that the child's fear is real, even if the object of the fear is not. Thus, it is not advisable to reinforce the child's fear of monsters in the bedroom with a pretend "search" for them. Having a consistent bedtime for the child, a regular pre-bedtime routine, avoidance of TV and videos before bedtime, and providing brief comfort and reassurance are all recommended techniques for managing this issue. *(Dixon, 421)*

66. **(C)** Many parents ask their child's physician if he or she should be kept back a year from beginning kindergarten. With a very few exceptions, the answer to this question is no. Children who may have actual special challenges need evaluation as soon as possible, and this is usually most appropriately performed within the school system. There is no evidence to suggest that delaying school entry is correlated with academic success once the child does enter school. The child's previous socialization and learning experiences should be reviewed. Generally, public schools have more access to specialized educational services than do private schools. Children short and/or small for their age should not delay kindergarten entry. *(Dixon, 464–465)*

67. **(D)** At term birth (40 weeks gestation), the percentage of fetal hemoglobin varies greatly from infant to infant but usually is between 60% and 90%. Fetal hemoglobin binds more tightly to oxygen than does adult hemoglobin, giving the newborn infant a relative advantage in picking up oxygen in the lung but a disadvantage in releasing oxygen to the tissues. The presence of significant amounts of fetal hemoglobin (which protects the sickle erythrocyte against sickling) is the major reason that young infants with sickle cell disease rarely are symptomatic. Oxygenated fetal hemoglobin is red, just like adult hemoglobin. Fetal hemoglobin does not predispose the red cell to hemolysis. *(Kliegman, 2001)*

68. **(D)** Both heart rate and respiratory rate are greater in infants and young children than in adults, reflecting the relatively larger surface area and higher metabolic rate of the youngsters. The respiratory rate of most normal 1-year-old children is between 20 and 30 times per minute. This is slower than a neonate and faster than an older child or adult. *(Kliegman, 389)*

69. **(A)** For the reasons explained in Answer 68 above, the infant normally has a more rapid heart rate than an adult. Rates of up to 180 beats per minute can be normal in the first year of life. This increased rate is associated with both a shorter respiratory rate and a shorter PR interval on the electrocardiogram. *(Kliegman, 1866-1868)*

70. **(D)** The blood pressure of a normal 2-year-old child averages about 95/60 mm Hg. There is almost no change in normal blood pressure values between 2 and 6 years, but after 6 years

there is a gradual increase to an average of 120/75 mm Hg at 16 years. It is generally recommended that routine measurement of blood pressure in children commence at 2–3 years of age; however, blood pressure should be measured in younger children, including neonates, whenever clinically indicated. *(Kliegman, 389)*

71. **(C)** The cerebrospinal fluid concentration of protein in the immediate newborn period normally may be as high as 125 mg/dL. The concentration gradually falls to "normal values" of less than 45 mg/dL by 6–8 weeks. *(Kliegman, 2441)*

72. **(A)** The physician needs to distinguish speech (pronunciation, articulation, and fluency) from language (content, meaning, vocabulary, and grammar) and to evaluate each separately. Normally, both speech and language are sufficiently developed by 4 years so that the child's verbal communications are fully understandable, even by strangers. Mispronunciations and grammatical errors, however, remain common until about 4½ years or even 5 years. *(Dixon, 438, 461)*

73. **(D)** Approximately 6%–9% of school-age children seen in primary care have symptoms consistent with attention-deficit hyperactivity disorder (ADHD). These children most commonly have a constellation of inattentive, hyperactive, and impulsive traits. Among these are fidgeting, excessive talking, apparent lack of attention when given directions, distractability, and symptoms reproducible in more than one environment (ie, school and home). *(Dixon, 482–488)*

74. **(E)** Approximately 50% of children will experience the divorce of their parents by midadolescence. Adverse effects may vary by age and gender, and include regressive behavior, depression, anger, anxiety, declining academic performance, and other externalizing and internalizing behaviors. At a time when children need their parents the most, parents may be emotionally unavailable to them as they process their own anger, grief, and other emotions. Boys in general appear to have a more difficult initial adjustment than do girls. However, as they

reach young adulthood, girls may experience a "sleeper" effect; though their initial adjustment occurred years before, they may undergo anxiety about male-female relationships. In a longitudinal study, nearly 40% of children were doing poorly (academic problems, behavior problems at school and/or home) 5 years after divorce. *(Dixon, 628–629)*

75. **(C)** Despite wide variations in size and rate of closure, it is generally accepted that the anterior fontanel closes sometime between 9 and 18 months. That is, by this time, it is composed of cartilage and bone and no longer is palpable as a soft spot. Early closure may be indicative of a disorder such as premature cranial synostosis. Late closure may be seen in conditions such as hypothyroidism, rickets, hypophosphatasia, hydrocephalus, or trisomy 18 syndrome. *(Kliegman, 2434)*

76. **(B)** An awareness of normal infant developmental milestones can assist providers in tailoring their guidance topics. It is appropriate to address rolling off elevated surfaces, as many infants begin rolling over at 3 months or slightly earlier. The typical 3-month-old infant is developmentally incapable of picking up small objects and putting them in his mouth. Infants who are growing well should be allowed to sleep through the night. Infants should be placed on their backs to sleep, as this sleeping position has been associated with fewer cases of sudden infant death syndrome. At this age, typically developing 3-month-olds are cooing, smiling and laughing spontaneously. *(Dixon, 255, 264)*

77. **(A)** Approximately 20% of sexually active teen girls become pregnant each year in the United States. Slightly more than half of these pregnancies result in a live birth, one-third are ended by abortion, and 15% end by miscarriage. Several factors have been associated with an increased risk of teen pregnancy, including lack of parental supervision, living in poverty, and drug or alcohol use. Adolescent girls with poor school performance are more likely to become pregnant than those with high academic performance. *(Dixon, 574)*

78. **(E)** About 50% of patients with isolated growth hormone (GH) deficiency grow normally during the first year of life. Growth then decelerates, and both height and weight fall further and further away from the normal curves. Bone age generally is delayed. By definition, in isolated GH deficiency other endocrine functions are normal; there is no associated disturbance of thyroid function. Before concluding that a child has isolated growth hormone deficiency, however, it is necessary to rule out physical destruction of the pituitary gland (eg, by a craniopharyngioma), or an associated pituitary abnormality such as ACTH deficiency. Isolated growth hormone deficiency can be sporadic or genetic. (Note: The astute student will realize that it is very unlikely that statements (C) and (E) are both correct and will concentrate on these, even if uncertain about the remaining choices.) *(Kliegman, 2295-2297)*

79. **(C)** Children with constitutional growth delay are initially short, but have a longer than normal period of growth and a later than normal adolescent growth spurt. Although there are some exceptions, ultimate height usually is normal, and ultimate weight is normal and proportionate to height. *(Kliegman, 2297)*

80. **(E)** Remarkable as it seems, American children spend an average of 30–40 h/week in front of the television set, whereas, in general, they spend only 25–30 h/week in school. Television has a major influence on children's knowledge, attitude, and behavior. The nature and quality of the program material is, of course, as much a problem as the volume. There are considerable concerns and some data that such excessive viewing adversely affects children's attitudes toward violence, gender roles, concepts of racial stereotypes, and commercialism. *(Dixon, 425)*

81. **(D)** Failure to thrive typically refers to children under the age of 5 whose growth parameters fall below the lower limits of the normal range set by the National Center for Health Statistics. There are many causes of failure to thrive, including psychosocial, medical (organic), nutritional, and developmental. Cystic fibrosis is an important cause of failure to thrive and should be excluded in such cases. Children with small atrial septal defects, acute bacterial meningitis, mild intermittent asthma, or recurrent otitis media generally do not fail to thrive unless they have another underlying condition. *(Parker, 183–187)*

82. **(E)** Adolescence is the period of psychosocial transition from childhood to adulthood. Puberty is a physiologic event. Adolescence is a psychosocial phenomenon, albeit strongly influenced by the child's reaction to the physical and physiologic changes of puberty. Adolescence cannot be defined by a fixed temporal relation to puberty. Often, adolescence appears to occur some time after the onset of puberty. *(Dixon, 535–536)*

83. **(E)** Although adolescence is characteristically a difficult period of psychosocial and emotional growth, change, and adjustment, current understanding of this period indicates that emotional turmoil, disruptive behavior, and family crises are not the norm and, when present, represent significant pathology. Declining scholastic grades are always worrisome. Such behavior warrants investigation and intervention rather than acceptance and reassurance. The differential diagnosis includes emotional problems, maladjustment, psychosis, drug abuse, and, rarely, organic disease. *(Dixon, 545)*

84. **(E)** Virtually all children bite sometime during their first 3 years of life. Boys are more likely to bite than girls, and children tend to bite others when they are in social situations beyond their coping abilities. In assessing the issue of biting, it is important to determine the age at which the biting began, the situations in which it occurs, how parents and daycare staff have managed biting, and if any concerns have been raised about the child's developmental progress. The age of first tooth eruption is not helpful. *(Parker, 136–138)*

85. **(C)** The average hemoglobin value at birth is about 17 g/dL. It then falls rapidly over the next 2–3 months to a low of about 11 g/dL in the term infant. Hemoglobin values then gradually

rise, although remaining below adult values until the early teen years. The mean value at 1 year of age is about 12 g/dL. *(Kliegman, 2003, 2025–2026)*

86. **(D)** Normal newborns have a surprising array of sensory abilities. They can sense pain and are also responsive to changes in their body position as they are moved by caregivers. They prefer their mother's face and voice over the faces and voices of other mothers. Newborns reflexively grasp the finger of an adult when the finger is placed in their palm. Although newborns can see objects 8–10 in away and can track slow-moving objects, they are nearsighted, and their visual acuity ranges from 20/200 to 20/400. The visual acuity of a child does not reach 20/20 until age 4. *(Davies, 120–122; Kliegman, 2569: 44; Dixon, 149)*

87. **(B)** Several techniques have been studied to improve childrens' behavior. Time in is "catching a child being good," providing mainly brief, nonverbal physical contact by the caregiver when the child is behaving well. Reinforcement refers to an item or activity for which a child works to gain access. Fading refers to gradually removing an object or activity from a child's environment rather than abruptly changing it. Rapprochement is defined as the normal transition from independent play to a period of clinging to the parent when the 18–24-month-old is around other children and adults. Incidental learning occurs when a child is in the presence of individuals who repeatedly practice the same behavior, such as smoking. Children of smokers are more likely to smoke themselves than children of nonsmokers. *(Parker, 55–57; Dixon, 367)*

88. **(C)** Although there is great variation within the normal range, the average infant roughly triples his or her birth weight by the first birthday. This means an increase from an average of 7 lb (3.25 kg) at birth to 22 lb (10 kg) at 1 year. Thus, the weight gain during the first year of life is about 15 lb (6 kg). *(Kliegman, 46)*

89. **(A)** As with weight gain, gain in height during the second year of life is considerably less than during the first year. During the first year, the child grows about 25 cm (10 in). Between the first and second birthdays, the youngster grows an average of only 13 cm (about 5 in), about half that of the first year. In the 4–6-year-old, the average height gain is 3 cm/yr. *(Kliegman, 54)*

90. **(C)** Head circumference increases relatively rapidly after birth, growing about 2 cm (1 in) the first month. Of course, this is related to the rapid growth of the brain that occurs during infancy. The rate of growth in head circumference in the first 2 months is 1 cm every 2 weeks. In the third through sixth month of life, the rate of growth is 1 cm/month. *(Dixon, 248)*

91. **(D)** Menarche usually occurs as, or shortly after, breast and pubic hair development reach SMR IV. Menarche generally follows rather than precedes the adolescent growth spurt. In fact, for most girls, menarche heralds the end of the adolescent growth spurt, and there is little further increase in height following menarche. *(Dixon, 538-53; Kliegman, 61, 64)*

92. **(E)** A child's temperament is an important concept to consider when evaluating parental concerns. It is not the parent's response to a tantrum, but a child's stable, individual modes of responding to his or her environment. Temperament types can be used to explain current and forecast future behavior. The emotional parent-child bond is known as attachment. A toddler exerts autonomy when acting independently. A toddler's emotional clinginess to the parent when faced with other children or adults is known as rapprochement. *(Dixon, 37, 356–357)*

93. **(A)** The Parents' Evaluations of Developmental Status (PEDS) consists of 10 questions for parents of newborns to 8-year-olds. The PEDS identifies levels of risk for various emotional and developmental problems and delays. *(Dixon, 729)*

94. **(D)** The Pediatric Symptom Checklist consists of 35 brief statements of problem behavior, including both externalizing (conduct) and internalizing (depression) behavior. It takes about 7 minutes to administer and has a high sensitivity rate. *(Dixon, 730).*

95. **(B)** One of the most widely used tools for detection of substance misuse in the pediatric office setting is the CAGE questionnaire. C stands for "Have you ever felt the need to CUT down on your alcohol (or drug) use?" A stands for "Have you ever felt ANNOYED by criticism about your use?" G stands for "Have you ever felt GUILTY about your use, or GUILTY about something you said or did while you were using?" Finally, E stands for "Have you ever needed an EYE-OPENER in the morning after a night of heavy use?" *(Dixon, 615-616)*

96. **(E)** In the United States, it is recommended that birth hospitals within all states perform a hearing screen before neonates are discharged. The otoacoustic emission test (OAE) is quick, easy to administer, inexpensive, and provides a sensitive indication of the presence of hearing loss. *(Kliegman, 2623)*

97. **(C)** The Vanderbilt Assessment Scale consists of questionnaires for teachers and parents as well as a primary care provider diagnostic tool. Teachers are prompted to observe and assess ADHD symptoms and the child's school and behavioral performance. The parent tools assesses 55 different behaviors and their occurrence over the past 6 months. *(Parker, 118)*

98. **(E)** Signs that a child is ready for toilet training usually appear between 18 and 24 months, and the process of becoming fully trained may take up to a year beyond initial signs of readiness. These clues include increased periods of daytime dryness and signs of interest in using the toilet. *(Dixon, 360)*

99. **(B)** Separation protest or "anxiety" typically surfaces between 6 and 9 months, and is marked by an infant's crying when his parent or caregiver leaves his presence. Most separation anxiety resolves naturally, as the infant develops cognitively and learns that absences are followed by reunions when parents return. *(Levine, 27–28)*

100. **(C)** Self-feeding, although messy and disorganized, represents a milestone in independence for the young toddler. Fine motor skills, hand-eye coordination, and learning to select different food textures and colors are several of the developmental skills enhanced by self-feeding. *(Dixon, 360–361)*

SELECTED READINGS

Hagan JF, Shaw JS, Duncan P, eds. *Bright Futures: Guidelines for Health Supervision of Infants, Children and Adolescents.* 3rd ed. Arlington, VA: National Center for Education in Maternal and Child Health; 2008.

Feeding and Nutrition

Sara Viessman, MD

Mary Stahl Levick, MD

William J. Klish, MD

Historically, as well as currently, the topic of feeding and nutrition has special importance in pediatrics because of the rapid growth and development of the pediatric patient, especially the infant. This rapid growth and development results in both quantitatively and qualitatively different nutritional needs than exist for the adult. Quantitatively, for example, newborns and young infants require more calories and more protein relative to body size than do older individuals. In a qualitative sense, for example, certain amino acids are essential for low-birth-weight and preterm infants but not for children or adults or even for normal term infants. Certain fats are essential for brain growth during the first few years of life but not thereafter.

Breastfeeding clearly is the healthiest choice for most babies. We currently are aware of many nutritional, psychologic, and immunologic advantages of breastfeeding. Further advantages likely will be uncovered in years to come. It is estimated that if all babies were breastfed for the first 12 weeks of life, the savings recognized by the United States would be about $3 billion per year. If all mothers in the WIC program breastfed their babies for only 4 weeks, an estimated $30 million would be saved. If all babies worldwide were breastfed for the first six months of life, hundreds of thousands of babies lives would be saved each year.

Malnutrition, secondary to medical or socioeconomic conditions, remains an important problem in infants and children in the United States. Self-inflicted malnutrition seen with eating disorders (or disordered eating) is increasingly prevalent. Obesity now is at epidemic proportions among children in the United States. At both ends of this spectrum, children are at risk for serious long-term medical and psychologic problems.

Although specific nutritional deficiencies, except for iron deficiency, are uncommon in developed countries, deficiencies of vitamins or protein remain a major problem among children in developing countries.

Questions

DIRECTIONS (Questions 1 through 34): For each of the multiple choice questions in this section select the one lettered answer that is the best response in each case.

1. A 3-year-old male child from South America is brought in for an adoption physical examination. He has a 4–5 mm, foamy, mildly vascular, conjuctival lesion next to the cornea on the medial side of both eyes. Which nutrient deficiency is most likely to cause this lesion?

   (A) vitamin A
   (B) vitamin B_6
   (C) thiamine
   (D) copper
   (E) riboflavin

2. Parents appear in your office to discuss their considerations for adopting their 11-month-old foster son. They state he has a history of failure to thrive at 6 months of age and they are concerned about the possibility of long-term problems. Undernutrition in the first year of life has which of the following effects?

   (A) has no permanent effect on physical growth or development of intelligence
   (B) can have permanent effects on physical growth but not on development of intelligence
   (C) can have permanent effects on development of intelligence but not on physical growth
   (D) can have permanent effects on both physical growth and development of intelligence
   (E) can have permanent effects on both physical growth and development of intelligence, but only if coupled with psychosocial deprivation

3. At a 4-month well child visit, a mother is distressed because her baby's grandmother believes she should have started feeding her baby solid food at 2 months of age. It is generally recommended that beikost (infant foods other than milk) be introduced into the infant's diet at about what age?

   (A) 3 weeks
   (B) 6 weeks
   (C) 3 months
   (D) 6 months
   (E) 1 year

4. A 23-month-old female is hospitalized for severe malnutrition. Which of the following problems is most likely to be the result of inappropriately rapid treatment of the severely malnourished child?

   (A) hyperkalemia
   (B) hyponatremia
   (C) hyperglycemia
   (D) congestive heart failure
   (E) renal failure

5. A 10-week-old child weighing 5 kg is being fed commercial infant formula. The mother is concerned she is underfeeding her baby. You tell her that, to satisfy both his fluid and caloric requirements, the daily intake ought to be at least how many ounces?

(A) 12 oz

(B) 18 oz

(C) 26 oz

(D) 36 oz

(E) 48 oz

6. A pregnant African-American woman plans to breastfeed her baby. She has read of the nutritional, psychologic, and immunologic advantages, but recalled breastfed babies might still require vitamin supplementation. The most current nutritional recommendations indicate she should supplement the baby's nutrition with which vitamin?

(A) vitamin A

(B) vitamin B

(C) vitamin C

(D) vitamin B_1

(E) vitamin D

7. You are in charge of the nutrition support service in the hospital where you are practicing. The company that makes the vitamin/mineral mixture for total parenteral nutrition (TPN) has gone out of business and for the past 2 months you have been trying to fortify the parenteral nutrition mixtures through other sources. An 8-month-old infant with short gut, who has been on TPN for the past 4 months, presents with a curious erythematous desquamating rash around his mouth, buttocks, and a small amount on his hands and feet. Which nutrient deficiency is the most likely cause?

(A) vitamin A

(B) thiamin

(C) riboflavin

(D) copper

(E) zinc

8. A physical examination of a 10-year-old Hispanic male reveals BMI greater than 95th percentile. Laboratory test results include fasting serum glucose of 98 mg/dL, fasting serum insulin of 30 μU/mL, an ALT of 60 U/L, total cholesterol of 128 mg/dL, and triglycerides of 130 mg/dL. You have great concern that he may have which of the following?

(A) diabetes

(B) prediabetes

(C) nonalcoholic steatohepatitis

(D) metabolic syndrome

(E) hyperlipidemia

Questions 9 through 11

At 1 year of age, a boy was at the 50th percentile for height and weight. At 2 years of age, he is at the 25th and 10th percentiles respectively. Review of systems reveals fussiness, loose stools, and possibly stomach aches all beginning after the mother stopped breastfeeding the boy and introduced table foods. Mother has consumed milk products lifelong, but her son does not drink cow milk.

9. Which is the most likely cause of these symptoms?

(A) toddler's diarrhea

(B) lactose intolerance

(C) celiac disease

(D) cow milk protein allergy

(E) chronic giardiasis

10. The most definitive test for this condition is which of the following?

(A) breath hydrogen test

(B) abdominal ultrasound

(C) serum antigliadin antibodies

(D) giardia antigen

(E) small bowel biopsy

11. Patients with this condition should avoid which of the following?

(A) corn

(B) barley and rye

(C) rice and legumes

(D) oats

(E) potatoes and legumes

Questions 12 and 13

A 5-year-old female presents with a 3-day history of crampy abdominal pain and a rash on her lower legs. On examination, she is cranky but nontoxic. Her abdomen is mildly diffusely tender with normal bowel sounds. A purpuric rash is located predominately on the extensor surface of lower legs. A complete blood count and urine analysis are normal.

12. Which of the following is the best next step?

    (A) intravenous corticosteroid therapy
    (B) intravenous antibiotics
    (C) hematology-oncology consult
    (D) sickle cell screening
    (E) colonoscopy

13. While hospitalized, the child's abdominal pain increases. She becomes pale and draws up her legs. On examination, distension of the right upper quadrant with palpable fullness is found. Which of the following is true of this complication?

    (A) recurrence occurs in at least 15% of children
    (B) rupture of the appendix may be an associated complication
    (C) usually starts with stool containing blood-stained mucus
    (D) ileoileal involvement is typical
    (E) highest occurrence is in this age group

14. Because her son prefers other beverages over milk, a school-age boy's mother is concerned he may not be getting enough calcium in his diet. As you recommend calcium-rich foods, you mention the calcium requirement for a school-age child is which of the following?

    (A) 0.1 g/day
    (B) 1.3 g/day
    (C) 10.5 g/day
    (D) 50.0 g/day
    (E) 100 g/day

15. During a preschool physical, the mother of a 5-year-old girl states the family follows a strict vegan diet (a diet excluding all animal products

including eggs, milk, and milk products, as well as meats and fish). In which of the following vitamins is this child likely to be deficient?

    (A) vitamin C
    (B) vitamin E
    (C) vitamin B_1
    (D) vitamin B_{12}
    (E) vitamin A

16. At a 2-month well child visit, a mother states her family has a history of cow milk protein allergies and wonders if soy formula would be better for her baby. Which of the following statements regarding soy formula is correct?

    (A) Infants fed exclusively with soy formula display growth comparable to infants fed cow milk protein formula.
    (B) The protein in soy formulas is essentially nonallergenic, and clinically significant soy protein hypersensitivity is extremely rare.
    (C) Soy formula is most useful in children with well-documented, severe, gastrointestinal allergic reactions to cow milk protein.
    (D) Soy formula should not be used by patients with a family history of celiac disease.
    (E) Infants fed soy formula should receive supplemental dietary calcium.

17. A 5-month-old male presents with poor weight gain. His diet consists only of goat milk. On examination, he appears tired and is mildly tachycardic. The laboratory value most likely to be elevated is which of the following?

    (A) serum albumin
    (B) red blood cell mean corpuscular volume
    (C) hemoglobin
    (D) serum vitamin B_{12} level
    (E) serum sodium

18. A 12-year-old female presents for her well-child visit with no complaints. However, she is concerned about her friend who counts calories and seems to be losing too much weight. During a discussion about this issue, you tell

her that the recommended energy intake for a 12-year-old female is which of the following?

(A) 1500 kcal/day

(B) 1800 kcal/day

(C) 2200 kcal/day

(D) 2500 kcal/day

(E) 3000 kcal/day

19. An 8-month-old female is hospitalized with failure to thrive. She has a 1-day history of fever and cough. On physical examination, you observe a very thin, well-hydrated alert infant in no acute distress. You obtain a complete blood count and order a chest x-ray for further evaluation of a one day history of fever and cough. You note the lung fields to be normal but also note an absence of a thymic shadow. Which of the following should be your next step?

(A) obtain an immunology consult

(B) order genetic karyotyping

(C) repeat the chest x-ray in 24 hours

(D) order a cardiac ultrasound

(E) feed the infant as tolerated, following weight and intake closely

20. A single, 35-year-old pregnant female has not been tested previously for HIV or hepatitis. While awaiting prenatal screening, she requests information regarding breastfeeding. You would most accurately tell her in the United States breastfeeding of infants is contraindicated in which of the following?

(A) an infant whose mother is seropositive for HIV antibody

(B) an infant whose mother is seropositive for hepatitis B surface antigen

(C) an infant whose mother is seropositive for hepatitis C antibody

(D) an infant whose mother was recently immunized with tetanus, diphtheria, acellular pertussis vaccine

(E) an infant whose mother was recently immunized with hepatitis B vaccine

21. A new mother at her baby's 2-week well visit is concerned that she may not be able to continue breastfeeding because her nipples are very sore and cracked, and have even bled. Inquiring about her feeding techniques, you discover she nurses her baby about 20–25 minutes on each breast each feeding. Which of the following offers the best supportive advice?

(A) Lengthen the time interval between every nursing by at least an hour.

(B) Nurse for a minimum of 30 minutes on each breast each feeding.

(C) Offer 1 oz of formula from a bottle before each breastfeeding so that her infant will not be as ravenous.

(D) Limit nursing to 5–10 minutes per breast per feeding.

(E) Substitute a bottle of formula for every other nursing just until her nipples are healed.

22. A mother is concerned because her 20-month-old son prefers to eat with his fingers rather than use a small spoon. Which of the following statements is correct?

(A) At 18 months of age, most toddlers prefer to feed themselves with a spoon.

(B) Most children learn to feed themselves independently during the second year of life.

(C) Self-spoon-feeding usually begins at 10 months of age when well-defined wrist rotation develops.

(D) Most children can feed themselves with a cup by 6 months of age.

(E) Most children prefer to feed themselves with a spoon by 12 months of age.

23. You are following a child with ADHD. His teacher requests information on diet and ADHD. In particular, she is interested in the role of ingestion of sugar in this condition. Which of the following statements is true regarding controlled studies of the effects of sucrose ingestion in children?

   (A) Sucrose ingestion has been linked to problem behavior in children with ADHD.
   (B) Sucrose ingestion has been linked to increased motor activity in children with ADHD.
   (C) Sucrose ingestion is associated with an increase in both motor activity and problem behavior in children with ADHD.
   (D) Sucrose ingestion is not associated with problem behavior or increased motor activity in children.
   (E) Sucrose ingestion is associated with decreased motor activity in children.

24. You are in a health clinic in Africa. An 18-month-old child is brought in for your help. On inspection you note that the child is edematous, has a dark desquamating skin rash over most of the pressure points on the body, has very thin hair, and what hair is left is reddish in color. Of the following, what laboratory test is most likely to be present?

   (A) serum albumin of 3.7 g/dL
   (B) serum sodium of 143 meq/L
   (C) serum albumin of 2.3 g/dL
   (D) serum potassium of 2 meq/L
   (E) serum prealbumin of 25 mg/dL

25. Recent concerns about the prevention of atherosclerotic heart disease have led to recommendations for reducing the fat content, and particularly the cholesterol content, of the diet early in life. This can include the use of skim milk. It is recommended that the use of skim milk begin no earlier what age?

   (A) 4 months
   (B) 6 months

   (C) 1 year
   (D) 2 years
   (E) 5 years

26. Because of her own success with a low carbohydrate diet, the mother of an overweight 9-year-old asks about a low carbohydrate diet for her son. As you discuss this with her, you point out that the greatest percentage of calories in the normal diet of the school-age child comes from which of the following?

   (A) carbohydrate
   (B) protein
   (C) fat
   (D) cholesterol
   (E) whey

27. A 3-month-old Caucasian female is brought to you for cold symptoms. On examination, you note her head circumference is at the 50th percentile, her length at the 25th percentile, and her weight less than the 5th percentile. She appears alert but very thin. She has skin folds on her arms, thighs, and buttocks. Parents state she drinks four 8 oz bottles of premixed formula each day. You feed the baby and she quickly drinks 7 oz. You decide to admit the infant. How many calories will she likely need for weight gain?

   (A) 60 kcal/kg/day
   (B) 80 kcal/kg/day
   (C) 100 kcal/kg/day
   (D) 150 kcal/kg/day
   (E) 200 kcal/kg/day

28. The mother of a headstrong 2-year-old is concerned that he insists on drinking six bottles of apple juice per day. Which of the following represents a serious nutritional concern in this situation?

   (A) development of obesity
   (B) development of diabetes mellitus
   (C) vitamin C deficiency
   (D) vitamin A toxicity
   (E) development of constipation

29. A 3-year-old male presents to your clinic for the first time for a well-child visit. You note macrocephaly, short fingers, and only six teeth. What additional finding is likely?

    (A) absent thumb
    (B) flat facial bones
    (C) hepatosplenomegaly
    (D) absent clavicles
    (E) absent radius

30. An 18-month-old Hispanic male presents for a well-child check. His parents report he drinks seven to eight bottles of cow milk each day and does not like solid foods. His weight is greater than the 95th percentile while height and head circumference are at the 25th percentile. His heart rate is 180 beats per minute and respiratory rate is 28 breaths per minute. On examination, you find a chubby, happy, pale, and otherwise normal baby. Which of the following tests will most likely be abnormal?

    (A) sweat test
    (B) serum sodium
    (C) eosinophil count
    (D) serum bicarbonate
    (E) hemoglobin

31. A 7-year-old male presents for a well-child visit. You note his height is at 75th percentile and weight is at greater than 95th percentile for age. His examination is otherwise normal. His father is overweight but his mother is thin. Which of the following is the most appropriate next step for you to take?

    (A) obtain T_4 and TSH levels
    (B) order serum chromosomes
    (C) refer to an endocrinologist
    (D) place on a diet of 75% of caloric needs for height
    (E) counsel the family on increasing exercise and eliminating target foods from diet

32. The most accurate method for assessing adiposity in the office setting is which of the following?

    (A) measurement of weight
    (B) calculation of percent above ideal body weight for height using age/sex norms
    (C) calculation of body mass index (weight/height^2)
    (D) measurement of subcutaneous fat thickness
    (E) use of densitometry

33. A 2-year-old Caucasian male presents with failure to thrive, chronic diarrhea, and recurrent pneumonia. Though his family history is negative for cystic fibrosis, a sweat test reveals a sodium concentration of 120 mg/dL. Which of the following is the appropriate next step in caring for this infant?

    (A) iron
    (B) vitamin B_{12} and folic acid
    (C) pancreatic enzyme supplementation
    (D) copper and magnesium
    (E) parenteral diuretics

34. A 15-year-old Caucasian female presents with the complaint that she is always cold. She has no history of illness, but she has not had a period for 4 months. Her mother states she is worried because although her daughter intermittently eats a large amount of food, she seems to be losing weight. On examination, the patient is extremely thin for her age. Which of the following is most likely?

    (A) She feels she is too thin, but likes it that way.
    (B) She feels she is too thin, and would like to gain weight.
    (C) She feels she is too fat, and wants to lose weight.
    (D) She feels she is too fat, but likes it that way.
    (E) She feels she is normal.

DIRECTIONS (Questions 35 through 39): The following group of questions is preceded by a list of lettered answer options. For each question, match the one lettered option that is most closely associated with the question. Each lettered option may be selected once, multiple times, or not at all.

Questions 35 through 37

   (A) carbohydrate
   (B) protein
   (C) fat
   (D) cholesterol
   (E) whey

35. The greatest percentage of calories in human breast milk

36. The greatest percentage of calories in unmodified cow milk

37. The greatest percentage of calories in skim milk

Questions 38 and 39

   (A) 2%
   (B) 10%
   (C) 15%
   (D) 25%
   (E) 40%

38. Percentage of all child deaths related to malnutrition in developing countries

39. Percentage of children in the world who are moderately to severely underweight

Answers and Explanations

1. **(A)** Vitamin A deficiency remains the leading cause of preventable childhood blindness worldwide. Though rare in the United States and other developed countries, this condition is prevalent in developing countries, especially in those with the highest burden of deaths among children under 5 years of age. The lesion described, a Bitot spot, is one of the early classic signs of vitamin A deficiency. As vitamin A deficiency symptoms progress, the eyes become dry and itchy (conjunctivitis sicca). Corneal ulcers subsequently can form. In the worst cases these ulcers can rupture allowing eye contents to avulse, resulting in permanent blindness.

Though most health care providers recognize that vitamin A deficiency can lead to blindness, most are unaware of the full impact of vitamin A deficiency on children's health worldwide. Before developing blindness, vitamin A deficient children face a 23% greater risk of dying from infectious diseases such as measles, malaria, and diarrhea. An estimated 100–140 million children live with vitamin A deficiency worldwide. UNICEF and other organizations are working to reduce this number as they work toward meeting the fourth Millennium Development Goal which is a two-thirds reduction in under-five mortality by 2015. (*McMillan, 113; UNICEF Statistics,* http://www.childinfo.org/areas/ vitamina; *UNICEF, The State of the World's Children*)

2. **(D)** Although somewhat controversial, serious undernutrition during the first year of life is felt to have deleterious and permanent effects on both mental and physical growth and development. This appears to be an organic effect independent of psychosocial deprivation, although exogenous undernutrition often is compounded by such deprivation. In follow-up, a high frequency of behavior problems and learning difficulties is found, despite adequate weight gain. The recognition of possible permanent effects of malnutrition during infancy and early childhood has led to increased efforts to avoid such undernutrition both in otherwise healthy children and those with chronic disease. (*Chase, 282:933–939, 1970; McMillan, 905*)

3. **(D)** It is recommended that the introduction of nonmilk foods (beikost) be delayed until the age of 4–6 months. Pancreatic enzymes, such as amylase and lipase, are low early in life but seem adequate to digest most nonmilk foods. The most compelling reason to delay introduction of solids relates to developmental readiness such as disappearance of tongue thrust (extrusor reflex), acquisition of head control, and ability to sit with support. More recently, the avoidance of overfeeding and overweight has become an argument for delaying the introduction of solids until after 4–6 months of age. Admittedly, it often is difficult to convince parents to refrain from introducing solids at an earlier age. (*AAP, 103–115*)

4. **(D)** Congestive heart failure is very easy to precipitate in a severly malnourished child particulary if colloid (blood) or crystalloid (sodium) is infused aggressively. Because the heart is malnourished, contractility and therefore cardiac output is already impaired. By increasing plasma volume which would occur by infusing either of the above substances, the preload to the heart would increase in the face of an impaired pump, resulting in congestive heart failure. During refeeding of severe malnutrition,

potassium and phosphate are rapidly taken up by the expanding body cell mass, resulting in low potassium and/or phosphate if not supplemented. Total body water increases in malnutrition resulting in a dilutional hyponatremia which slowly corrects with refeeding. Glycogen stores are depleted in severe malnutrition and hypoglycemia can easily occur if the malnourished child is stressed. *(Tsang, 93–95)*

5. **(C)** An infant's fluid requirements are 120–140 mL/kg/day. Yet, to get sufficient calories for growth, an infant must take in 150–180 mL/kg/day. It generally is accepted that the caloric requirements of a newborn are about 120 cal/kg/day falling to 110 cal/kg/day by 12 months of age. The most recent Dietary Reference Intakes published by the National Academy of Sciences has decreased this slightly and has proposed age, weight, and physical activity based estimated energy requirements (EER) derived from regression equations. For this age group (0–3 months) the equation is EER = (89 × weight in kg − 100) + 175 kcal. This 10-week-old, 5-kg infant has a caloric requirement of about 500–600 cal/day. Most milks (human and cow) and prepared formulas contain 20 cal/oz. Therefore, it would take 25–30 oz of milk or formula to provide the 500–600 calories required each day. *(AAP, 241–246)*

6. **(E)** To the best of our current knowledge, formulas are fortified with the necessary vitamins and minerals. Breast milk contains quantitatively small amounts of vitamin D. However, this is sufficient for many babies. Exclusively breastfed infants who are at risk for vitamin D deficiency include infants with inadequate maternal intake of vitamin D (eg, mothers who are strict vegans), infants with inadequate sunlight exposure (eg, dark skin pigmentation, cold climates, urban environments, clothing practices, and more recently the overuse of sun-blocking agents), and older infants still exclusively breastfed. Therefore, vitamin D supplementation is recommended for most babies who are exclusively breastfed. Too much vitamin D can be toxic and just as dangerous as too little. The major target organ of vitamin D poisoning is the kidney. *(McMillan, 112–116; AAP, 71)*

7. **(E)** The rash described is called acrodermatitis which means dermatitis of the acral or outer points of the body. This is the classic rash associated with zinc deficiency. This rash is also associated with a rare genetic disease called acrodermatitis enteropathica. Infants with acrodermatitis enteropathica cannot absorb zinc well. They typically present in the first 2 years of life with this skin rash, diarrhea, and failure to thrive. Treatment is zinc supplementation. *(McMillan, 856, 1999)*

8. **(C)** This obese child has an elevated ALT at 60 IU/L (normal <40 IU/L) and is at risk of nonalcoholic steatohepatits (NASH), a form of nonalcoholic fatty liver disease. Male Hispanics of Mexican origin seem to be most susceptable to this disease in childhood. If the ALT is greater than 150% normal, the chance of an obese child to have steatohepatitis is about 85%. Though patients with NASH generally are asymptomatic, their condition may lead to fibrosis and even cirrhosis. Treatment of NASH in an obese child primarily includes weight loss and exercise.

Other important comorbidities for obesity in childhood include type 2 diabetes, hyperlipidemia and the metabolic syndrome, sleep apnea, hypertension, skeletal and psychological issues. The screening test for diabetes is a fasting serum glucose. A serum glucose greater than 100 mg/dL is diagnostic of prediabetes and greater than 127 mg/dL is diagnostic of diabetes. A fasting serum insulin greater than 17 μU/mL is consistent with insulin resistance and the potential for developing diabetes in the future. *(McMillan, 2020–2021)*

9. **(C)** Of the choices listed, all may cause diarrhea and abdominal pain in this age and context, but celiac disease and cow milk protein allergy are most likely to cause failure to thrive. Celiac disease, or gluten-sensitive enteropathy, typically presents at 6 months to 2 years of age, after the introduction of gluten into the diet. The estimated incidence of celiac disease in the United States is about 1:250, and can range as high as 1:50 in selected populations. A significant cow milk protein allergy would have manifested earlier in life with exposure through breast milk. Cow milk allergy usually resolves

by 1–3 years of age. Toddler's diarrhea, due to excessive juice/fluid intake, is the most common cause of diarrhea in toddlers under 3 years of age, and is due to the osmotic effect of sorbitol and fructose found in fruit juices and the limited reabsorptive capacity of the colon. Although common, lactose intolerance and chronic giardiasis (in an immunocompetent host) should not cause growth deceleration. (*McMillan, 1992–1993, 2700–2701*)

10. **(E)** The most definitive test for celiac disease is small bowel biopsy, although the sensitivity of antiendomysial antibodies (IgA) approaches 100% and the specificity 98%. The tissue transglutaminase (IgA and IgG) assay, which is easier to standardize, has a sensitivity of 92%–94% and a specificity of 95%–98%. Antigliadin antibodies (IgA and IgG) can be present in cow milk protein enteropathy, Crohn disease, tropical sprue, IgA nephropathy, eosinophilic enteritis, and dermatitis herpetiformis, accounting for its lower specificity of 86% (IgG) and 95.5% (IgA). An important limitation of all the IgA antibody assays is the fact that 2%–3% of patients with celiac disease are IgA deficient. (*McMillan, 1992–1993*)

11. **(B)** Treatment of celiac disease involves strict lifelong avoidance of gluten, found in wheat, barley, and rye. Oat products may be contaminated with gluten during processing, but the allergenicity of oat itself is still debated. Corn, rice, potatoes, and legumes are not implicated in gluten-associated enteropathy. (*McMillan, 1992–1993*)

12. **(A)** Although controversial, the use of a short course of 1–2 mg/kg/day prednisone may hasten resolution of the abdominal pain in Henoch-Schöenlein Purpura (HSP). An estimated 75% of children with HSP develop gastrointestinal involvement, often as the first manifestation. Vomiting is reported in 25% of cases. The abdominal pain typically resolves within 3–7 days. (*McMillan, 2562*)

13. **(D)** Acute worsening of the abdominal pain in a child with HSP warrants close attention. This patient displays signs and symptoms characteristic of intussusception which occurs in 3% of

patients with HSP. Intussusception often results in pooling of fluid in the gut with subsequent hypovolemic shock. Among patients with HSP, intussusception occurs most frequently in the older age group and most frequently (65%) is ileoileal. Remember, sporadic cases of intussusception most commonly are ileocolic occurring in children younger than 3 years of age. Intussusception recurs in approximately 5% of patients. (*McMillan, 2559–2562; Lissauer, 264*)

14. **(B)** The multiplicity of factors affecting calcium metabolism, not the least of which is the effect of other dietary factors, makes it difficult to give an exact figure for the daily requirement of calcium. For a school-age child it is estimated to be about 1.3 g/day. (Contrast this with the amount of protein required, which for this age group is nearly 1 g per kg of body weight per day!) This amount of calcium is easily provided by most ordinary diets, and calcium supplementation usually is not necessary, even for the child who drinks little or no milk. Eggs, molasses, nuts, and many fish and vegetables are good sources of calcium. A variety of products (specific brands of cereal, bread, orange juice, and even ice cream) are fortified with calcium. (*McMillan, 110*)

15. **(D)** A vegan or strict vegetarian diet provides almost no vitamin B_{12} as well as marginal levels of calcium, vitamin D, and iron. The relatively low caloric density of vegetables also means that a large bulk of food must be ingested to provide adequate calories. However, the content of vitamins other than B_{12} and D is apt to be adequate. (*Shinwell, 70:582–586, 1982; AAP, 191–208*)

16. **(A)** Soy protein based commercial infant formulas presently available provide adequate nutrition (including calcium), and infants fed these formulas exhibit normal growth. Soy formulas often are prescribed for infants with personal or family history of allergy in the hope of avoiding the development of milk-protein allergy. Unfortunately, severe gastrointestinal allergic reactions to soy protein in infants are well recognized and are not rare. For this reason, soy formula is not recommended for infants or children already demonstrating significant gastrointestinal hypersensitivity to cow

milk protein. These patients are best prescribed a protein hydrolysate formula. Soy-based formulas are not recommended for premature infants. *(AAP Committee on Nutrition, 72:359–363, 1983; AAP, 92–93)*

17. **(B)** Goat milk contains little folate. Infants fed primarily goat milk are at risk to develop a megaloblastic anemia from folate deficiency. Therefore, the mean corpuscular volume (MCV) will be elevated. The metabolism of folic acid and vitamin B_{12} is interrelated. Hematologic problems caused by a deficiency in one can be improved with supplementation of either. The neurologic complications of vitamin B_{12} deficiency, however, will not be improved with treatment with folic acid. Therefore, it is important to carefully sort the child's deficiencies. Large doses of folic acid should not be given until vitamin B_{12} deficiency has been excluded. *(AAP, 938, McMillan, 1694–1695)*

18. **(D)** Based on the new dietary reference intakes (DRIs), the estimated energy requirement (EER) of an average weight and height, mildly active 12-year-old girl would be about 2500 calories. This is based on the newly published regression equations by the National Academy of Sciences. For girls 9–18 years the equation is EER = 135.3 − [30.8 × age in years] + [PA × (10.0 × weight in kg) + (934 × height in meters)] + 25 kcal. PA is a factor for physical activity where sedentary is 1, low activity is 1.13, average activity is 1.31, and very active is 1.56 and taking into account individual ages, weights, heights, and physical activities, these new guidelines are more accurate. For this girl the equation would read: EER = 135.3 − [30.8 × 12] + [1.31 × (10 × 44)] + [934 × 1.52] + 25 or EER = 2524. *(Dietary Reference Intakes at Institute of Medicine website:* http://www.iom.edu/CMS/3788/4574.aspx*)*

19. **(E)** The thymus dramatically decreases in size during periods of undernutrition. Therefore, it is not uncommon to see loss of thymic shadow on the chest x-ray of infants admitted for failure to thrive. Involution of the thymus during starvation accounts for some of the increased susceptibility to infection in these children. The combination of thymic dysplasia and failure to thrive could bring to mind DiGeorge anomaly (or 22q11 deletion syndrome). These infants, however, typically present with cardiac disease or symptoms related to abnormal calcium metabolism during early infancy. *(Katz, 59:490–494, 1977)*

20. **(A)** The human immunodeficiency virus can be transmitted from mother to baby via breast-feeding. In the United States, where other means of infant nutrition are readily available, HIV-infected women should be advised *not* to feed their breast milk to babies. According to WHO recommendations, in developing countries, the risk of HIV transmission from breast-feeding must be weighed against the risk of contaminated or nutritionally incomplete replacement feeding, therefore at the time of this writing, it is still recommended that HIV-positive women from developing countries breastfeed their babies until 6 months of age. UNICEF reports only 37% of babies in developing countries are being breastfed. Suboptimal breastfeeding is responsible for an estimated 1.4 million child deaths worldwide.

Although hepatitis B surface antigen has been detected in breast milk, studies indicate this does not significantly increase the risk of transmission of hepatitis among breastfed infants. Transmission of hepatitis C virus via breast-feeding is theoretically possible but not clinically documented in anti-HCV-positive, HIV-negative women. *(AAP:Red Book 2006: 126)*

21. **(D)** Normal infants will ingest most of the available milk from a breast within 3–5 minutes. Additional sucking stimulates future milk production, which is necessary for continued successful breastfeeding. Prolonged nursing, especially during the first few weeks, can result in extremely sore or cracked nipples, which can result in early cessation of breastfeeding. Early introduction of bottles can undermine attempts to breastfeed. *(McMillan, 116)*

22. **(B)** Children do learn to feed themselves independently during the second year of life. However, this will not necessarily include the use of utensils. Holding and manipulating a spoon to scoop food and then bring it to the mouth requires complex development. Most

2-year-old children are *able* to use a spoon to feed themselves, but many still *prefer* to use their fingers. *(McMillan, 596–597)*

23. **(D)** Despite public belief, sucrose alone has not been determined to be a cause of problem behavior or increasing hyperactivity in children. Controlled, double-blind studies have not shown a difference in behavior measures, motor activity, or cognitive performance of children receiving sucrose compared to those receiving a control substance. *(Wolraich, 330:301–307, 1994)*

24. **(C)** The child described has many of the classic signs of Kwashiorkor or protein calorie malnutrition. By definition, the serum albumin has to be less than 2.5 mg/dL to make this diagnosis therefore C is most correct. Patients with Kwashiorkor have a dilutional hyponatremia with serum sodium usually around 130–133 meq/L. Serum potassium is usually normal during the acute phase, but can become low during rehabilitation if adequate potassium is not in the diet. Prealbumin is an index of protein intake and functionally is thyroxin-binding protein or transthyretin. Since it has a very short half-life of about 3.5 days, it is a fairly sensitive indicator of protein intake. The lower limits of normal is 20 mg/dL. *(Tsang, 93–95)*

25. **(D)** Skim milk is essentially free of all fat. If it is used at a time when the infant receives most or all of his calories from milk (as seen in most children < 12 months of age and many children < 2 years of age), this could lead to essential fatty acid deficiency. Fats, especially saturated fats, are essential for myelination and brain growth. Additionally, since skim milk contains only 10 cal/oz, the infant would need to consume twice the volume in order to obtain sufficient calories for growth. (*Note*: There is a difference between skim milk and low-fat milk. The former has zero fat, whereas the latter has $1/2$%–2% fat. Two percent fat milk would be permissible at an earlier age than skim milk. The question specified skim milk.) *(AAP Committee on Nutrition, 72: 253–255, 1983; AAP, 265–268)*

26. **(A)** The average school-age child ingests about 30%–35% of their calories from fat, 15% of their calories as protein, and the rest as carbohydrate.

Carbohydrates are the major source of calories in the normal diet throughout life except in the newborn period, when more than half of ingested calories are derived from fat. Excessive carbohydrate intake as well as excessive fat intake can result in obesity because of the resulting increase in caloric intake. Inadequate intake of carbohydrate (<5% of the calories) not only results in caloric deprivation and weight loss but also the excessive combustion of fat, a rise in fatty acid and ketone bodies in the blood, and occasionally acidosis. This is not conducive to healthy growth. This child would be better encouraged to increase activity levels and eat a balanced diet. *(McMillan, 109–118)*

27. **(D)** In healthy infants, the nutritional requirements average 100 kcal/kg/day. However, infants who are failing to thrive most often will need more than 100 kcal/kg/day to gain weight. Their intake requirements typically are as much as 50% higher than normal, or 150 kcal/kg/day. *(McMillan, 904)*

28. **(A)** Fruit juice is almost pure carbohydrate, mostly sugar rather than starch. Less than 5% of the calories are derived from protein and fat. Excessive intake of fruit juices by a young infant increases the caloric intake and can result in obesity. Another problem associated with excessive intake of juice is the development of chronic diarrhea due to the relative malabsorption of sorbitol or fructose, both naturally found in many juices. Inadequate protein intake is also possible despite adequate total calories if protein is not provided by other sources such as milk. *(AAP, 131 and 1134)*

29. **(D)** Dental eruption correlates with bone maturation. This process begins at about 4–6 months of age. Eruption usually is symmetric and tends to occur in the mandibular arch just ahead of the maxillary arch. Twenty primary teeth usually erupt in children during the first 3 years of life. Although lack of dentition by 12 months of age is defined as delayed, this finding is a normal variation is a small percentage of children. In this scenario, macrocephaly, short fingers, and the history of dental eruption delay strongly suggest an inherited disorder

such as cleidocranial dysostosis. Absent or hypoplastic clavicles are a common finding in this autosomal dominant disease. *(McMillan, 782–783, 2523)*

30. **(E)** Milk contains very little iron, only about 1.2 mg/L. The average infant requires 1–1.5 mg/kg of iron daily. A diet predominantly consisting of milk is a common cause of iron deficiency anemia in the older infant and the toddler. This is especially true when the milk is unmodified cow milk. The iron in cow milk is less well absorbed than that in breast milk. Also, a large intake of unmodified cow milk often is associated with microscopic gastrointestinal blood loss in infants less than 12 months of age. Cow milk, of course, contains adequate amounts of protein and calories, so the child described would grow well. *(McMillan, 1692–1693)*

31. **(E)** Childhood obesity is a growing problem in the United States. It is estimated that around 20% of children in the United States are obese with obesity rates as high as 30% in some regions. Obesity places these children at risk for life-long health problems, psychologic issues, and discrimination. There will be an underlying definable cause in less than 5% of children with obesity. This child's adequate linear growth and family history along with an otherwise normal physical examination suggest no further workup is necessary. It generally is not recommended or very successful to severely restrict calories in a child who is overweight. The best outcome for an obese child includes a plan that involves the entire family's eating habits and physical activity. It is important to increase the physical activity of the child. This needs to be tailored to the child's interests and should take into account the activities readily available. Clearly, this requires commitment on the part of the family, child, and practitioner. *(AAP, 551–592; Rudolph, 12–16)*

32. **(C)** Although all of the mentioned methods have roles in the assessment of obesity, the best and what is now considered standard for the office-based measurement of adiposity is to calculate the BMI and compare it to the published reference values. A BMI greater than the 85th percentile on the CDC reference charts is considered overweight and greater than the 95th percentile is considered obese. The use of skin-fold measurements although useful are very hard to do accurately in the obese. Measuring weight alone does not allow for various-size body frames. Using weight for height is useful and is the standard for children less than 3 years of age. Weight for height standards do not exist for children greater than 12. Densitometry is still the gold standard for body composition measurements, that is, body fatness, but requires total submersion in water and therefore is impractical for obvious reasons. *(AAP, 407–423)*

33. **(C)** A sweat chloride greater than 40 is consistent with the diagnosis of cystic fibrosis (CF). This child presents with CF—the most common genetically transmitted lethal disease among Caucasians (1/3300). This multisystem disease leads to pancreatic insufficiency in about 85% of patients. This causes fat malabsorption with resultant malabsorption of the fat-soluble vitamins (A, D, E, K). Therefore, all CF patients should receive pancreatic enzyme supplementation. CF patients also are at risk for iron deficiency anemia. Only when anemia or low serum ferritin levels are documented should they receive iron supplementation. *(McMillan, 1431; Rudolph, 717–719)*

34. **(C)** Adolescents with anorexia nervosa typically perceive themselves as too fat and hope to lose weight, even in the face of emaciation. The degree of distortion of their body image corresponds to the difficulty encountered in treating the patients. This adolescent with anorexia nervosa seems, by history, to have difficulty with bingeing. Because her weight is low for her age, she is likely purging with self-induced vomiting. Therefore, she would be classified as anorexia nervosa, bulimic type or what is called bulimia nervosa. *(McMillan, 657)*

35. **(C)** Since fat yields about 9 cal/g, whereas protein and carbohydrate yield only 4 cal/g, more than 50% of the calories in human breast milk are in the form of fat even though carbohydrate is more abundant by weight in human milk. Of all mammals known, seals have the richest fat content in their milk, which is the consistency of mayonnaise. The milk of seals

contains 12–20 times more fat than human milk and does not contain lactose. This allows short lactation times and high pup growth rates. While human infants will double their birth weight by 4 months of age, seal pups quadruple their birth weight by 2 weeks of age. *(McMillan, 115; Miller, 40)*

36. **(C)** Fat also accounts for about half of the calories in unmodified cow milk. Cow milk contains significantly higher amounts of protein than human milk. Protein accounts for 22% of calories in cow milk as compared to 8% of calories in human breast milk. Of note, the protein nitrogen concentration in the ileocecal contents of 1–5-month-old infants fed cow milk formula is three times higher than that found in infants fed breast milk. *(McMillan, 115; AAP, 87–97)*

37. **(A)** Skim milk is essentially free of fat. About 60% of the calories are provided as carbohydrate, and the other 40% as protein. *(AAP Committee on Nutrition, 72:253–255, 1983; McMillan, 115)*

38. **(E), 39. (B)** Worldwide, undernutrition is the single biggest factor for nearly half of all deaths of children under the age of 5 years. UNICEF is calling for an increased effort in addressing the health-related Millennium Development Goals, most of which directly or indirectly call for improvement in nutrition of children and their mothers. In order to reach a target indicator, the number of under-five deaths in the world must decline from 9.7 million in 2006 to less than 5 million in 2015. UNICEF states, "It is clear that meeting all of these goals will require political will, resources, and sound strategies on an unprecedented scale." It seems obvious this should be a priority for all nations. Jonas Salk said, "Children are the message we send to a future we will never see." *(UNICEF, The State of the World's Children; http://www.un.org/millenniumgoals)*

SELECTED READINGS

Bhatia J, Greer F, and the Committee on Nutrition. Use of soy protein-based formulas in infant feeding. *Pediatrics.* 2008;121:1062–1068.

Fomon SJ, Filer LJ, Anderson TA, et al. Recommendations for feeding normal infants. *Pediatrics.* 1979;63:52–59.

————————————— CHAPTER 6 —————————————

Fluids, Electrolytes, and Metabolic Disorders

Joseph T. Cernich, MD

Angela L. Turpin, MD

This chapter covers very common abnormalities as well as very rare abnormalities. Disorders of fluids and electrolytes often occur with common illnesses such as vomiting and diarrhea and are encountered frequently. Knowledge of fluid and electrolyte requirements for all ages of pediatric patients is vital. Specific metabolic derangements are more commonly associated with certain age groups. For instance, neonates frequently experience hypoglycemia, hyponatremia, and hypocalcemia nonspecifically with illnesses. Older infants and young children commonly develop dehydration and/or electrolyte abnormalities from gastroenteritis.

In contrast to fluid and electrolyte abnormalities, genetic inborn errors of metabolism are rare. Inborn errors of metabolism are relatively unique to pediatrics in their presentation and management. It is important to be aware of common presentations of these uncommon disorders as early recognition and treatment can significantly improve the patient's outcome. Because of this, these metabolic abnormalities are well reviewed in many texts and are well tested on examinations. This section will attempt to focus the material and to review the more commonly encountered defects in each area of metabolism (eg, carbohydrates, amino acids, lipids).

Questions

DIRECTIONS (Questions 1 through 36): For each of the multiple choice questions in this section select the one lettered answer that is the best response in each case.

1. A new mother asks you how much formula her 3 kg infant should be consuming daily. To give her an idea on how much fluid the child should be taking, you calculate out the approximate daily fluid requirement. Which of the following most closely resembles this child's daily fluid requirements?

   (A) 900 mL
   (B) 700 mL
   (C) 500 mL
   (D) 300 mL
   (E) 100 mL

2. A 30 kg child you are taking care of in the hospital is receiving IV fluids in preparation for surgery. You are trying to determine if the fluids are running at an appropriate rate for daily maintenance. What do you determine is the approximate daily fluid requirement for this child?

   (A) 3000 mL
   (B) 2400 mL
   (C) 1700 mL
   (D) 1200 mL
   (E) 1000 mL

3. A 50 kg child you are taking care of has just received replacement for her fluid deficit. You are now trying to determine the hourly fluid rate needed to supply maintenance fluid requirements. Which number below most accurately reflects the correct mL/h?

   (A) 125 mL/h
   (B) 115 mL/h
   (C) 100 mL/h
   (D) 90 mL/h
   (E) 80 mL/h

4. An infant presents with a weight of 8 kg and a 3-day history of diarrhea and vomiting. He appears severely dehydrated with decreased sensorium, sunken fontanelle, poor skin turgor, and decreased urine output. Which of the following most closely estimates the fluid deficit of this child?

   (A) 1900–2000 mL
   (B) 1300–1500 mL
   (C) 900–1100 mL
   (D) 400–500 mL
   (E) 200–250 mL

5. A child with diabetic ketoacidosis has the following serum values: glucose 500 mg/dL, Na^+ 126 meq/L, K^+ 4 meq/L, Cl^- 80 meq/L, BUN 16 mg/dL, and $HCO3^-$ 6 meq/L. Which of the following most approximates this patient's serum osmolality?

   (A) 285 mOsm/L
   (B) 295 mOsm/L
   (C) 310 mOsm/L
   (D) 270 mOsm/L
   (E) 260 mOsm/L

6. An infant with diarrhea is 10% dehydrated. Before the onset of illness, the weight was 5 kg and the surface area 0.3 m². The child's serum sodium concentration is normal. Assuming the child will not be fed and the diarrhea ceases, what is the approximate total amount of fluid you should deliver to meet maintenance needs and restore the child to a state of normal hydration in the first 24 hours?

    (A) 750 mL
    (B) 1000 mL
    (C) 1250 mL
    (D) 1500 mL
    (E) 1750 mL

7. A 6-year-old girl has vomiting, headache, and irritability. She does not appear dehydrated. But when reviewing her vitals you notice her weight is up 3 kg from just 3 weeks ago. Laboratory findings are: Na^+ 112 meq/L, K^+ 4.0 meq/L, Cl^- 75 meq/L, HCO_3^- 19 meq/L, BUN 10 mg/dL, and creatinine 0.4 mg/dL. A spot urine sodium concentration is 100 meq/L. Which of the following is the most likely cause of these findings?

    (A) decreased glucocorticoid production
    (B) decreased mineralcorticoid production
    (C) increased oral intake of water
    (D) decreased antidiuretic hormone secretion
    (E) increased antidiuretic hormone secretion

8. A 14-year-old with type 1 diabetes is admitted with diabetic ketoacidosis. Initial laboratory values are as follows: glucose 563 mg/dL, sodium 136 meq/L, potassium 4.3 meq/L, chloride 107 meq/L, CO_2 9 meq/L, BUN 18 mg/dL, creatinine 0.6 mg/dL, and calcium 9.7 mg/dL. She receives a 10 cc/kg bolus of normal saline followed by IV fluids consisting of $1/2$ normal saline, as well as IV insulin. Eight hours into therapy, she develops muscle weakness. In addition, her electrocardiogram shows flat T waves as well as U waves. What is the most likely cause of her symptoms?

    (A) cerebral edema
    (B) hyponatremia

    (C) hypoglycemia
    (D) hypokalemia
    (E) hypocalcemia

9. A 10-month-old male infant had multiple episodes of vomiting and diarrhea over the last 24 hours. The infant now has slightly sunken eyes, mildly decreased activity, and dry skin. Vital signs are stable. Which of the following is the generally preferred method for rehydration for this patient?

    (A) oral administration of a solution containing 75 meq/L of sodium and 5 g/dL of glucose
    (B) oral administration of a solution containing 50 meq/L of sodium and 2 g/dL of glucose
    (C) oral administration of a solution containing 35 meq/L of sodium and 10 g/dL of glucose
    (D) intravenous administration of a solution containing 154 meq/L of sodium and 5 g/dL of glucose
    (E) intravenous administration of a solution containing 35 meq/L of sodium and 10 g/dL of glucose

10. A 16-year-old male is brought to the emergency room by his friends. They relate they were drinking alcohol and that their friend "passed out" about 2 hours ago and is increasingly difficult to arouse. Which of the following is *most* useful in your immediate management of this patient?

    (A) serum sodium
    (B) serum glucose
    (C) blood alcohol level
    (D) serum calcium
    (E) serum drug screen

11. You are discussing the family history with the father of a boy who is new to your practice. During your discussion the father reports that the family had a daughter who died at age 9 months from complications associated with glycogen storage disease. That child had muscle weakness, hypotonia, and severe cardiomegaly. She did not have significant hyperlipidemia, gout, skeletal involvement, or frequent bacterial infections. Which glycogen storage disease was most likely in the deceased child?

    (A) type Ia (von Gierke disease)
    (B) type Ib (glucose-6-phosphatase microsomal transport defect)
    (C) type II (Pompe disease)
    (D) type III (debranching enzyme deficiency)
    (E) type IV (branch enzyme deficiency)

12. A 3-day-old infant with severe jaundice, hypoglycemia, and anemia is further noted to have liver nodules and cirrhosis. Serum tyrosine and methionine levels are markedly elevated. What enzyme defect is causing this child's liver failure?

    (A) tyrosine aminotransferase
    (B) phenylalanine hydroxylase
    (C) fumarylacetoacetate hydrolase
    (D) malylacetoacetate isomerase
    (E) carbinolamine dehydratase

13. In counselling a family regarding the diagnosis of alcaptonuria, you state that is a metabolic disease caused by a defect in or lack of homogentisic acid oxidase. The excess homogentisic acid leads to which clinical finding?

    (A) kinky hair
    (B) absent patella
    (C) black urine and darkly pigmented sclera, cornea, and ears
    (D) blue sclera
    (E) absent radii

14. A 4-year-old female presents to the emergency department complaining of pain and weakness in her extremities. She has a cabbage-like odor. Her mother reports that her daughter's

symptoms developed acutely today despite the child taking nitisinone and complying with a diet free of phenylalanine, tyrosine, and methionine. Which of the following is most likely to cause future death in this child?

    (A) renal failure
    (B) hepatic failure
    (C) diabetes
    (D) respiratory failure
    (E) infection

15. A child with mental retardation is also noted to have severe myopia. On examination, subluxation of the ocular lens (ectopia lentis) is found. This generally occurs after 3 years of age in children with which of the following?

    (A) hawkinsinuria
    (B) tyrosinemia
    (C) phenylketonuria
    (D) isovaleric acidemia
    (E) homocystinuria

16. An 8-month-old Caucasian male is brought with concerns of a 4-day history of fever and decreased food intake. The mother states that he has slept most of the day. On examination, the patient is febrile with otherwise normal vital signs. He does not open his eyes during the examination. The liver is noted to be slightly enlarged. His laboratory values show normal electrolytes without acidosis. The serum glucose is 33 mg/dL. Liver enzymes as well as ammonia are slightly elevated. Serum insulin is undetectable. A simultaneous urine sample is negative for ketones. Which of the following conditions is the most likely diagnosis?

    (A) sulfonylurea ingestion
    (B) glycogen storage disease type I
    (C) accelerated starvation
    (D) primary adrenal insufficiency
    (E) medium-chain acyl-CoA dehydrogenase deficiency

17. A febrile infant with poor feeding and moderate respiratory distress due to pneumonia is being admitted to your inpatient service. With regard

to sodium content, which of the following intravenous fluids would be the maintenance fluid of choice of a 12 kg infant?

(A) 0.9% NaCl
(B) 0.2% NaCl
(C) 0.45% NaCl
(D) plasmalyte
(E) Ringer lactate

18. A 15-kg toddler with group A coxsackievirus infection is refusing to drink. His serum potassium is normal. For maintenance of intravenous fluids, what concentration of KCl should be added?

(A) 5 meq KCl/L
(B) 10 meq KCl/L
(C) 25 meq KCl/L
(D) 40 meq KCl/L
(E) 50 meq KCl/L

19. A 15-month-old male presents with moderate dehydration. Resuscitation proceeds with assessment of airway, breathing, and circulation. An isotonic intravenous fluid bolus of 20 cc/kg is administered. Laboratory studies reveal a serum sodium of 165 meq/L and a normal serum potassium. Which of the following is the most appropriate plan for rehydration?

(A) correct the hypernatremia over 8 hours with 0.45% NS without maintenance potassium
(B) correct the hypernatremia over 8 hours with D_5W with maintenance potassium
(C) correct the hypernatremia over 24–48 hours with D_5 0.45% NS with maintenance potassium
(D) correct the hypernatremia over 12 hours with D_5 0.45% NS with maintenance potassium
(E) correct the hypernatremia over 24–48 hours with $D_{10}W$ without maintenance potassium

20. A 12-year-old male is brought to your office for concerns regarding excessive drinking. The family states that the excessive drinking is also causing him to urinate frequently. His weight has decreased 6 kg in the past 5 months. His current medications include albuterol as needed as well as lithium. A urine analysis shows no glucose, ketones, or evidence of a urinary tract infection. The specific gravity is less than 1.005. Further work-up shows the serum sodium to be 163 meq/L, with a normal potassium and glucose. BUN is mildly elevated. Urine osmolality is less than serum osmolality. The urine concentrates only minimally when parenteral DDAVP is administered. What is the most helpful treatment for the patient's condition?

(A) fludrocortisone
(B) fluid restriction
(C) intranasal DDAVP
(D) hydrochlorothiazide
(E) insulin

21. One of your patients recently underwent splenectomy due to an autosomal recessive glycolytic enzyme deficiency. Which of the following is a common clinical sign in neonatal presentation of this disorder?

(A) sepsis
(B) jaundice
(C) hepatomegaly
(D) hypertonia
(E) seizures

22. What is the most likely clinical finding in an 8-year-old with Wilson disease?

(A) hepatitis-like illness
(B) acral cyanosis
(C) polyuria
(D) behavioral changes
(E) poor visual acuity

23. A 2-month-old infant is noted to have bilateral cataracts. The remainder of the infant's examination is normal; and developmentally she is on target. What early dietary adjustment could have prevented the development of cataracts in this child?

    (A) eliminating gluten
    (B) providing low iron formula
    (C) eliminating milk and milk products
    (D) providing increased amounts of milk and milk products
    (E) providing increased amounts of folate

24. A 10-month-old male infant with a history of umbilical hernia repair is noted to have coarse facial features and is diagnosed with Hurler disease. This condition is the most severe of which of the following groups of inherited diseases?

    (A) glycogen storage diseases
    (B) glycoproteinoses
    (C) mucopolysaccharidoses
    (D) sphingolipidoses
    (E) mucolipidoses

25. You are obtaining the history of a 7-year-old male, who presents to your office with a several-week history of ataxia and visual changes. Previously he has been treated for attention deficit disorder. As you are about to examine the child he begins to seize. An X-linked peroxisomal disease is suspected. Plasma elevation of which of the following substances confirms your suspicions?

    (A) lead
    (B) iron
    (C) short chain fatty acids
    (D) long chain fatty acids
    (E) very long chain fatty acids

26. An 8-month-old Caucasian male is brought into your pediatric clinic for a routine check up. Upon examination you note severely bowed legs and flaring of both wrists. Feeding history reveals he is formula fed and receives a daily multivitamin supplement. Laboratory results demonstrate the following: high $25(OH)_2D$, low $1,25(OH)_2D$, low calcium, and normal phosphorous. What diagnosis is most consistent with these findings?

    (A) vitamin D refractory rickets type I
    (B) hypophosphatemic rickets
    (C) vitamin D deficiency rickets
    (D) 22q11 deletion syndrome
    (E) cystic fibrosis

27. Pyruvate dehydrogenase complex deficiency is an autosomal recessive disease and leads to the development of an anion gap acidosis. Which of the following accumulates to result in an elevated anion gap?

    (A) beta-hydroxybutyric acid
    (B) acetoacetic acid
    (C) lactic acid
    (D) hydrochloric acid
    (E) fumaric acid

28. You are evaluating a 10-month-old infant for recurrent fractures following relatively minor trauma. You note deep blue sclera and bowing of the lower extremities. X-ray examination reveals generalized osteopenia. Which of the following is the most likely diagnosis?

    (A) achondroplasia
    (B) histiocytosis X
    (C) osteogenesis imperfecta
    (D) osteopetrosis
    (E) rickets

29. A 2-week-old infant has a 12-hour history of recurrent episodes of bilious vomiting. A firm, tender abdomen is noted on physical examination. Flat plate of the abdomen demonstrates a large dilated loop of distended bowel consistent with midgut volvulus. Which of the following best corresponds with this patient's condition?

Serum pH		Serum Electrolytes					
		[Na+] (meq/L)	[K+] (meq/L)	[Cl⁻] (meq/L)	[HCO3⁻] (meq/L)	[BUN] (mg/dL)	[Cr] (mg/dL)
(A)	7.28	128	5.8	88	16	25	0.2
(B)	7.35	130	2.8	90	21	18	0.1
(C)	7.50	130	3.6	88	34	18	0.1
(D)	7.45	140	4.0	100	22	9	0.1
(E)	7.32	140	3.0	112	18	13	0.2

30. A 4-month-old male with failure to thrive ingests greater than 175 cal/kg/day during 72 hours of hospitalization, but does not gain weight. Laboratory values are serum Na^+ 138 meq/L, K^+ 3.5 meq/L, Cl^- 111 meq/L, HCO_3^- 12 meq/L, BUN 2 mg/dL, Cr 0.2 mg/dL, glucose 112 mg/dL, serum pH 7.30, and urine pH 8.0 (under oil). The serum phosphate level is 2.4 meq/L. Which of the following is the most likely condition of this infant?

    (A) nonorganic failure to thrive
    (B) congenital adrenal hyperplasia
    (C) cystic fibrosis
    (D) renal tubular acidosis
    (E) diabetes insipidus

31. A 5-week-old male presents with poor feeding, poor growth, a peculiar odor, hypertonia, and hyperactive reflexes. He is afebrile. History reveals no problems with labor and delivery and early hospital discharge at 24 hours of age. He has not seen a physician since that time. Which of the following is the most likely etiology of this infant's condition?

    (A) sepsis
    (B) pyloric stenosis
    (C) overfeeding
    (D) phenylketonuria (PKU)
    (E) hypothyroidism

32. The most important part of management of the infant described above is to restrict consumption of which of the following?

    (A) iron
    (B) complex carbohydrates

    (C) short chain fatty acids
    (D) phenylalanine
    (E) all proteins

33. A 2-week-old female is admitted to the hospital for jaundice, hypoglycemia, and acidosis. She has also recently been febrile and blood cultures are positive for *Escherichia coli*. The patient is most likely deficient in which enzyme?

    (A) galactokinase
    (B) galactose-1-phosphate uridyl transferase
    (C) pyruvate dehydrogenase
    (D) galactose-1-phosphate dehydrogenase
    (E) uridyl diphosphogalactose-4-epimerase

34. You are seeing a 10-month-old Caucasian female whose mother brought her in for wheezing. This is the child's third visit in the past 2 months for the same complaint. Today you also notice that her weight is less than the 3rd percentile while her length is at the 25th percentile. What is the first choice for diagnosing the suspected disease?

    (A) pancreatic biopsy
    (B) molecular genetics
    (C) evaluate stool sample for fecal fat
    (D) sweat chloride test
    (E) obtain blood sample for endomysial antibodies

35. A 6-week-old presents with a history of frequent, nonbilious vomiting, which the parents state "shoots clear across the room." Examination reveals a thin, alert baby. Gastric peristaltic waves are present as well as a small epigastric mass. Which of the following sets of electrolytes, with values in meq/L, is most consistent with this infant's probable condition?

    (A) Na^+ 142, K^+ 4.0, Cl^- 110, HCO_3^- 22
    (B) Na^+ 140, K^+ 3.8, Cl^- 96, HCO_3^- 22
    (C) Na^+ 138, K^+ 3.5, Cl^- 88, HCO_3^- 38
    (D) Na^+ 145, K^+ 2.5, Cl^- 110, HCO_3^- 30
    (E) Na^+ 128, K^+ 6.0, Cl^- 110, HCO_3^- 18

36. The parents of a 3-day-old male infant present to the emergency department with their child. They report that he was born without complication and was previously doing well. Today, he became very lethargic and started vomiting feeds. Mother reports that she had a brother who died suddenly as a neonate. An ammonia level was drawn and was noted to be markedly elevated. You suspect ornithine transcarbamylase deficiency. What is the probability of these parents having future offspring effected by this disease?

    (A) 50% of males would be severely affected.
    (B) 25% of males and 25% of females would be affected.
    (C) All offspring would be affected.
    (D) 50% of males and 50% of females would be severely affected.
    (E) No increased risk compared to general population.

Questions 37 through 39

A 5-month-old male infant, previously well, is admitted to the hospital following 2 days of severe diarrhea. There is no history of fever or vomiting. The infant has been fed unmodified cow milk, orange juice, tea, rice water, and plain water. The child is lethargic and dehydrated with sunken eyes, depressed fontanelle, dry mucous membranes, and poor skin turgor. Pulses are "thready," and capillary refill time is 4 seconds. Blood pressure is 70/30 mm Hg, heart rate is 190 beats per minute, T is 102°F, weight is 6.3 kg. The remainder of the examination is within normal limits.

37. The child should immediately be given a rapid intravenous infusion (bolus) of what amount of normal saline?

    (A) 1 mL/kg
    (B) 5 mL/kg
    (C) 20 mL/kg
    (D) 50 mL/kg
    (E) 100 mL/kg

38. The initial intravenous fluid bolus given to this child should contain which of the following?

    (A) 140 meq/L of sodium
    (B) 100 meq/L of sodium
    (C) 75 meq/L of sodium, D_5
    (D) 35 meq/L of sodium, D_5
    (E) no sodium, $D_{25}W$

39. This initial intravenous bolus should also contain which of the following?

    (A) 60 meq/L of potassium
    (B) 40 meq/L of potassium
    (C) 20 meq/L of potassium
    (D) 10 meq/L of potassium
    (E) no potassium

Questions 40 through 42

A 1-week-old female infant was admitted because of vomiting, weight loss, and poor feeding. The infant weighed 2.8 kg at birth. Vomiting and poor feeding started the fourth day of life and loose stools were a problem since birth. The infant was fed a standard prepared cow milk formula. On examination, the child was found to be poorly nourished and mildly dehydrated. Weight was 2.1 kg. The clitoris was large and the posterior aspects of the labia majora were fused. The remainder of the physical examination was normal. Serum electrolytes were Na^+ 110 meq/L, Cl- 82 meq/L, K^+ 7.2 meq/L, BUN 31 mg/dL, and glucose 56 mg/dL.

40. The most likely cause of this clinical picture is which of the following?

    (A) viral gastroenteritis
    (B) obstructive uropathy

(C) adrenal insufficiency

(D) inappropriate feeding

(E) inappropriate secretion of ADH

41. This patient's chromosomal analysis would most likely show which of the following karyotypes?

(A) XX

(B) XY

(C) XO

(D) XXY

(E) XYY

42. Therapy for this child should include which of the following?

(A) peritoneal dialysis

(B) low protein diet

(C) fluid restriction

(D) low salt diet

(E) glucocorticoid and mineralcorticoid replacement

Questions 43 through 45

An 8-day-old male infant is brought to clinic for a routine postdelivery evaluation. On examination, the child weighs 6 kg. Multiple pits are present on the posterior helix of the ears. The neonate is excessively jittery. Pregnancy history, labor, and vaginal delivery were unremarkable. The mother states the baby is feeding well.

43. Evaluation of which of the following would be most beneficial in an infant with these physical findings and history?

(A) calcium

(B) thyroid

(C) magnesium

(D) glucose

(E) sodium

44. Additional family history is obtained and the siblings examined. There is a history of mental retardation in the family. Some of the siblings are large for their age and have the same lines or pits seen on the posterior helix of their ears. Which of the following genetic disorders does this family most likely have?

(A) Prader-Willi syndrome

(B) neurofibromatosis

(C) 22q11 deletion syndrome

(D) Sotos syndrome

(E) Beckwith-Wiedemann syndrome

45. Based on your diagnosis, the most likely etiology of this child's jitteriness and abnormal laboratory study is which of the following?

(A) hyperinsulinism

(B) thyrotoxicosis

(C) SIADH

(D) adrenal insufficiency

(E) excess growth hormone

Questions 46 and 47

A 3-year-old, formerly healthy male toddler is seen in clinic with an acute onset of vomiting. On physical examination the child is tachypneic (respirations of 60 breaths per minute), febrile (temperature of 102°F), sleepy, and difficult to arouse. The parents explain they are visiting the child's grandparents. Serum laboratory results are Na^+ 150 meq/L, K^+ 2.9, Cl^- 99, HCO_3^- 18 meq/L, glucose 45 mg/dL, anion gap 26, BUN 16 mg/dL, creatinine 0.3 mg/dL. Blood gas pH 7.25, Pco_2 15, Po_2 88, BE –18.0.

46. This child most likely ingested which of the following?

(A) ethanol

(B) ibuprofen

(C) acetaminophen

(D) organophosphate

(E) oil of wintergreen

47. Treatment beyond acute supportive care should focus on which of the following?

(A) alkalization of the urine

(B) administration of a cathartic

(C) administration of N-acetylcystiene

(D) peritoneal dialysis

(E) antibiotic administration

DIRECTIONS (Questions 48 through 56): The following group of questions is preceded by a list of lettered answer options. For each question, match the one lettered option that is most closely associated with the question. Each lettered option may be selected once, multiple times, or not at all.

Questions 48 through 52

- (A) citrullinemia
- (B) porphyria
- (C) abetalipoproteinemia
- (D) familial hypercholesterolemia
- (E) hypertrophic pyloric stenosis
- (F) Gaucher disease (MPS II)
- (G) Wilson disease

48. A 3-year-old presents to your office for evaluation of recurrent rash with sun exposure. This sun sensitivity seems to be worsening with age. Examination of his skin reveals areas of resolving damage and new areas of exposure which are red, swollen, and excoriated. Additional physical findings are splenomegaly and brownish teeth.

49. A 4-month-old child presents with diarrhea and poor growth since birth. The child has adequate oral intake but recurrent large malodorous stools. He has been evaluated for cystic fibrosis but tests were negative. Stool studies reveal an increased amount of fecal fat. Celiac sprue is considered and the child undergoes colonoscopy. Intestinal biopsy, however, demonstrates normal-appearing villi.

50. A 16-year-old male comes to clinic for a routine sports physical examination. His physical examination is unremarkable except for the skin findings of multiple pale masses which appear to be xanthomas. Additional family history is remarkable for the sudden early deaths of two paternal uncles with myocardial infarction.

Questions 51 through 54

- (A) familial hypercholesterolemia
- (B) Tay-Sachs disease
- (C) Wilson disease
- (D) Menkes syndrome

51. Kayser-Fleischer rings

52. cherry red macular spots

53. kinky hair

54. Arcus juvenilis

Questions 55 and 56

- (A) hypercalcemia
- (B) hypocalcemia
- (C) hypercholesterolemia
- (D) hypomagnesemia

55. An 11-month-old male infant presents with abdominal distention and vomiting. His oral intake is three times his daily maintenance requirement of formula and his urine output is 10 mL/kg/h. The child is small for age and has abnormal "elfin" facies. Physical examination is remarkable for a loud grade IV/VI systolic ejection murmur at the left sternal border. Echocardiography reveals supravalvular aortic stenosis.

56. A 3-month-old female with a history of seizures develops cyanosis and dyspnea. A grade IV/VI systolic murmur is present. A chest x-ray shows a boot-shaped heart. No thymic shadow is noted on the radiograph.

Answers and Explanations

1. **(D)** Infants weighing less than 10 kg expend an average of 100 cal/kg of body weight. A 3-kg infant has a basal caloric requirement of 300 calories. The infant needs approximately 100 mL of water per 100 calories metabolized. This translates to a fluid requirement of 300 ml. This concept is an important one to remember since fluid and caloric calculations for adults are different from those for children. *(McMillan, 67; Behrman, 242–245)*

2. **(C)** There is a simple method for calculating the fluid (and caloric) requirements for an infant or child: 100 mL/kg for the first 10 kg of body weight, 50 mL/kg for the second 10 kg of body weight (between 11 and 20 kg), and 20 mL/kg for each kg of body weight greater than 20 kg. Using this method, the fluid requirements for this child are calculated as follows:

   For the first 10 kg
   $$100 \text{ mL/kg} \times 10 \text{ kg} = 1000 \text{ mL}$$
   For the second 10 kg
   $$50 \text{ mL/kg} \times 10 \text{ kg} = 500 \text{ mL}$$
   For the remaining 10 kg
   $$20 \text{ mL/kg} \times 10 \text{ kg} = 200 \text{ mL}$$

   This gives the child a total fluid requirement of 1000 mL + 500 mL + 200 mL = 1700 mL. Notice that this child does not require 10 times as much fluid as the 3-kg child. *(McMillan, 67–68; Behrman, 242–245)*

3. **(D)** Calculate the daily fluid requirements of the patient.

   For the first 10 kg
   $$10 \text{ kg} \times 100 \text{ mL/kg} = 1000 \text{ mL}$$
   For the next 10 kg
   $$10 \text{ kg} \times 50 \text{ mL/kg} = 500 \text{ mL}$$
   For the remainder of the body weight
   $$30 \text{ kg} \times 20 \text{ mL/kg} = 600 \text{ mL}$$

   Adding these together (1000 mL + 500 mL + 600 mL) gives a daily total of 2100 mL. This daily maintenance requirement divided over 24 hours (2100 mL/24 h) gives you 88 mL/h, or approximately 90 mL/h. *(Behrman, 242–245)*

4. **(B)** The infant described is probably about 15% (severely) dehydrated. In classifying infants and young children, dehydration is divided into mild (5%), moderate (10%), and severe (15%) based on clinical examination. (For an older child and adult, comparable figures would be 3%, 6%, and 9%.) An infant that is mildly (5%) dehydrated has a normal to slightly increased heart rate, slightly dry mucous membranes, poor tear production, and slightly decreased urine output. An infant moderately (10%) dehydrated demonstrates worsening of the previous signs along with decreased skin turgor and sunken anterior fontanelle. An infant with severe (15%) dehydration presents with symptoms of hypovolemic shock with decreased blood pressure, delayed cap refill, Kussmaul respiration, and depressed sensorium. Many students and physicians would calculate a rough estimate of total body fluid deficit as $8 \text{ kg} \times 15\% = 1200$ mL deficit. However, this calculation is not entirely correct, or accurate, as dehydration and percent dehydration are related to a premorbid weight (wt_{pre})—in this case, the infant's weight before he became dehydrated. Current weight = $wt_{pre} \times (1 - \text{percent dehydrated}/100)$.

Therefore, the deficit is 15% of 9.4 kg, or 1400 mL. (Note: Total fluid deficit is not the same as total fluid requirement. Daily total fluid requirements in a dehydrated child includes deficit fluid replacement in addition to routine daily fluid requirements and any abnormal ongoing losses such as continued diarrhea.) *(Behrman, 245–249)*

5. **(A)** Total serum osmolality in this patient is normal (285–295 mOsm/L). The elevated serum glucose increases osmolality, but this is compensated by the lowered sodium concentration which decreases osmolality. By using the calculation $2(Na) + BUN/2.8 + glucose/18$, the estimated osmolality is figured as $2(126) + 16/2.8 + 500/18$, or 285 mOsm/L. The actual measured osmolality might be a little lower than this calculated figure because some of the ionic material is protein bound and therefore does not actually contribute to osmolality. When managing a patient in diabetic ketoacidosis the abnormalities in osmolarity are

important, and warrant slow correction of serum glucose and careful monitoring of serum electrolytes and mental status changes. (Note: It is important to recognize that a patient is not necessarily hyperosmolar with a blood glucose of 500 mg/dL or hypoosmolar with a low serum sodium.) *(Behrman, 193)*

6. **(B)** A child's maintenance requirements might be calculated either on a caloric (weight) basis ($5 \text{ kg} \times 100$ mL (calories)/kg = 500 mL) or on a surface area basis ($0.30 \text{ m}^2 \times 1600 \text{ mL/m}^2 = 480$ mL). For children weighing less than 10 kg, the preferred method is the use of the caloric basis, or the Holliday-Segar method. The deficit, however, must be calculated on the basis of weight (not surface area): $5 \text{ kg} \times 100 \text{ mL/kg} = 500$ mL. Adding deficit and maintenance: 500 mL + 500 mL = 1000 mL. *(Robertson, 283–285; Behrman, 245–249).*

7. **(E)** The diagnosis of the syndrome of inappropriate antidiuretic hormone secretion (SIADH) is made in this patient with a low serum sodium, normal renal function, and inappropriately elevated urine sodium concentration. This increase in the extracellular fluid volume occurs from the action of antidiuretic hormone or vasopressin on the renal collecting tubule, resulting in retention of water and loss of sodium into the urine. Management involves fluid restriction and treating the underlying cause of the SIADH which includes, among others, central nervous system lesions, pulmonary diseases, and medications.

All of the listed answers are possible causes of hyponatremia, defined as a serum sodium less than 130 meq/L. Symptomatic hyponatremia (eg, weight gain, nausea, confusion) is not seen until serum sodium concentration is near 120 meq/L. Seizures and coma occur when the serum sodium value drops quickly or becomes less than 110 meq/L. Adrenal insufficiency, with deficiency of glucocorticoid/mineralcorticoid, as a cause of hyponatremia often will be accompanied by acidosis and hyperkalemia. Psychogenic polydypsia can cause a dramatically low serum sodium, but urine is diluted with a low sodium level. Depending on the laboratory method used, hypertriglyceridemia can result in a fictitiously low sodium;

it is a rare cause of hyponatremia in children. SIADH is the most likely etiology of this child's hyponatremia. *(Behrman, 199–202, 2043–2044)*

8. **(D)** Deficiency of insulin resulting in diabetic ketoacidosis (DKA) can be associated with several metabolic derangements. Insulin acts to drive potassium intracellularly and deficiency of insulin decreases this movement of potassium from the extracellular space to the intracellular space. In addition, as acidosis develops secondary to excessive ketone production, potassium is further shifted extracellularly in exchange for a hydrogen ion which moves in the opposite direction. With hyperglycemia, osmotic diuresis ensues and extracellular potassium is lost in the urine. Therefore, patients with DKA are depleted of potassium even if serum levels are normal or elevated. Patients are at risk for developing hypokalemia as treatment is initiated. Both insulin administration and correction of acidosis shift potassium back to the intracellular compartment, therefore dropping serum levels. Symptoms and signs of hypokalemia include muscle weakness that may progress to paralysis, cardiac dysrhythmias, as well as flat or absent T waves and the presence of a U wave on ECG. Potassium levels should be monitored closely and potassium replacement started as long as hyperkalemia is not present and the patient has voided.

Cerebral edema is the most common cause of morbidity related to DKA and most often occurs after treatment is initiated. It is not associated with weakness or ECG changes. Hyponatremia can also complicate therapy for DKA. Hyponatremia is not associated with the patient's symptoms or ECG changes. It should be noted that for every 100 mg/dL increase in serum glucose, the serum sodium will decrease by roughly 1.6 meq/L. Therefore, the patient's original sodium would correct to nearly 142 meq/dL if the hyperglycemia is considered. Hypocalcemia is associated with neuromuscular excitability and prolonged QT interval. Hypoglycemia is another possible complication of DKA and blood sugars must be monitored closely. *(McMillan, 67–69, 2110–2112)*

9. **(A)** Infants that present with these physical findings are mildly to moderately dehydrated and are candidates for oral rehydration therapy. Consistent administration of small volumes is effective in correcting dehydration even with continued diarrhea. Composition of the oral replacement fluid should be designed to optimize repletion of the ECF space and provide some carbohydrate to give minimal calories in order to avoid catabolism. The relationship of sodium concentration to carbohydrate concentration is important for appropriate absorption of sodium without worsening the fluid losses from an osmotic diarrhea caused by overadministered and/or inappropriate carbohydrate solutions. Most household liquids (tea and kool-aid) are inappropriate because of their hypotonic (low sodium) content. However, commercially available rehydration formulas (ie, Pedialyte) are useful. Intravenous therapy is necessary only when the child refuses fluids orally or has severe dehydration with impending circulatory collapse. *(Behrman, 246–250)*

10. **(B)** In an obtunded or comatose patient, regardless of suspected etiology, a serum glucose measurement is useful in directing acute management efforts. The change in sensorium can be a result of the direct effects of alcohol or a result of hypoglycemia which occurs secondary to the effect of alcohol on gluconeogenesis. Gluconeogenesis is impaired in two ways. First, ethanol is an acid in the blood stream and creates a metabolic acidosis which directly reduces the activity of the metabolic pathway responsible for glucose mobilization. Second, the depletion of NADH in the system by the metabolism of alcohol to acetaldehyde (via reduction of NAD by alcohol dehydrogenase) indirectly stops glucose production, as NADH depletion halts gluconeogenesis. The other pathway of alcohol metabolism, which utilizes the microsomal system, results in the abnormal clearance of other drugs metabolized by this same pathway in the body. The preferential metabolism of ethanol by this system often causes the clearance of other drugs to be slowed and their blood levels to rise, resulting in their additive toxic effects to ethanol toxicity. *(Behrman, 515)*

11. **(C)** Pompe disease is an abnormality of carbohydrate metabolism with autosomal recessive inheritance. Clinically normal at birth, the infants have a deficiency of acid maltase that leads to a build-up of glycogen products in cells. This in turn leads to marked muscle weakness, hypotonia, and severe cardiomegaly. Children with Pompe disease often die within the first 2 years of life from cardiac or respiratory failure. *(Behrman, 474)*

12. **(C)** A deficiency in the enzyme fumarylacetoacetate hydrolase results in moderate elevations of tyrosine. This is thought to lead to accumulation of intermediate metabolites, primarily succinylacetone, leading to damage of the liver, kidney, and central nervous system. *(Behrman, 347–349)*

13. **(C)** The defect seen in alcaptonuria leads to increased amounts of homogentisic acid which is excreted in the urine. Alkaline urine appears black secondary to oxidation and polymerization of the homogentisic acid. This unusually colored urine helps establish the diagnosis. Additionally, the sclera, cornea, and ear cartilage of patients with alcaptonuria become darkly pigmented (ochronosis) secondary to the black polymer of homogentisic acid. Later in life they develop arthritis, which is the only disabling aspect of the illness. *(Behrman, 347–349)*

14. **(B)** Tyrosinemia primarily affects the liver, peripheral nerves, and kidneys. Early death most often is a result of hepatic failure. Affected infants may become symptomatic as early as 2 weeks of age, or may appear normal during the first year of life. Commonly, affected infants will first present with an acute hepatic crisis precipitated by an intercurrent illness and resultant catabolic state. Chronic renal failure, respiratory failure, and paralysis can also occur, but are less likely to be the cause of death. Diabetes and infection are not associated. *(Behrman, 402–405)*

15. **(E)** Subluxation of the ocular lens known as ectopia lentis occurs generally after 3 years of age in homocystinuria, leading to severe myopia and iridodonesis (quivering of the iris). These patients lack the enzyme cystathionine synthase and have multiple problems including severe mental retardation, increased thromboembolic events, psychiatric disorders, skeletal abnormalities resembling Marfan disease, generalized osteoporosis, and seizures. None of the other choices is associated with suluxation of the lens. *(McMillan, 1833–1834)*

16. **(E)** The patient has hypoketotic hypoglycemia without acidosis. Of the possible diagnoses, medium-chain acyl-CoA dehydrogenase deficiency (MCADD) is most likely. MCADD is the most common disorder of fatty acid oxidation. Deficiency of the enzyme results in decreased ability to convert medium-chain fatty acids into acetyl-CoA in mitochondria. During hypoglycemia, acetyl-CoA is used to produce ketone bodies and is used as a source of energy via the tricarboxylic acid cycle. Therefore patients with MCADD present with hypoketotic hypoglycemia. Patients usually present between the ages of 5–24 months and symptoms often occur in conjunction with an intercurrent illness. Clinical presentation can vary from incidentally discovered hypoglycemia to encephalopathy. Some patients may be misdiagnosed with Reye syndrome. Treatment consists of avoiding prolonged fasting. l-Carnitine can be used in symptomatic patients.

Adrenal insufficiency, accelerated starvation, and glycogen storage disease type I result in hyperketotic hypoglycemia, which is not consistent with the patient's presentation. Accidental ingestion needs to be considered in cases of hypoglycemia. Sulfonylureas act to increase insulin secretion by the beta cells of the pancreas. Insulin acts to decrease lipolysis which then decreases production of fatty acids. This in turn, decreases ketone body (as ketones are synthesized from fatty acid breakdown) formation resulting in hypoketotic hypoglycemia. The patient's insulin level is appropriately low in this case, making sulfonylurea ingestion unlikely. *(McMillan, 2176–2178)*

17. **(B)** Sodium and chloride requirements are approximately 3 meq/kg/day, or 36 meq NaCl in a 12 kg infant. Requirements for fluids in a 12 kg infant are approximately 1100 mL/day. Therefore, 36 meq of NaCl must be provided in 1100 mL of fluid each day to meet requirements $(36/1100 \times 1000 = 32$ meq NaCl/L IVF). Of the

choices listed, 0.9% NaCl contains 155 meq NaCl/L, 0.45% NaCl contains 77 meq NaCl/L, 0.2% NaCl contains 35 meq NaCl/L, LR contains 130 meq NaCl/L, and plasmalyte contains 140 meq NaCl/L. Thus, the best choice for intravenous fluids in this child is 0.2% NS. *(McMillan, 68; Robertson, 284)*

18. **(C)** Potassium requirement generally is calculated at 2–2.5 meq KCl/kg/day. For this 15 kg child that would be 30–37 meq KCl/day. Using the Holliday-Segar method, the child's maintenance fluid requirement is 1250 cc/day; 30 meq KCl/1.250 L = 24 meq KCl/L, or approximately 25 meq KCl/L. *(McMillan, 68; Robertson, 284)*

19. **(C)** Evaluation of dehydration must always include the "ABCs" to evaluate for hypovolemic shock. Following initial fluid resuscitation, the serum sodium should be corrected over 24–48 hours. The duration of the hypernatremic state determines the body's level of compensation of osmolality. The brain has been found to make "idiogenic osmoles" in order to preserve cerebral oncotic pressure and to prevent neuronal shrinkage. Administering too much free water (such as D_5W) too quickly can lead to cerebral edema and seizures, thus the hypernatremic dehydration must be corrected slowly. *(Rudolph, 1651–1652)*

20. **(D)** The patient is presenting with diabetes insipidus (DI). This condition can be divided into two forms: central or nephrogenic. Central DI is due to lack of antidiuretic hormone from the pituitary gland and responds to DDAVP. Nephrogenic DI is due to renal unresponsiveness to antidiuretic hormone. As this patient's urine did not concentrate upon administration of DDAVP, nephrogenic DI is the diagnosis. Nephrogenic DI can be treated with hydrochlorothiazide. Although it may seem paradoxical to treat polyuria with a diuretic, depletion of sodium (due to diuretic therapy) results in increased reabsorption of sodium and water in the proximal tubule. This results in a decrease in the water, lost due to the defect of ADH action, on the collecting ducts. Nephrogenic DI can be congenital or acquired. The congenital form is x-linked and presents in infancy in males. Acquired nephrogenic DI can

be due to renal failure, obstructive lesions of the urinary tract, vesicoureteral reflux, nephrocalcinosis, hypokalemia, hypercalcemia, or drugs such as lithium or amphotericin.

Fludrocortisone is a mineralocorticoid agonist used to treat deficiency of aldosterone. Aldosterone deficiency presents with hyponatremia with hyperkalemia. Fluid restriction is dangerous in the face of diabetes insipidus as it can lead to severe dehydration in a short period of time. Nephrogenic DI will not respond to DDAVP, whether it is given parenterally, orally, or nasally. Insulin has no benefit in this patient, although diabetes mellitus usually also presents with polyuria, polydipsia, and weight loss. *(McMillan, 1901–1904)*

21. **(B)** Pyruvate kinase deficiency causes a congenital nonspherocytic hemolytic anemia with resultant hyperbilirubinemia. The breakdown may be so severe as to put the neonate at risk for bilirubin encephalopathy and require exchange transfusion. Blood transfusion may be indicated for the anemia. Splenectomy improves the anemia but does not cure the underlying defect. Sepsis is not a common initial presentation. Gallstones may occur causing hepatomegaly in those with pyruvate kinase deficiency. However, this typically occurs in adults rather than neonates. Seizures and hypertonia are not associated. *(Rudolph, 1542; McMillan, 1455)*

22. **(A)** Wilson disease is an autosomal recessive disorder associated with progressive accumulation of intracellular copper in the liver, brain, kidneys, and eyes. This accumulation of copper results from impaired incorporation of copper into ceruloplasmin and decreased biliary copper excretion. The gene for Wilson disease is located on the long arm of chromosome 13 and is designated ATP7B. Typically, the first organ to demonstrate signs of dysfunction from copper deposition is the liver. Undiagnosed young adults usually present with neurologic findings. Deposition of copper in Descemet membrane, known as Kayser-Fleischer rings, may be absent in young children. Polyuria is not a common symptom, but renal dysfunction can occur causing Fanconi syndrome. *(McMillan, 2021–2022; Rudolph, 1491–1492)*

23. **(C)** Strict elimination of mammalian milk, which is the natural source of lactose (and therefore galactose) is the treatment for galactokinase deficiency. Avoidance of milk products and other products, such as some medications or candy that contain lactose, is important. If started early in the neonatal period, this diet can prevent the formation of nuclear cataracts, usually the sole manifestation of this disease. Once formed, the cataracts are not reversible. The disease is autosomal recessive with gene coding located on chromosome 17q24. Eliminating gluten would be the treatment for celiac disease, while providing increased amounts of folate may be helpful in pyruvate kinase deficiency. *(Rudolph, 641)*

24. **(C)** The mucopolysaccharidoses (MPS) form a group of diseases associated with lysosomal accumulation of partially degraded acid mucopolysaccharides. Hurler disease, the most severe of the MPS disorders, is autosomal recessive and occurs in about 1:100,000 births. It is associated with coarse facial features, clouding of the corneas, deafness, airway obstruction, hydrocephalus, thickening of the cardiac valve leaflets, cardiomyopathy, congestive heart failure, poor growth and development, mental retardation, and early death often secondary to cardiopulmonary problems. *(McMillan, 2201–2202; Rudolph, 657–658)*

25. **(E)** ALD is an X-linked disease characterized by progressive neurologic degeneration and adrenal insufficiency. Patients with ALD have elevated plasma levels of very long chain fatty acids (VLCFAs), which accumulate in cerebral white matter and adrenal cortex. Treatment includes hormone replacement for adrenal insufficiency, restriction of dietary VLCFAs, provision of C18:1 and C22:1 fatty acids, and bone marrow transplant. The dietary supplements and bone marrow therapy seem to be more successful when instituted prior to onset of neurologic symptoms. Death generally occurs 3–5 years after onset of symptoms. High plasma levels of short or long chain fatty acids are typically associated with hyperinsulinism and hypoglycemia, not ALD. Elevated plasma lead and iron levels are not associated with ALD. *(Rudolph, 2324)*

26. **(A)** Vitamin D refractory rickets type I is a rare cause of rickets. It results from impaired 1-hydroxylation of $25(OH)_2D$ to $1,25(OH)_2D$ (the active form of vitamin D) and causes low calcium levels in the face of normal vitamin D intake and absorption. Phosphate levels may be normal or slightly decreased in this disorder. Levels of $25(OH)_2D$ are usually normal or elevated while $1,25(OH)_2D$ levels are low. Hypophosphatemic rickets is characterized by low serum phosphate caused by abnormal renal phosphate loss. It is an X-linked autosomal dominant disorder. Vitamin D deficiency rickets results from poor absorption and/or poor intake of vitamin D. Both forms of vitamin D would be low in such children. Dark-skinned, breastfed individuals born in the winter are at particular risk for vitamin D deficiency rickets. Breast milk is known to have insufficient vitamin D; and supplementing breastfed children is recommended. Sunlight exposure causes production of vitamin D in the skin. Therefore inadequate exposure to light may compound this problem. Children with cystic fibrosis may also have vitamin D deficiency rickets caused by poor vitamin D absorption due to pancreatic insufficiency. Finally, children with 22q11 deletion syndrome may have hypocalcemia, but this is typically due to the congenital absence of parathyroid glands. Vitamin D levels are normal. *(Rudolph, 798, 2156–2160)*

27. **(C)** Pyruvate is converted to acetyl-CoA during glycolysis via the pyruvate dehydrogenase complex, which consists of five enzymes. Babies with this defect may have a severe lactic acidosis with resultant tachypnea, hypotonia, lethargy, and coma in the first few days of life, or the disease may not manifest itself for months to years until the child is stressed by infection, prolonged fasting, or other conditions requiring increased gluconeogenesis. Treatment centers on reducing gluconeogenesis (the major pathway is through pyruvate) by providing a high-fat, low-carbohydrate diet, normalizing blood sugars, and administering sodium bicarbonate and carnitine. Beta-hydroxybutyrate and acetoacetate are ketone bodies and play a prominent role in diabetic ketoacidosis. *(McMillan, 2334)*

28. **(C)** The child described probably has osteogenesis imperfecta, a disorder characterized by osteoporotic bones that fracture easily. Blue sclera, present in infancy, is a common feature. Some patients also have opalescent dentin (dentinogenesis imperfecta), and many develop conductive hearing loss in adolescence. At least four types have been described, with differing modes of inheritance and varying degrees of severity. Osteopenia is not seen with achondroplasia. Phenotypically, people with achondroplasia have rhizomelic short stature, flat nasal bridge, and prominent forehead. Those with histiocytosis X demonstrate sharply demarcated osteolytic lesions on x-ray rather than osteopenia. Osteopetrosis radiographs show extreme bone density. Children with rickets may have leg bowing and/or flared wrists noted on x-ray in addition to osteopenia. Osteogenesis imperfecta is the only choice that has blue sclera associated with it. *(Rudolph, 2161)*

29. **(B)** Bilious vomitus consists of gastric and duodenal (pancreatic secretions and bile) contents. Pancreatic secretions contain sodium at 120–140 meq/L, potassium at 5–15 meq/L, chloride at 100–150 meq/L, bicarbonate at 100 meq/L; bile contains sodium at 120–140 meq/L, potassium at 5–15 meq/L, chloride at 80–120 meq/L, and bicarbonate at 40 meq/L. Knowledge of body fluid composition is useful in understanding the metabolic derangement seen. Typically, bilious vomiting results in isotonic dehydration and either a neutral pH or acidic pH. This contrasts with pure gastric losses, such as those seen in pyloric stenosis, where the dehydration typically results in a hypochloremic, metabolic alkalosis. *(Rudolph, 1400–1402; Robertson, 288)*

30. **(D)** This patient most likely has renal tubular acidosis (RTA), described as Fanconi or a Fanconi-like syndrome. This is a proximal RTA heralded by urinary losses of bicarbonate and phosphate. Classic findings are aminoaciduria, phosphaturia, and glycosuria with resultant hyperchloremic metabolic acidosis with normal anion gap. There are multiple causes of this disorder including inborn errors of metabolism (cystinosis, galactosemia, tyrosinemia, and Wilson disease), and acquired forms from heavy metal toxicity and drug toxicity (ie, gentamicin, valproic acid, cisplatin). The metabolic acidosis and phosphate loss seen in this disorder lead to growth failure and vitamin D-resistant rickets. Nonorganic failure to thrive would not be expected with this calorie intake. Congenital adrenal hyperplasia typically demonstrates hyperkalemia and hypernatremia. Diabetes insipidus usually exhibits hypernatremia. *(Rudolph, 1708–1709)*

31. **(D)** Classic phenylketonuria results from the lack of, or near complete lack of, phenylalanine hydroxylase. Impaired metabolism of the common essential amino acid phenylalanine to tyrosine leads to build-up of phenylpyruvic acid and phenylethylamine. These products as well as excess phenylalanine lead to central nervous system damage. Newborns are routinely screened for PKU. The screening is performed by collecting blood spots on filter paper at the time of discharge from the hospital to home and before 7 days of life. Infants discharged at less than 24 hours of age should have the screening test repeated prior to 14 days of life. Unfortunately, this baby did not have adequate newborn screening. For PKU, presymptomatic diagnosis allows control of the disease through control of the diet of the infant. Though further CNS damage can be prevented in this case with dietary control, the signs and symptoms this baby displays are, for the most part, irreversible. The other choices are not associated with this constellation of symptoms. *(Rudolph CD, 579, 609–611)*

32. **(D)** Treatment of phenylketonuria consists of a very strict diet low in phenylalanine. Reducing phenylalanine in the diet will then reduce the serum levels and help reduce the consequences of the disease, which include brain damage, mental retardation, seizures, athetosis, hyperactivity, and behavioral problems. The diet is difficult to adhere to, and creates increased stress on the child and the family, which adds to the complexity of the disease. *(Behrman, 344–346)*

33. **(B)** Classic galactosemia occurs in 1 in 60,000 newborns. Defective or total lack of galactose-1-phosphate uridyl transferase causes an inability to convert galactose into glucose. Normally galactose converts to galactose-1-phosphate by galactokinase. Galactose-1-phosphate is then converted to glucose-1-phosphate by the enzyme in question. Without the enzyme, galactose-1-phosphate accumulates, causing parenchymal damage to the kidneys, liver, and brain. Indirect hyperbilirubinemia, acidosis, and urosepsis (classically due to *E coli*), frequently are seen at presentation. Other manifestations include hypoglycemia, hepatomegaly, vomiting, seizures, and cataracts. With time, cirrhosis and mental retardation can develop. *(Rudolph, 640–641)*

34. **(D)** The incidence of cystic fibrosis (CF) in Caucasians is about 1 in 3,300 live births; incidence in African-Americans and Asians is significantly lower. CF is an autosomal recessive disease causing an abnormality in the cystic fibrosis transmembrane conductance regulator resulting in abnormal transport of sodium and chloride across epithelial cell membranes. CF affects primarily the pulmonary and gastrointestinal systems with varying degrees. Pulmonary symptoms include chronic cough and sputum production, persistent radiographic changes (hyperinflation, atelectasis), wheezing, nasal polyps, and digital clubbing. GI symptoms include meconium ileus, prolonged jaundice, hepatic disease due to biliary cirrhosis, and failure to thrive (deficiency of fat-soluble vitamins and protein). Patients suspected of having CF are first evaluated by a sweat chloride test. A sweat chloride concentration of 60 mmol/L or greater is consistent with a diagnosis of CF. Concentrations of 40 mmol/L or greater in infants aged 3 months or younger is highly suggestive of CF. DNA analysis can detect the majority of mutations that cause CF and may be done for further confirmation or when results of a sweat chloride test are borderline. There are capabilities to do newborn screening, but this is not in widespread use at this time. Children with CF may have increased fecal fat due to pancreatic insufficiency. However, measuring fecal fat alone is not diagnostic. Pancreatic biopsy is not considered a diagnostic measure. Endomysial antibodies are a useful screen for celiac disease, but not helpful in CF. *(Rudolph, 1967–1973; McMillan, 1992)*

35. **(C)** Pyloric stenosis with persistent vomiting leads to loss of hydrochloric acid. The resultant hypochloremic metabolic alkalosis can be profound, and must be corrected prior to surgery. The incidence is approximately 1/150 male infants and 1/750 female infants and the risks are greatly increased in male infants born to mothers who had pyloric stenosis. *(Rudolph, 722:1402)*

36. **(A)** Ornithine transcarbamylase (OTC) deficiency is the most common of the urea cycle disorders. It is an X-linked trait with affected males typically presenting as neonates with extreme hyperammonemia while citrulline levels are significantly reduced. Therapy includes a restricted dietary protein intake and special foods with only essential amino acids, l-citrulline, and sodium phenylbutyrate. Many individuals die during the neonatal period even with aggressive therapy. Because the disorder is X-linked, male offspring have a 50% chance of having severe OTC deficiency, though female carriers can have varying degrees of usually much milder symptoms. *(McMillan, 2162–2163)*

37. **(C)** In this child, immediate treatment indicated is a 20 mL/kg rapid infusion of fluid to quickly expand the extracellular fluid volume. Such aggressive fluid resuscitation is the mainstay of preventing and treating shock. Only isotonic fluids should be used. Use of hypotonic fluids results in loss of fluid intracellularly, cell lysis, and potentially life-threatening cerebral edema. Other fluids such as albumin and blood can be used for volume expansion, but usually are not as readily available as crystalloid solutions in emergent rehydration situations. Depending on the degree, severity, and nature of the volume loss, two to three isotonic fluid boluses of normal saline (154 meq/L of sodium and chloride) may be required. *(Rudolph, 1644–1646)*

38. **(A)** The initial hydrating solution should contain 135–154 meq/L of sodium for two reasons.

One reason is that sodium will effectively stay in the intravascular space and help to expand the intravascular volume because it does not readily cross intracellularly. The second reason is the record of safety in administering isotonic fluid as opposed to hypertonic or hypotonic fluid. Even in cases of severe hypernatremic or hyponatremic dehydration, the additional sodium and free water provided with even two to three boluses of the isotonic fluid is negligible in its impact on the serum sodium level, especially when repleting the intravascular space of a patient in shock or near shock. *(Rudolph, 650–653)*

39. **(E)** Because of the concern about renal impairment/damage from the dehydration and hypoperfusion of the kidneys, potassium should be withheld from the rehydration solutions until the patient has voided or the serum potassium level is known. In addition, potassium chloride should be administered as a bolus only in specific situations and in a carefully controlled manner because of the possibility of precipitating EKG abnormalities, arrythmias, and muscle weakness. *(Rudolph, 1645–1646)*

40. **(C)** The history of vomiting and diarrhea, the weight loss greater than 10% of birth weight, low serum sodium, and elevated serum potassium are highly suggestive of adrenal insufficiency. The findings on physical examination of a prominent clitoris and labial fusion are suggestive of virilization, and further support the diagnosis of adrenal insufficiency. Congenital adrenal hyperplasia (CAH) could explain all of these findings. CAH is a condition resulting from an inherited defect in cortisol synthesis. Ninety to ninety-five percent of cases are caused by 21-hydroxylase deficiency. Most forms of this disorder are associated with virilization and/or salt wasting. Although a viral gastroenteritis could explain the dehydration in an older infant or child, it would be less likely in a neonate of this age. Those affected by inappropriate secretion of ADH also have low sodium, but often experience abnormal increases in weight secondary to fluid retention. *(Rudolph, 2038–2041)*

41. **(A)** Congenital adrenal hyperplasia is an autosomal recessive genetic disorder associated with either XX or XY genotype. However, because of the virilization associated with CAH, many affected XX females are evaluated for ambiguous genitalia in the newborn period. Males and females are affected equally, though diagnosis in males is often delayed outside the newborn period until they experience a "salt-losing" crisis (usually in the second week of life after maternal mineralocorticoids are metabolized) or show evidence of increased masculinization. Many states have added 17-hydroxyprogesterone levels to the newborn screening in order to detect those male infants without ambiguous genitalia. Prenatal diagnosis is available for at risk families. Screening methods include HLA typing, DNA probe hybridization, and measurements of 17-hydroxyprogesterone in the amniotic fluid. *(Behrman, 1909–1913)*

42. **(E)** Therapy for the salt-losing form of adrenal hyperplasia requires replacement of both mineralcorticoids and glucocorticoids. In stressed children (ie, those experiencing illness or salt-losing crisis) a "stress" dosage should be administered of the glucocorticoid that is two to three times the daily calculated replacement. A high salt intake is also useful depending on the degree of salt wasting. For infants, NaCl is added to the formula (1 g NaCl/10 kg of weight). *(Behrman, 1735)*

43. **(D)** Although jitteriness in neonates can result from abnormalities of each of the possible answers, this infant has qualities that make hypoglycemia the most likely cause. The size of the infant is well above the 90th percentile for newborn males. Many causes of macrosomia (eg, previous large-for-gestational age infants and maternal diabetes) are associated with abnormal glucose metabolism. The additional findings of ear anomalies could implicate a calcium abnormality (eg, DiGeorge anomaly/sequence), but the child has no heart murmur and is not failing to thrive at this point, making this a less likely diagnosis. *(McMillan, 346–347)*

44. **(E)** There is a well-known association of Beckwith-Wiedemann syndrome (BWS) with hypoglycemia affecting up to 50% of children with the disorder. Physical findings are characterized by macrosomia, microcephaly, visceromegaly, and macroglossia. Other associated anomalies are an increased incidence of hemihypertrophy, omphaloceles, cryptorchidism, and renal tumors. The ear pits or creases are not always present in affected patients but are highly characteristic of BWS. Transmission is often from a sporadic mutation on chromosome 11p15, although autosomal dominant inheritance is also seen. The frequency of occurrence is 1:15,000, with variable expression. Mild to moderate mental deficiency has been reported in this disorder and is thought to be related to neonatal hypoglycemia. The other syndromes are not associated with hypoglycemia. *(McMillan, 2641)*

45. **(A)** The exact etiology of hypoglycemia in a neonate can be difficult to determine and involves a differential that is very different from that seen in an older infant, child, or adult. Small–for-gestational-age infants and premature infants both have increased incidence of symptomatic hypoglycemia. A majority of their glucose problems are related to deficient glycogen stores, muscle protein, and body fat needed for metabolization to meet energy requirements. Infants born to diabetic mothers also experience an increased incidence of hypoglycemia. However, hypoglycemia in infants of diabetic mothers is not due to insufficient stores, but is due to hyperinsulinemia and low glucagon levels. Beckwith-Wiedemann syndrome infants also experience hyperinsulinemia which causes hypoglycemia. Their increased insulin secretion is caused by pancreatic islet cell hypertrophy. Treatment for these infants is the same as for other causes of hyperinsulinism; supportive administration of intravenous glucose at a rate of 6–8 mg/kg/min. At times, more aggressive treatments are warranted (eg, increased rates of glucose administration and supplementation of regulatory hormones by injections of steroids and growth hormone). *(McMillan, 346–347)*

46. **(E)** Oil of wintergreen is a solution containing methylsalicylate, a form of salicylic acid. When ingested, a small quantity can cause a rather toxic ingestion because one teaspoon (5 cc) of this liquid contains an amount of salicylate equivalent of 22 adult aspirin. Salicylate ingestions are impressive in the unique metabolic derangements comprised of a mixed respiratory alkalosis with metabolic acidosis. Initially, the salicylate is absorbed rapidly and directly stimulates the respiratory center causing tachypnea and a respiratory alkalosis. Eventually, lactic acid levels, along with other metabolic acid levels, begin to rise in the serum resulting in a severe acidosis. Oxidative phosphorylation is uncoupled by the salicylate and the patient's acidosis worsens. Symptoms of hyperpnea, tachycardia, lethargy, vomiting, dehydration, and coma can occur. Treatment is directed at primarily supportive care until the toxicity has been corrected. Organophosphate poisoning leads to cholinergic symptoms. Acetaminophen overdose leads to initial nonspecific symptoms, followed by liver dysfunction. Acidosis is rare in ibuprofen ingestion as this usuallly presents with GI complaints. Ethanol ingestion is not associated with a respiratory alkalosis but is associated with a metabolic acidosis. *(Behrman, 2367–2368; McMillan, 755–758)*

47. **(A)** The mainstay of management with any ingestion is (1) preventing further absorption of the toxic material, (2) facilitating removal of the toxin from the system, and (3) administering an antidote to the toxin/poison if one is available. These management steps along with good supportive care will minimize the duration of toxicity and facilitate rapid recovery of the patient with the least amount of adverse effects.

    Patients with salicylate toxicity typically are approximately 5%–10% dehydrated and have experienced losses of potassium and hydrogen via the urine. Therapy includes both aggressive rehydration and alkalinization of the urine with administration of sodium bicarbonate. Unfortunately, no antidote is available for salicylate poisoning. In severe ingestions, hemodialysis may be necessary if the quantity of ingestion, level of salicylates, and observed toxicity are not responding to conventional measures. *(Behrman, 2367–2368; McMillan, 757–758)*

48. **(B)** This child is suffering from one of the porphyrias, a group of relatively rare inherited disorders that result in defects in heme biosynthesis and a build-up of heme precursors. These precursors exist in elevated amounts in the skin creating the reactions to ultraviolet light. Some forms cause repetitive attacks of abdominal pain (neurovisceral attacks). *(McMillan, 1999–2003)*

49. **(C)** This patient's history is most suggestive of abetalipoproteinemia, or Bassen-Kornsweig disease. This disease is an autosomal recessive disorder resulting in absence of the betalipoproteins in the plasma. The resultant features are fat malabsorption (due to failure to form chylomicrons in the intestine), failure to thrive, cerebellar ataxia, retinitis pigmentosa, and changes in red blood cell morphology (acanthocytosis). Management includes supplementation of fat-soluble vitamins (ADEK) and maintenance of a low-fat diet. *(McMillan, 1998)*

50. **(D)** This patient's history is most suggestive of familial hypercholesterolemia, an autosomal dominant disorder with a prevalence of 1/500 individuals. Additional evaluation of a fasting serum cholesterol level (with HDL and LDL levels), triglyceride levels, and 12-lead ECG is indicated. Dietary reduction of cholesterol can be effective treatment; however, cholesterol-lowering agents such as cholysteramine (ion exchange resin) or lovastatin (HMG-CoA reductase inhibitor) are usually necessary. *(McMillan, 1865–1866)*

51. **(C)** Wilson disease is an autosomal recessive disorder associated with increased deposition of copper into tissues, primarily the liver initially, then other parts of the body. The basic defect appears to be an inability to excrete hepatic copper into bile and an inability to incorporate copper into apoceruloplasmin. Storage of copper in the cornea may result in brownish green granular copper deposits in Descemet membrane, given the name Kayser-Fleischer rings. The presence of these often correlates with neurologic involvement. *(McMillan, 2355–2357)*

52. **(B)** Tay-Sachs disease is one of the sphingolipidoses and produces disease secondary to abnormal lysosomal accumulation of glycosphingolipids, gangliosides, and sphingomyelin. Faulty degradation due to absent or deficient lysosomal acid hydrolases is the defect. Tay-Sachs is associated with storage of G_{M2} ganglioside in the nervous system. Cherry red spots represent a normal red macular area of the eye surrounded by a white area of storage material. Later, the spots will turn darker as macular degeneration progresses. The disease is associated with progressive CNS degeneration, seizures, blindness, respiratory problems, and death, usually by 3 or 4 years of age. *(McMillan, 1875)*

53. **(D)** Menkes syndrome is an X-linked recessive disease associated with faulty copper transport. In part, the basic defect includes an impaired ability to incorporate copper into certain enzymes that need it as a cofactor. Children with the disease develop progressive neurologic deterioration, seizures, and eventual death (primarily from infection). The most characteristic aspect of the disease is the "kinky hair" which is brittle, depigmented, dull, short, and brush-like. *(McMillan, 2355; Jones, 216–217)*

54. **(A)** Arcus juvenilis is the appearance of an opaque ring close to the periphery of the cornea associated with hypercholesterolemia and hyperlipidemia. Other ocular findings are xanthomas of the eyelids and pale deposits in the retina (lipemia retinalis). Familial hypercholesterolemia results in accelerated cholesterol synthesis, leading to increased risk of atherogenesis which results in peripheral vascular disease, heart attack, or stroke. The disease is also associated with the more commonly known xanthomas of the skin. *(McMillan, 1865–1866)*

55. (A) This patient shows symptoms of hypercalcemia (increased drinking and voiding) commonly associated with Williams syndrome. Williams syndrome is an autosomal dominant genetic disorder that commonly results from sporadic mutations on chromosome 7 (a microdeletion of the elastin gene). The syndrome is characterized by its unique facial features of prominent lips and thin philtrum, as well as cardiac anomalies (eg, supravalvular aortic stenosis). Infantile hypercalcemia often is noted and can lead to problems of nephrocalcinosis, constipation, and mental status changes. The hypercalcemia rarely persists into adulthood. *(Rudolph, 2153; Robertson, 301; Jones, 120–123)*

56. (B) The patient presents with findings of tetralogy of Fallot. The absence of a thymic shadow indicates thymic aplasia. These findings are consistent with 22q11 deletion syndrome. This condition is due to developmental defects in the 3rd and 4th pharyngeal arches and is associated with conotruncal heart defects, thymic aplasia (leading to immunodeficiency), and hypoparathyroidism. Initial presentation is often due to hypocalcemic seizures. *(McMillan, 1547–1548, 2075–2076, 2462–2463)*

SELECTED READINGS

Clayton PT. Diagnosis of inherited disorders of liver metabolism. *J Inherit Metab Dis.* 2003;26:135–146.

Kliegman RM, Behrman RE, Jenson HB, Stanton BF. *Nelson Textbook of Pediatrics.* 18th ed. Philadelphia, PA: Saunders Elsevier; 2007: 267–319.

McMillan JA, Feigin RD, DeAngelis CD, Jones MD. et al. *Oski's Pediatrics: Principles and Practice.* 4th ed. Philadelphia, PA: Lippincott Williams & Wilkins; 2006: 2145–2175, 2181–2217.

Nassogne MC. Urea cycle defects: Management and outcomes. *J Inhert Metab Dis.* 2005;28:407–414.

Prietsch V, Lindner M, Zschocke J, Nyhan WL, Hoffmann GF. Emergency management of inherited metabolic diseases. *J Inherit Metab Dis.* 2002;25:531–546.

CHAPTER 7

Infectious Diseases

Emily A. Thorell, MD

Angela Myers, MD, MPH

As many as 80% of child health visits relate to infectious disease. Public health programs directed toward improvements in water, nutrition, and immunization against communicable diseases has resulted in significant declines in infant mortality of up to 200-fold between the mid-1800s and late 1990s. Still half of all postneonatal deaths in the United States are caused by potentially preventable causes including infections and injuries. The advent of Haemophilus influenzae type b vaccine in the late 1980s virtually eradicated the most important pathogen of sepsis and meningitis in the infant population. However, the persistence of such pathogens as tuberculosis, HIV, and malaria and the emergence of new infectious agents offset the gains of the last century and continue to underscore the importance of the study of infectious diseases, particularly for those involved in the care of children. The following questions address appropriate knowledge of pediatric infections with focus on specific etiologic agents, epidemiology of disease, clinical manifestations, diagnostic tests, treatment, and control measures.

Questions

1. A 13-year-old female presents to the emergency department with a 3-day history of fever above 104°F (40°C); vomiting; diarrhea; and diffuse, erythematous rash. She is found to have orthostatic hypotension. Laboratory evaluation reveals decreased platelets and elevated liver and renal function tests. The mother of the child informs you that the child is currently menstruating. You suspect that this child has a toxin mediated infection. What is the most likely etiology of this toxin mediated infection?

   (A) *Streptococcus pyogenes*
   (B) *Staphylococcus aureus*
   (C) *Neisseria gonorrhoeae*
   (D) *Streptococcus agalactiae*
   (E) Shiga-toxin-producing *Escherichia coli*

2. What are additional features commonly associated with the toxin-mediated process described in Question 1?

   (A) pneumonia and pleural effusion
   (B) arthritis and myositis
   (C) exudative tonsillitis and cervical adenitis
   (D) thrombocytopenia and conjunctival hyperemia
   (E) intraabdominal abscess and ascites

3. Hilar lymphadenopathy is noticed on the chest x-ray obtained for a 6-year-old male known to have mild intermittent asthma. The child is from rural Ohio and lives on a farm with chickens. Tuberculin skin testing is negative and the family denies history of exposure to tuberculosis. You suspect histoplasmosis infection. What is the most likely mode of transmission of the spores?

   (A) ingestion
   (B) direct contact from another person
   (C) inhalation
   (D) skin inoculation
   (E) contaminated fomites

4. You are seeing a healthy, full-term infant just after delivery. The mother plans on breast-feeding the baby and asks you how long immunity transferred to the baby from the pregnancy would be present. When does passively transferred maternal IgG antibody reach a nadir?

   (A) 1–2 months
   (B) 3–6 months
   (C) 12–18 months
   (D) 18–24 months
   (E) 24 months

5. The mother from Question 3 also tells you that she has read that breast-feeding immunity is different than that acquired in utero. What is the major source of immunity conferred in breast milk?

   (A) T-cell mediated
   (B) complement mediated
   (C) IgM
   (D) IgA
   (E) IgD

6. The mother of a 3-year-old child in your office for a well-child visit mentions that her child has been scratching his bottom lately. The mother reports to you that on a few occasions she has seen what appears to be rice in his diaper. Which of the following is the most likely explanation?

(A) *Enterobius vermicularis* infection.
(B) The child has malabsorption disorder.
(C) The child eats rice frequently.
(D) *Strongyloides stercoralis* infection.
(E) *Taenia solium* infection.

7. You were called to the neonatal nursery to see an infant with the following features: growth retardation, rash, and absent red reflexes. On your examination, the baby is very small, with bluish purpuric skin lesions, and obvious cataracts. The baby also has a heart murmur. You suspect congenital infection. What is the most likely etiology?

(A) HIV
(B) toxoplasmosis
(C) CMV
(D) parvovirus
(E) rubella

8. A 6-year-old unimmunized child has fever of 104°F (40°C) and cropped vesicles on the trunk with scattered scabbed lesions. Which of the following infections is the likely diagnosis?

(A) measles
(B) smallpox
(C) HHV-6
(D) herpes simplex virus
(E) varicella

9. The mother of a 6-month-old child seeing you for a well visit, requests immunization against measles as she has heard it is present in the community. At what age should the first dose of live attenuated measles vaccine (as MMR) be routinely administered in the absence of a community measles outbreak?

(A) 6 months of age
(B) 9 months of age

(C) 12–15 months of age
(D) 18–24 months of age
(E) At the time of school entry

10. A 12-month-old child presents to your office for a well-child visit. The mother informs you that at the 6 month visit the child had fever and localized arm swelling after diphtheria-tetanus-acellular pertussis (DTaP) vaccine. She is wondering if this vaccine should be held. Which of the following is a contraindication to receiving DTaP immunization?

(A) encephalopathy within 7 days of previous dose
(B) family history of seizures
(C) for a preterm infant who is 2 months of age
(D) an internationally adopted child
(E) a prior dose associated with temperature > 103.1°F (39.5°C)

11. An 8-year-old child presents to the emergency department with a 3-day history of fever and new altered mental status. Her parents report that they have been camping several times and she has sustained a lot of mosquito bites. Mosquitoes are recognized as vectors in the transmission of encephalitis of which of the following viruses?

(A) arbovirus
(B) coxsackievirus
(C) enterovirus
(D) influenza virus
(E) mumps virus

12. A malnourished 3-year-old child from Mexico has a positive tuberculin skin test (TST > 10 mm for this age). Which of the following would be most concerning for extra-pulmonary disease?

(A) fever
(B) hilar lymphadenopathy on roentgenograph
(C) night sweats
(D) weight loss
(E) hepatosplenomegaly

13. A 15-year-old female comes to your office with 4-day history of fever and cough. Chest x-ray findings include bilateral patchy infiltrates. Oxygen saturation is normal. What is the most likely etiology of her pneumonia?

    (A) *Streptococcus pneumoniae*
    (B) *Staphylococcus aureus*
    (C) *Mycoplasma pneumoniae*
    (D) *Chlamydophila psittaci*
    (E) *Pneumocystis jiroveci*

14. A 3-month-old infant has had upper respiratory symptoms for a few days and presents to the emergency department with respiratory distress, wheezing, and hypoxia. You diagnose bronchiolitis. What is the most common cause of acute bronchiolitis in infants?

    (A) respiratory syncytial virus
    (B) parainfluenza virus
    (C) cytomegalovirus
    (D) influenza virus
    (E) human metapneumovirus

15. On tuberculin skin testing, a well 5-year-old who traveled last year to Mexico is found to have 8 mm of induration to 5 tuberculin units (TU) of purified protein. There is no history suggestive of contact with tuberculosis. What does this reaction likely indicate?

    (A) sensitivity to the diluent
    (B) subcutaneous rather than intradermal injection of test material
    (C) cross-sensitivity to nontuberculous mycobacteria
    (D) tuberculosis infection
    (E) tuberculosis disease

16. A 4-year-old child presents with fever, night sweats, weight loss, and cough. A diagnosis of pulmonary tuberculosis infection was made based on chest x-ray and tuberculin skin testing. The mother of the child asks when her child may return to day care. When can a child diagnosed with pulmonary tuberculosis infection return to day care or school?

    (A) as soon as effective therapy has been instituted
    (B) 2 weeks after therapy is initiated
    (C) once negative sputum smears are confirmed
    (D) once therapy is completed
    (E) whether they are receiving therapy or not

17. A 7-year-old child who recently traveled with her family to India presents to your office with a 2-day history of fever, diarrhea, and tenesmus. Stool examination reveals blood and leukocytes. You suspect infection with *Salmonella typhi* as the cause of her symptoms. What additional signs/symptoms are typically found with this infection?

    (A) rectal prolapse
    (B) hepatosplenomegaly and abdominal pain
    (C) intensely pruritic skin rash
    (D) cough and lymphadenopathy
    (E) toxic megacolon and perforation

18. You are seeing an 8-month-old child in your office for recurrent thrush, candida diaper dermatitis, and multiple recent skin pustules. In addition, he was recently hospitalized with a hepatic abscess. You suspect that this child may have chronic granulomatous disease. Which of the following defense mechanisms is defective and the cause for recurrent infections in chronic granulomatous disease?

    (A) leukocyte migration
    (B) synthesis of collagen
    (C) capillary permeability
    (D) tissue repair following injury
    (E) phagocyte oxidative burst

19. A mother brings her 11-month-old infant along with her 3- and 9-year-old children into your office for a several day history of pruritic rash. You note the rash is similar in the two older children with burrows characteristic of scabies in between the fingers, and on the flexor surfaces of the wrists. Which of the following represents the typical manifestation in infants?

(A) a maculopapular rash

(B) concentration of burrows in the anterior axillary folds

(C) characteristic sparing of the face

(D) initial fever

(E) a papulovesicular rash

20. You are seeing a 4-year-old child in the emergency department with abdominal pain, and acute onset of bloody diarrhea. Due to a recent outbreak in the community related to a popular fast food restaurant, you suspect *E coli* 0157:H7. Which of the following is seen most commonly as a complication of Shiga-toxin-producing *E coli* (formerly known as enterohemorrhagic *E coli*) diarrhea?

(A) meningitis

(B) hemolytic-uremic syndrome

(C) chronic diarrhea

(D) endocarditis

(E) pneumonia

21. A full-term infant is born to a mother without previous prenatal screening. Laboratory evaluation obtained at delivery reveals a positive RPR at 1:32. You carefully examine the infant after birth to evaluate for cutaneous manifestations of congenital syphilis. Which of the following cutaneous findings would be most characteristic of congenital syphilis?

(A) that the lesions are sterile

(B) that lesions are most numerous on the trunk

(C) a fleeting pink macular rash

(D) a papular purpuric eruption on the legs and buttocks

(E) vesiculobullous lesions of the palms and soles

22. The parents of a 1-month-old female infant bring their daughter to the emergency department for febrile illness. The parents deny any localizing symptoms, but report fussiness. You proceed with laboratory evaluation including complete blood count, urinalysis with culture, blood culture, and CSF examination. The most common serious bacterial infection encountered in a febrile 1-month-old infant is

(A) *Escherichia coli* urinary tract infection

(B) *Salmonella* enteritis

(C) group A streptococcal bacteremia

(D) meningococcemia

(E) *Haemophilus influenzae* type b meningitis

23. A 10-year-old female presents to the emergency department for forensic examination after sexual abuse. Cultures are obtained for *Neisseria gonorrhoeae* and *Chlamydia trachomatis*. What is the most common manifestation of infection with *N gonorrhoeae* in a prepubertal girl?

(A) arthritis

(B) conjunctivitis

(C) peritonitis

(D) salpingitis

(E) vaginitis

24. A 16-year-old female presents to your office with complaints of vague abdominal discomfort and vaginal discharge. Pelvic examination is performed and *N gonorrhoeae* grows on chocolate agar. What is the most common clinical presentation for primary symptomatic gonococcal disease in the adolescent female?

(A) hematuria

(B) cervicitis

(C) fever and shaking chills

(D) arthritis

(E) painless chancre

25. In reviewing for your microbiology final examination, you learn that staphylococcal food poisoning is caused by a heat-stable, preformed enterotoxin. What are the clinical characteristics associated with this disease process?

(A) high fever

(B) onset of symptoms within minutes of ingestion of the toxin

(C) concurrent staphylococcal bacteremia

(D) vomiting and abdominal cramps, followed by diarrhea

(E) frequently accompanied by a rash

26. You are seeing a school-age child in your office for fever and sore throat. You diagnose streptococcal pharyngitis based on a positive rapid streptococcal antigen test. The mother is concerned that her 1-year-old child may also be infected. You inform her that group A streptococcal infection in this age group is likely to present as which of the following?

    (A) meningitis
    (B) scarlet fever
    (C) fever and peritonsillar abscess
    (D) acute rheumatic fever
    (E) fever and serous rhinitis

27. A 12-year-old presents to the emergency department in August with fever 102.2°F (39°C) and intense headache. A lumbar puncture (LP) is performed, and your suspicion of aseptic meningitis is confirmed. Which of the following CSF findings is most likely 48 hours into the course of enteroviral meningitis?

    (A) 5,000 WBC, 90% polymorphonuclear leukocytes
    (B) 100 WBC, 90% eosinophils
    (C) 150 WBC, 80% lymphocytes
    (D) 50 WBC, 90% polymorphonuclear leukocytes
    (E) 50 WBC, 70% monocytes

28. It is the middle of the winter and you have seen many children of different ages in your clinic with upper respiratory symptoms. Which of the following children is most likely to have group A streptococcal infection?

    (A) exudative pharyngitis in a 1-year-old
    (B) tonsillitis, rash, and fever in a 5-year-old
    (C) cough and pharyngitis in a 15-year-old
    (D) "slapped cheek" appearance in a 5-year-old
    (E) fever, congestion, cough, and pharyngitis in a 3-year-old

29. A 4-year-old child presents to your office with fever, and increased work of breathing manifested by tachypnea and retractions. A chest x-ray confirms lobar pneumonia. What is the most likely etiology of pneumonia in this child?

    (A) *Mycoplasma pneumoniae*
    (B) *Streptococcus pyogenes*
    (C) *Chlamydophila pneumoniae*
    (D) *Streptococcus pneumoniae*
    (E) *Staphylococcus epidermidis*

30. A 2-year-old presents to the emergency department with temperature of 104°F (40°C) and generalized erythema that is exquisitely tender. On close examination you notice large superficial bullae. You suspect a toxin-mediated infection. Which of the following toxins is the cause of these manifestations?

    (A) exfoliatoxin A and B
    (B) toxic shock syndrome toxin-1
    (C) Shiga toxin
    (D) lipopolysaccharide
    (E) enterotoxin A

31. A 3-year-old child is admitted to the hospital in February with temperature of 101.3°C (38.5°C), vomiting, and diarrhea. The mother describes the stools as watery, green, and very foul smelling. The most common organism causing this presentation is

    (A) adenovirus
    (B) rotavirus
    (C) *Salmonella enteriditis*
    (D) *Shigella sonnei*
    (E) enterovirus

32. A 12-year-old male who just returned from Boy Scout camp comes to your office after 2 days of fever, vomiting, headache, and myalgias. You note a petechial rash predominately on his extremities including his palms and soles (see Figure 7-1). You suspect Rocky Mountain spotted fever. Which of the following laboratory findings would be consistent with that diagnosis?

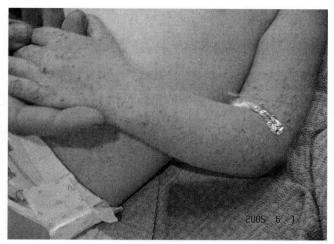

Figure 7-1
(*Courtesy of Emily A. Thorell, MD*)

(A) leukocytosis, anemia, and thrombocytosis
(B) leukopenia, hypernatremia, and thrombocytopenia
(C) leukopenia, hyponatremia, and thrombocytosis
(D) leukopenia, hyponatremia, and thrombocytopenia
(E) leukocytosis, erythrocytosis, and thrombocytosis

33. There has been a recent increase in cases of pertussis in your community. When counseling a family who declines immunization, you should inform them of the common manifestations of pertussis. Which of the following is a typical presentation of pertussis infection?

(A) 4 or 5 days of high fever followed by croupy cough
(B) sudden onset of fever and cough
(C) gradual onset of cough, followed by abrupt onset of fever and whooping
(D) mild upper respiratory symptoms followed by paroxysmal cough
(E) protracted fever and paroxysmal cough

34. The mother of the family in the previous question develops paroxysmal cough a few weeks later. Her infant is subsequently admitted to the hospital with apneic episodes. Which of the following white blood cell counts is most suggestive of pertussis?

(A) 3,000/mm^3 with 75% lymphocytes
(B) 20,000/mm^3 with 65% lymphocytes
(C) 7,000/mm^3 with 65% polymorphonuclear leukocytes
(D) 25,000/mm^3 with 65% polymorphonuclear leukocytes
(E) 12,000/mm^3 with 20% eosinophils

35. A 12-year-old child developed fever about 1 week after visiting relatives in India. The fever has persisted for about 10 days. Diarrhea was present for a few days, and then cleared. The child is now constipated. The child appears moderately acutely ill. The liver and spleen are enlarged. There are palpable, small (2–4 mm) erythematous spots on the trunk only. What is the most likely cause of this child's infection?

(A) measles
(B) typhoid fever
(C) *Neisseria meningitidis* bacteremia
(D) rat-bite fever
(E) leptospirosis

36. You are working in a clinic in rural Mexico and examine an 8-year-old boy who has a rectal temperature of 100°F (38°C), bilateral tender parotid swelling, and pain when you flex his neck. He has been complaining of a headache. His immunization history is unknown. What is the most likely cause of this child's infection?

(A) brucellosis
(B) cysticercosis
(C) Epstein-Barr virus infection
(D) mumps
(E) leukemia

37. A previously well 3-year-old child has a temperature of 104°F (40°C), headache, and stiff neck. He has a 2-day history of upper respiratory tract symptoms and is now vomiting. This clinical presentation most likley represents which of the following diagnoses?

(A) brain tumor
(B) optic neuritis
(C) subarachnoid hemorrhage
(D) meningitis
(E) bacterial sepsis

38. The child in the previous question has a CSF evaluation which revealed 4000 WBCs which are 95% polymorphonuclear leukocytes. Culture grows *S pneumoniae* and he is treated with ceftriaxone to which the organism is susceptible. He is noted to have subdural effusions on CT scan of his head. Which of the following is true concerning subdural effusions with bacterial meningitis?

    (A) They are the result of inadequate treatment.
    (B) They are indicative of a bleeding disorder.
    (C) Finding them is a poor prognostic indicator.
    (D) They are caused by incidental trauma rather than the infection itself.
    (E) They are a common occurrence.

39. A 16-year-old adolescent presents with temperature of 103.1°F (39.5°C) and purpuric skin lesions. The child is found to have a blood pressure of 60/30 and heart rate of 180 with bounding pulses and a respiratory rate of 40. What infectious agent is the most likely to cause the above symptoms?

    (A) *Neisseria meningitidis*
    (B) *Haemophilus influenzae*
    (C) *Streptococcus pneumoniae*
    (D) *Staphylococcus aureus*
    (E) Group B beta-hemolytic streptococcus

40. Of the choices below, what is the first priority in management of the child in question #39?

    (A) intravenous immune globulin infusion
    (B) CSF examination
    (C) intravenous fluid resuscitation
    (D) taking an exposure history
    (E) complete blood count and blood culture

41. A 3-year-old child presents with fever for 8 days, lymphadenopathy, splenomegaly, and numerous reactive or atypical lymphocytes on peripheral blood smear. The monospot test is negative. A likely cause of this clinical picture is infection with which of the following?

    (A) adenovirus
    (B) respiratory syncytial virus
    (C) herpesvirus
    (D) Epstein-Barr virus
    (E) rubella virus

42. Which of the following drug regimens is the most appropriate chemoprophylaxis for adult household contacts of a child with meningococcal meningitis?

    (A) single-dose ciprofloxacin
    (B) penicillin for 2 days
    (C) ceftriaxone IM
    (D) trimethoprim-sulfamethoxazole for 7 days
    (E) penicillin and rifampin for 2 days

43. You are counseling a mother who is 37 weeks into her second pregnancy. Group B streptococcal screening was negative with her prior pregnancy 2 years ago, but she was positive on testing this time. She understands that she will receive antibiotics during labor, but is concerned about possible risk of infection in her newborn. Which of the following is true regarding early-onset group B streptococcal infection in the neonate?

    (A) It is more common in infants born at less than 37 weeks gestation.
    (B) It usually presents with meningitis.
    (C) It is associated with good prognosis if treated promptly.
    (D) It generally presents with osteomyelitis.
    (E) It is frequently associated with recurrent disease.

44. A 24-year-old primigravid woman presents to labor and delivery with fever, malaise, abdominal pain, and back pain. She is found to be in labor and subsequently delivers a full-term infant with tachypnea, grunting, and tachycardia. Blood culture evaluation of the infant reveals *Listeria monocytogenes*. Which maternal exposure is considered a risk factor for development of listeriosis?

(A) ingestion of washed raw vegetables

(B) exposure to cat feces

(C) ingestion of unpasteurized dairy or prepared meat

(D) ingestion of shellfish

(E) exposure to bird droppings

45. A 17-month-old nonimmunized child has had fever for 4 days and now has a maculopapular rash. She is seen in clinic and diagnosed as having measles. There is a 4-month-old sibling at home. What is the appropriate management for the sibling?

(A) immediate immunization with live attenuated measles vaccine

(B) immediate immunization with killed measles vaccine

(C) a single dose of immune globulin (IG)

(D) IG plus live attenuated measles vaccine

(E) no treatment necessary

46. A young child with fever, cough, hepatosplenomegaly, and eosinophilia has 3 negative examinations of the stool for ova and parasites. What is the most likely parasite to cause this combination of symptoms?

(A) *Ascaris lumbricoides*

(B) *Toxocara canis*

(C) *Dracunculus medinensis*

(D) *Enterobius vermicularis*

(E) *Trichuris trichiura*

47. You are working in a hospital in Africa on an international elective. A 2-year-old child presents with vomiting and a distended abdomen. Abdominal radiographs reveal acute obstruction of the small intestine with air fluid levels. Eosinophilia is found on complete blood count. Of the following parasitic infections, which is most likely to present with intestinal obstruction?

(A) *Enterobius vermicularis*

(B) *Necator americanus*

(C) *Ascaris lumbricoides*

(D) *Strongyloides stercoralis*

(E) *Trichuris trichiura*

48. A 3-year-old child presents with 5 days of fever; conjunctivitis; red, cracked lips; polymorphous rash; and an isolated 2 cm cervical lymph node. You diagnose Kawasaki syndrome based on clinical findings. Which of the following sequelae of Kawasaki syndrome is most common?

(A) fulminant hepatitis

(B) coronary artery aneurysm

(C) recurrent pericarditis

(D) cerebral edema

(E) renal failure

49. A 15-month-old child presents to your office with a high fever, and an intense, red rash on the cheeks with circumoral pallor. What is the most likely etiology of this febrile exanthem?

(A) enterovirus 71

(B) adenovirus

(C) parvovirus B19

(D) rubeola virus

(E) coxsackievirus A16

50. A 2-week-old infant presents to the pediatric intensive care unit in shock with vesicular rash, pneumonitis, hepatitis, and coagulopathy. The prenatal and birth history were uneventful and the mother was healthy. What is the most likely etiology of this illness?

(A) group B streptococcus

(B) herpes simplex virus

(C) varicella virus

(D) *Treponema pallidum*

(E) human immunodeficiency virus

51. Which of the following tests should be included in the initial workup of the infant in the previous question?

(A) long bone x-ray

(B) liver biopsy

(C) MRI head

(D) CSF evaluation

(E) abdominal ultrasound

52. You are working in the local health department and receive a phone call regarding a hepatitis A outbreak in a day care center. The teachers ask you if they will be able to identify infected children. What percentages of infected children less than 6-years-old are symptomatic?

    (A) <1%
    (B) 15%
    (C) 30%
    (D) 50%
    (E) 75%

53. A family has recently moved to your area from China. The mother tells you that her hepatitis B screen was positive on arrival to the United States. She has a 2-month-old child and asks you what signs of infection would be in the child. What is the most common presentation of congenital hepatitis B?

    (A) jaundice
    (B) arthritis
    (C) asymptomatic infection
    (D) papular acrodermatitis (Gianotti-Crosti syndrome)
    (E) vomiting and diarrhea

54. In regard to the mother of the child in the previous question, the presence of which of the following serologic markers for hepatitis B represents an increased risk of transmitting infection?

    (A) HBsAg
    (B) HBeAg
    (C) IgM anti-HBc
    (D) antibody to HBc
    (E) antibody to HBs

55. A 10-month-old child has a temperature of 104°F (40°C) for 4 days without other signs. On the fourth day a rose pink, maculopapular rash appears and the temperature returns to normal. What is the most likely diagnosis?

    (A) echovirus
    (B) human herpes virus 6
    (C) measles virus

    (D) group A streptococcus
    (E) typhus

56. An 18-month-old child presents to your office with a 2-day history of fever. He is not eating well and the mother tells you that she thinks his mouth hurts. On examination you see 3 mm vesicles on erythematous bases on the soft palate and tonsils. What is the most likely etiology of this infection?

    (A) streptococcal pharyngitis
    (B) herpangina
    (C) herpes simplex virus
    (D) human herpes virus 6
    (E) candida pharyngitis

57. The child in the above question also has small vesicular lesions on his palms and soles. You suspect hand, foot, and mouth syndrome. What virus is the most likely causative agent of this disease?

    (A) adenovirus
    (B) group A streptococcus
    (C) *Arcanobacterium haemolyticum*
    (D) coxsackievirus A16
    (E) herpes simplex virus

58. You are taking care of a 26-month-old child with bacterial meningitis. Blood and spinal fluid cultures are positive for *N meningitidis*. The child's household consists of the parents, one grandparent, a 6-month-old sibling, a 5-year-old sibling, and a 14-year-old exchange student who has been living with the family for about 1 month. Which members of the household should receive chemoprophylaxis?

    (A) everyone in the household
    (B) everyone except the grandparent
    (C) everyone except the grandparent and the visiting student
    (D) the siblings only
    (E) the 6-month-old sibling only

59. A 4-year-old child presents with temperature of 101.3°C (38.5°C) and a sore throat. On examination, you notice exudative pharyngitis and bilateral, anterior cervical lymphadenopathy. Rapid streptococcal antigen testing is negative. What is the most likely etiology of this presentation?

(A) Kawasaki syndrome
(B) Behçet syndrome
(C) adenovirus
(D) parainfluenza virus
(E) respiratory syncytial virus

60. A previously well 12-year-old presents with fever, sore throat, and general malaise. On physical examination, you notice generalized lymphadenopathy, exudative pharyngitis, and splenomegaly. Laboratory evaluation reveals elevated serum transaminase levels. What is the organism most likely responsible for these findings?

(A) *Treponema pallidum*
(B) hepatitis B virus
(C) rubella virus
(D) Epstein-Barr virus
(E) toxoplasmosis

61. A 15-year-old presents with pain, photophobia, and blurred vision in one eye. Examination reveals chemosis of the affected eye and small vesicular lesions below the eye and on the nose. Application of fluorescein dye reveals branching, dendritic lesions on the cornea. What is the most likely cause of this clinical picture?

(A) cytomegalovirus
(B) adenoviral infection
(C) rubella virus
(D) herpes simplex infection
(E) trauma

62. A 4-month-old infant born with perinatally acquired HIV infection presents with fever, grunting, and hypoxia. Influenza and RSV testing are negative. Which of the following is the likely opportunistic infection in this infant with perinatally acquired HIV infection?

(A) *Pneumocystis* pneumonia
(B) disseminated cytomegalovirus infection
(C) disseminated toxoplasmosis
(D) cryptococcal meningitis
(E) giardiasis

63. A newborn infant has microcephaly, periventricular calcifications, jaundice, and thrombocytopenia. You suspect congenital infection. Which of the following is most likely?

(A) Epstein-Barr virus
(B) cytomegalovirus
(C) coxsackievirus B
(D) human immunodeficiency virus
(E) human parvovirus B-19

64. A 12-year-old who went camping 2 weeks ago in Oklahoma now presents with fever and headache. Laboratory studies demonstrate leukopenia, thrombocytopenia, elevated liver enzymes, and hyponatremia. Of the following, what is the most likely causative agent?

(A) *Rickettsia prowazekii*
(B) *Rickettsia typhi*
(C) *Ehrlichia chaffeensis*
(D) *Coxiella burnetii*
(E) *Borrelia burgdorferi*

65. A 12-year-old child presents to the pediatric intensive care unit in shock with evidence of disseminated intravascular coagulation. Blood culture reveals lancet-shaped, gram-positive cocci in pairs. You suspect *S pneumoniae* infection. Which of the following underlying diseases places them at increase risk for invasive pneumococcal infection in terms of incidence and severity?

(A) underlying liver disease
(B) sickle cell disease
(C) valvular cardiac disease
(D) cystic fibrosis
(E) end stage renal disease

66. A 7-year-old unimmunized child presents with fever and vesicular rash. You notice about 300 lesions, some of which were crusted. You suspect varicella infection. Which of the following is a TRUE statement about varicella?

    (A) It has an incubation period of 5–7 days.
    (B) The rash is confluent, centrifugal, and pustular.
    (C) It is associated with Koplik spots.
    (D) There is a high risk of shingles.
    (E) It can cause visceral dissemination in the immunocompromised host.

67. You are counseling a primigravid woman who has been found to be rubella nonimmune on prenatal laboratory evaluation. She asks you if her fetus is at risk for malformations. When is maternal infection with rubella virus most commonly associated with congenital defects?

    (A) in the first 4 weeks of gestation
    (B) in the second month
    (C) in the third or fourth month
    (D) in the last trimester
    (E) anytime during pregnancy

68. A 15-year-old has exudative tonsillitis, cervical adenitis, and splenomegaly. His monospot test is positive. Which of the following is the most common complication encountered?

    (A) chronic fatigue lasting greater than 6 months
    (B) hemorrhage
    (C) pneumonia
    (D) encephalitis
    (E) airway obstruction

69. An 8-year-old male presents to the emergency department with an erythematous, swollen hand. He sustained a dog bite to the hand the day prior which broke the skin and was treated with irrigation. Purulent material drains from the bite site with palpation. What is the most likely organism causing this infection?

    (A) *Pasteurella multocida*
    (B) *Eikenella corrodens*
    (C) *Streptobacillus moniliformis*
    (D) group A streptococcus
    (E) *Staphylococcus aureus*

70. A 15-year-old presents with fever, acute pharyngitis, and rash. Rapid streptococcal antigen testing is negative. Three days later the laboratory informs you that *A haemolyticum* is growing on culture. Which of the following is the most accurate description of the rash associated with this infection?

    (A) It has a rough, sandpaper-like texture.
    (B) It has a tendency to involve the palms and soles.
    (C) It has a tendency to become vesicular within 24 hours.
    (D) It is pustular.
    (E) It has a predilection for the face.

71. A 3-year-old child travels with his family to Mexico, where he dines on the local cuisine. One month after return, he develops fever, anorexia, myalgias, and abdominal pain. Serologic testing is positive for *Brucella* infection. Which of the following is a common manifestation of brucellosis in children?

    (A) hepatosplenomegaly
    (B) glaucoma
    (C) meningitis
    (D) endocarditis
    (E) osteomyelitis

72. A 3-year-old child in day care develops abdominal pain with diarrhea and malaise. His class recently had a field trip to the local petting zoo. Stool culture subsequently grows *Campylobacter jejuni*. Which of the following is the most common clinical manifestation that follows infection with *Campylobacter*?

    (A) Guillain-Barré syndrome
    (B) polyarticular arthritis
    (C) encephalitis
    (D) inguinal lymphadenitis
    (E) anterior uveitis

73. You see a 5-year-old child in your office with a palpable lymph node in her right axilla that is progressing in size over the last 3 days. It has become erythematous and warm. On examination, the node is indurated. You also note many scratches on the child's arms. On further questioning, you discover that the family has recently adopted a new kitten. What is the most likely etiology of the child's adenopathy?

(A) *Coxiella burnetii*
(B) *Streptobacillus moniliformis*
(C) *Bartonella henselae*
(D) *Mycobacterium avium* complex
(E) *Mycobacterium tuberculosis*

74. A 3-month-old infant is admitted to the hospital with respiratory distress. He has had cough and congestion for the last 2 days and is now breathing too fast to eat effectively. You suspect bronchiolitis and respiratory syncytial virus (RSV) antigen testing is positive. Which of the following roentgenographic findings is most commonly seen in infants with bronchiolitis caused by RSV?

(A) hyperinflation
(B) hilar adenopathy
(C) multilobar infiltrate
(D) lower lobe infiltrates
(E) pleural effusion

75. An 8-year-old was hiking with his Boy Scout troop a few days ago. He now presents to your office with 2 days of abdominal pain. On further history, you realize he drank from the stream on his hike. You suspect *Giardia intestinalis* infection. What additional symptom would you see most commonly in a child with giardiasis?

(A) fever
(B) watery diarrhea
(C) bloody diarrhea
(D) failure to thrive
(E) vomiting

76. After confirmation of giardiasis by antigen testing on the stool, you initiate therapy on the child in the previous question. What is the most appropriate therapy for giardiasis?

(A) trimethoprim-sulfamethoxazole
(B) ketoconazole
(C) mebendazole
(D) nitrofurantoin
(E) metronidazole

77. A 3-year-old child from Somalia presents to the emergency department with a 2-week history of low-grade fever, headache, and irritability. This morning he was difficult to arouse and subsequently had a seizure. On examination, he has a temperature of 102.2°F (39°C), nuchal rigidity, and somnolence. You discover that he and his parents had positive tuberculin skin tests on arrival to the United States and suspect tuberculous meningitis. Which of the following is characteristic of the cerebrospinal fluid in tuberculous meningitis?

(A) The color is usually blood tinged.
(B) Protein is normal.
(C) Culture reveals tuberculous organisms within 1 week.
(D) Glucose is low.
(E) Neutrophils predominate.

78. A 3-month-old African American infant presents to the emergency department on Thanksgiving weekend with fever and hematochezia. From the history, you discover that the family prepared chitterlings for the Thanksgiving meal. Fecal leukocytes are present. Stool cultures are positive. What is the most likely etiology of this infant's infection?

(A) *Salmonella enteritidis*
(B) *Salmonella typhi*
(C) *Escherichia coli*
(D) *Shigella flexneri*
(E) *Yersinia enterocolitica*

79. A 16-year-old sexually active male presents to your office with a painful ulcer on his penis and fluctuant, tender lymph nodes in his left inguinal area. You aspirate the most fluctuant node and Gram stained smear is negative. What is the most likely etiology of this presentation?

    (A) lymphogranuloma venereum
    (B) herpes simplex virus
    (C) syphilis
    (D) chancroid
    (E) granuloma inguinale

80. The mother of a newborn infant brings her 2-week-old child in for his first checkup in November. The mother has heard reports on the local news of influenza in the community and that young infants are at very high risk if they contract the disease. She asks you if her child can be immunized. At what age can a child first receive influenza vaccine?

    (A) birth
    (B) 2 months
    (C) 4 months
    (D) 6 months
    (E) 12 months

81. A 13-year-old male is taking inhaled steroids for his moderate intermittent asthma. On examination, you find white plaques on his buccal mucosa. You suspect thrush caused by *Candida albicans*. Which of the following would be most appropriate for treatment?

    (A) itraconazole
    (B) amphotericin B
    (C) metronidazole
    (D) nystatin
    (E) mebendazole

82. A 3-year-old female with perinatally acquired human immunodeficiency virus has history of medical nonadherence to therapy. Her most recent CD4 count was less than 100. She presents to your clinic with fatigue, abdominal cramping, vomiting, and diarrhea. She has not been eating and has had significant weight loss since her last visit. Upon further questioning, you realize that she has had diarrhea for over a month. Stool examination reveals 4–6 μm spherical cysts. What is the most likely etiology of this presentation?

    (A) *Giardia lamblia*
    (B) *Entamoeba histolytica*
    (C) *Cryptosporidium parvum*
    (D) *Isospora belli*
    (E) *Cryptococcus neoformans*

83. A 9-month-old presents to your office with 2-day history of temperature of 101.6°F (38.7°C) and fussiness. Mother reports that the child has been pulling at her ear. On physical examination, you note an erythematous, bulging, right tympanic membrane with purulent effusion. You diagnose otitis media. What organism is the most likely cause of this infection?

    (A) *Streptococcus pyogenes*
    (B) *Streptococcus pneumoniae*
    (C) *Haemophilus influenzae type B*
    (D) *Staphylococcus aureus*
    (E) *Pseudomonas aeruginosa*

84. A 14-year-old presents to your office with 2 week history of cough and purulent rhinorrhea. He now has 2-day history of fever and frontal headache. On examination he is tender to palpation over his maxillary sinuses and his mother tells you that he appears swollen over that area. You make the clinical diagnosis of acute sinusitis. He has no allergies to medication. What is the first-line therapy for this child?

    (A) ceftriaxone
    (B) cephalexin
    (C) clindamycin
    (D) amoxicillin
    (E) azithromycin

85. A 15-year-old male just returned from a hunting trip with his father. He has an abrupt onset of fever, chills, myalgia, and headache. He develops painful anterior cervical chain lymphadenopathy. On examination, you see an ulcer under his arm. His father tells you that they removed a tick from that spot a few days

prior. What is the most likely diagnosis for this patient?

(A) tularemia
(B) Lyme disease
(C) Rocky Mountain spotted fever
(D) ehrlichiosis
(E) Q fever

86. A 7-year-old child was grabbing at a neighbor dog's tail and was bitten on the arm. He presents to the emergency department for wound management. The dog's behavior is normal and it is in custody of animal control, but the owner's do not have record of the last rabies vaccine. The health department has not had reports of rabies in the county where the child was bitten. Besides local wound care, what is the most appropriate intervention regarding possible rabies exposure?

(A) Euthanize the dog and send brain tissue for rabies antigen testing.
(B) Give the child the rabies vaccine series as well as rabies immune globulin and observe the dog for 10 days for signs of rabies.
(C) Give the child rabies vaccine alone and observe the dog for 10 days for signs of rabies.
(D) Give the child rabies immune globulin alone and observe the dog for 10 days for signs of rabies.
(E) Observe the dog for 10 days for signs of rabies.

87. A 5-year-old unimmunized child fell while playing in an old barn and sustained a laceration to his leg. After local wound care, what would be the most appropriate management regarding tetanus prophylaxis?

(A) give Td only
(B) give DTaP only
(C) give Td and tetanus immune globulin
(D) give DTaP and tetanus immune globulin
(E) give tetanus immune globulin only

88. A family is visiting their summer home in New England. Their 8-year-old child presents to your office with a rash over his back. The rash started as a small, erythematous macular area and is expanding to form an annular, erythematous lesion with a distinct border that is more than 10 cm in diameter. What is the causative agent of this child's infection?

(A) *Rickettsia rickettsiae*
(B) *Borrelia burgdorferi*
(C) *Anaplasma phagocytophilia*
(D) *Rickettsia typhi*
(E) *Rickettsia prowazekii*

89. What is the term used to describe the exanthem in the patient in the above question?

(A) erythema nodosum
(B) erythema marginatum
(C) erythema migrans
(D) erythema toxicum
(E) erythema multiforme

90. A 2-year-old African American child presents to your office with areas of alopecia. On examination you note a boggy, inflammatory mass with some purulent drainage over the scalp and occipital lymphadenopathy. Cultures are obtained via skin scraping and grow *Trichophyton tonsurans*. What is the best initial treatment for tinea capitis?

(A) topical nystatin
(B) oral griseofulvin
(C) topical miconazole
(D) oral itraconazole
(E) ketoconazole shampoo

91. You are attending in the newborn nursery and are informed that a baby was born to a mother with human immunodeficiency virus (HIV). What is the best test to diagnose HIV infection in this infant?

(A) Enzyme immunoassay (ELISA)
(B) RNA PCR
(C) Western blot
(D) DNA PCR
(E) HIV p24 antigen

92. A 5-month-old child is admitted with severe hypoxia and respiratory failure to the pediatric intensive care unit. A diagnosis of *P jiroveci* pneumonia (PCP) is made on silver staining of bronchoalveolar lavage fluid. You suspect immunodeficiency in this patient, and HIV testing is negative. What is the most likely immunodeficiency?

    (A) Bruton agammaglobulinemia
    (B) adenosine deaminase deficiency
    (C) common variable immunodeficiency
    (D) Job syndrome
    (E) asplenia

93. A 9-year-old child is hospitalized with her second episode of meningococcemia. Immunodeficiency is suspected. What is the most likely immune deficiency which would predispose this child to recurrent *N meningitidis* infection?

    (A) X-linked agammaglobulinemia
    (B) Chediak-Higashi syndrome
    (C) human immunodeficiency virus
    (D) Wiskott-Aldrich syndrome
    (E) terminal complement deficiency

94. You are seeing a 6-month-old for well-child visit and immunizations. Anticipatory guidance is given. What immunizations would you prescribe if the child were up to date at that point?

    (A) hepatitis B, DTaP, HIB, IPV, PCV
    (B) hepatitis A, hepatitis B, DTaP, HIB, PCV
    (C) DTaP, HIB, IPV, PCV, MMR
    (D) hepatitis A, DTaP, HIB, IPV, PCV
    (E) DTaP, HIB, MMR, varicella, PCV

95. A 6-year-old child has recently emigrated from sub-Saharan Africa. For the last 2 weeks, he has had fever every other day along with nausea, vomiting, arthralgia, and abdominal pain. On further questioning, the mother tells you that the child has rigors with fever and sweats when the fever breaks. You suspect malaria. What is the best diagnostic method for this illness?

    (A) aerobic and anaerobic blood culture
    (B) serologic testing
    (C) thick and thin blood smear preparations

(D) PCR on serum
(E) liver biopsy

96. You diagnose group A streptococcal pharyngitis in an 8-year-old child and treat appropriately. The mother of the child asks how long she must stay home from school. When can the child return to school?

    (A) as soon as therapy is initiated
    (B) 24 hours after the initiation of therapy
    (C) 48 hours after the initiation of therapy
    (D) 72 hours after the initiation of therapy
    (E) the full length of therapy

97. An 18-year-old male comes home from college for winter break and comes to your office complaining of malaise, knee pain, and rash. On examination, you find generalized, polymorphic, maculopapular rash including the palms and soles, generalized lymphadenopathy, and splenomegaly. When questioned about his sexual history, he tells you he has had multiple partners. Of the following, what is the most likely etiology of his illness?

    (A) primary syphilis
    (B) secondary syphilis
    (C) chancroid
    (D) lymphogranuloma venereum
    (E) gonococcal infection

98. In regard to the patient in the above question, what is the most appropriate antimicrobial therapy for his treatment?

    (A) penicillin
    (B) ceftriaxone
    (C) cephalexin
    (D) azithromycin
    (E) ciprofloxacin

99. A 3-year-old child is in your office for the second time with otitis media that is not responding to antibiotics. He has been on standard-dose amoxicillin for the last 10 days and his tympanic membrane is still bulging with purulent effusion. You perform a tympanocentesis and recover *S pneumoniae*. The parents ask you why the initial

antibiotic did not work. What is the most likely cause of pneumococcal resistance to amoxicillin?

(A) mutation in *mef* (membrane efflux pump) gene
(B) mutation in *erm* (erythromycin ribosome methylation) gene
(C) beta-lactamase
(D) point mutation in DNA gyrase
(E) penicillin-binding protein mutation

100. You are seeing a 5-year-old child with recurrent furunculosis secondary to methicillin-resistant S aureus (MRSA). Susceptibility testing confirms the isolate is clindamycin susceptible and that D-zone testing is negative. You elect to treat with clindamycin. What is the mechanism of action of clindamycin?

(A) inhibitor of cell wall synthesis
(B) inhibitor of protein synthesis
(C) inhibitor of bacterial DNA synthesis

(D) inhibitor of bacterial enzyme
(E) interferes with cell membrane permeability

101. An 18-month-old child presents to the emergency department with fever. The parents inform you that they think the child has been limping on the right leg for the last week. On examination, the only focal finding is that the right knee seems swollen and a little warm. Arthrocentesis is performed and synovial fluid shows 75,000 WBC with 90% neutrophils. Gram stain is negative. After 5 days, the culture grows a gram-negative coccobacillus. What is the most likely etiology of the septic arthritis in this child?

(A) *Staphylococcus aureus*
(B) *Streptococcus pyogenes*
(C) *Kingella kingae*
(D) *Salmonella enteritidis*
(E) *Fusobacterium necrophorum*

Answers and Explanations

1. **(B)** Manifestations of staphylococcal toxic shock syndrome, which include fever, mental status changes, conjunctivitis, diffuse macular erythroderma, and multiple organ failure, are caused by a toxin elaborated by the staphylococci rather than by tissue invasion of the organism. The name of the toxin is toxic shock syndrome toxin-1 (TSST-1), and is produced by *S aureus*. The organism usually can be cultured from skin or mucous membrane and only rarely from the blood. It has been recovered from the vagina and has been associated with the use of tampons, especially those designed to be changed infrequently. Streptococcal toxic shock syndrome is cause by *S pyogenes* (group A streptococcus). The incidence is highest among young children, particularly those with concomitant varicella. The organism can be isolated from blood about 50% of the time. Both *N gonorrhoeae* and *S agalactiae* can be found in the genital tract (the former as a pathogen and the latter as normal flora); neither is associated with toxin-mediated disease. Shiga toxin produced by *E coli* causes diarrhea and can be associated with hemolytic uremic syndrome. *(Long, 110–112; American Academy of Pediatrics, 660–661)*

2. **(D)** The case definition of staphylococcal toxic shock syndrome includes five to six of the following findings: fever; diffuse rash; desquamation 1–2 weeks after onset; hypotension; if obtained, negative results for blood (except S aureus approximately 5% of the time), throat, and CSF cultures, and negative serologic testing for Rocky Mountain spotted fever, measles, or leptospirosis; and multisystem organ failure. Organ involvement must include three or more of the following: gastrointestinal symptoms, muscular symptoms such as myalgia, mucous membrane involvement such as conjunctival hyperemia, vaginal or oropharyngeal involvement, hepatic dysfunction, renal dysfunction, platelet count less than 100,000/μL, or central nervous system dysfunction such as altered mental status. *(American Academy of Pediatrics, 662)*

3. **(C)** *Histoplasma capsulatum* is the most common primary systemic mycosis in the United States, and most often occurs in the Ohio and Mississippi river valleys. The organism grows in moist soil and is facilitated by bird droppings. As in adults, the respiratory tract is the portal of entry for histoplasmosis in essentially all cases in children. Inoculation other than by inhalation is exceedingly rare, and person to person transmission does not occur. *(Long, 11198; American Academy of Pediatrics, 371–372)*

4. **(B)** Passively transferred maternal IgG decreases commensurate with the half-life, which is approximately 30 days. Therefore the nadir occurs in infants at the age of 3–6 months. *(Long, 92)*

5. **(D)** Human milk provides optimal nutrition for the growing infant. It contains lactose and other carbohydrates that are substrates for protective microflora, such as *Bifidobacterium* and *Lactobacillus spp*. The major immunoglobulin present in breast milk is secretory IgA, and is available to act at the mucosal surface of the small intestine. Immunity is conferred against many specific enteropathogens and toxins. It also has been shown to inhibit binding of *H influenzae* and *S pneumoniae* to pharyngeal cells. *(Nelson, 158)*

6. **(A)** *Enterobius vermicularis* infection (Pinworms) occurs from ingestion of embryonated eggs which hatch intraluminally and mature as they descend the GI tract. An adult female deposits eggs on the perianal skin at night causing pruritus ani. It is considered the most common helminthiasis in the United States and other developed countries. Most infections occur in children with documented transmission in child care centers and elementary schools. The most reliable diagnosis is made via transparent tape preparation. Malabsorption disorders and ingestion of rice do not cause pruritus. *Strongyloides stercoralis* is a round worm and *T solium* is the pork tape worm. Both may cause abdominal pain, vomiting, and diarrhea, but typically not pruritus ani. *(Long, 1301–1302; American Academy of Pediatrics, 520–522, 629–630, 644–645)*

7. **(E)** Infants congenitally infected with rubella excrete the virus in urine and pharyngeal secretions and can be infectious for many weeks or months. Such infants pose a definite hazard to nonimmune family members, caretakers, as well as medical and nursing personnel. Pregnant females who are not certain of their rubella immunity status should not handle these infants or their secretions. Infants with perinatally acquired HIV are generally asymptomatic at birth. An infant with congenital CMV and toxoplasmosis may have a similar presentation to congenital rubella, although cataracts and congenital heart disease are not typical manifestations. In addition, patients with toxoplasmosis may have scattered cerebral calcifications, while patients with CMV may have periventricular calcifications. *(American Academy of Pediatrics, 574–579, 666, 273–274)*

8. **(E)** Of the so-called common childhood diseases listed in this question, primary varicella infection (or chickenpox) is most likely to present with a generalized, pruritic vesicular rash and mild fever. The typical exanthem appears first on the scalp, face, or trunk. New crops of lesions develop over a 1–7 day period. Progression from vesicle to pustule to crusted scab occurs quickly such that lesions of all stages are present after the first 48 hours. *(American Academy of Pediatrics, 711; Long, 1021–1022).*

9. **(C)** Ordinarily, the first dose of live attenuated measles vaccine (combined with mumps and rubella as the MMR vaccine) should be administered between 12 and 15 months of age to maximize the likelihood that transplacentally acquired antibodies have disappeared completely from the child's blood. Otherwise, these antibodies may blunt the infant's immunologic response to the vaccine. On the other hand, administration of the vaccine should not be delayed much beyond 15 months because of the seriousness of measles infection. It is recommended that a second dose of the vaccine be given when the child enters elementary school. In areas where, or at times when, measles is epidemic, it is recommended that an initial dose of monovalent measles vaccine be given as early as 6 months of age, followed by the two MMRs as noted. *(American Academy of Pediatrics, 447, 448; Long, 1126)*

10. **(A)** The use of a combined diphtheria-tetanus-acellular pertussis (DTaP) vaccine is routine and is the method of choice for the primary immunization of infants and young children. There are two contraindications to pertussis immunization: an immediate anaphylactic reaction or encephalopathy within 7 days of a prior dose manifested by major alterations in consciousness or protracted generalized or focal seizures without recovery within 24 hours. *(American Academy of Pediatrics, 40, 510–513)*

11. **(A)** Mumps virus, enterovirus, coxsackievirus, and influenza virus are spread primarily by direct contact (eg, respiratory droplets, hands) and not through an arthropod vector. A number of viruses, notably the arboviruses, are spread by mosquito vectors, as well as ticks and sandflies. Examples in North America include eastern and western equine encephalitis, St. Louis encephalitis, and LaCrosse and West Nile encephalitis. *(Long, 1084)*

12. **(E)** Fever, cough, hilar lymphadenopathy, and elevated sedimentation rate are seen commonly in uncomplicated primary pulmonary tuberculosis. Hepatosplenomegaly is generally not seen in uncomplicated primary pulmonary tuberculosis, but does occur in more than 50% of children with disseminated disease. *(Long, 776)*

13. **(C)** *Mycoplasma pneumoniae* has long been known to cause pneumonia, bronchitis, otitis media, myringitis bullosa, and nonspecific upper respiratory infection. More recently, this organism also has been recognized as a cause of various non-respiratory manifestations such as polymorphous mucocutaneous eruptions including Stevens-Johnson syndrome, encephalitis, and meningitis. Other neurologic manifestations reported with *M pneumoniae* infection include transverse myelitis, psychosis, poliomyelitis-like syndrome, and Guillain-Barré syndrome. *Streptococcus pneumoniae* and *S aureus* typically cause lobar pneumonia, oftentimes with empyema. While chest radiograph findings in *M pneumoniae* infection often include patchy alveolar infiltrates with small pleural effusion, the accompanying chest radiograph which shows a white out of one lung would be most likely associated with empyema. While *C psittaci* may have the same clinical presentation as mycoplasma, there will typically be a history of bird exposure. *Pneumocystis jiroveci* is considered a pathogen in the immunocompromised host (see Figure 7-2). *(Long, 979–981; American Academy of Pediatrics, 251, 468)*

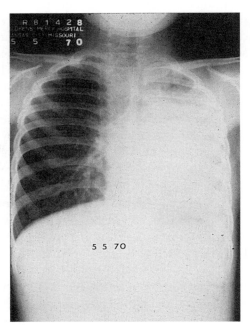

Figure 7-2

14. **(A)** Infants with bronchiolitis can have varying presentations, from mild tachypnea to severe cough, retractions, tachypnea, and wheezing.

RSV is the most common cause, and infection is universal in the first 2 years of life. Parainfluenza, influenza, and human metapneumovirus are all recognized causes of bronchiolitis. However, they are not as common as RSV. CMV is not a cause of bronchiolitis. *(Long, 1113; American Academy of Pediatrics, 560–561)*

15. **(C)** In healthy children over age 4 years, reactions of less than 5-mm induration to 5 TU are considered negative. Reactions between 5 and 15 mm are considered doubtful and usually represent infection with nontuberculous mycobacteria. Reactions of 15 mm or more induration generally are considered positive and indicative of infection with *M tuberculosis* but do not necessarily mean clinically evident disease. The point to remember is that the threshold for interpreting a tuberculin skin test as positive is lower for children with signs or symptoms suggestive of tuberculosis or with a history of contact with tuberculosis. *(American Academy of Pediatrics, 660; Long, 772)*

16. **(A)** In general, children with uncomplicated primary pulmonary tuberculosis are noninfectious and do not require isolation. This is believed to relate to the scanty sputum production, lack of expectoration, and the small number of organisms that can be recovered from sputum or gastric culture. In contrast, children with laryngeal involvement, with cavitary pulmonary tuberculosis, extensive pulmonary infection, positive sputum AFB smears, or suspected congenital tuberculosis should be considered contagious and appropriate precautions should be taken. Children with tuberculosis disease can attend school or child care if they are receiving therapy. *(American Academy of Pediatrics, 696)*

17. **(B)** In enteric Salmonella infections, fever is characteristic; diarrhea may or may not be present. Some features highly suggestive of Salmonella infection include leukopenia and a relative bradycardia; that is, the heart rate is slower than would be anticipated for the degree of fever present, though this is seen more commonly in adults than in children. Clinical manifestations such as fever, abdominal pain, hepatomegaly, splenomegaly, rose spots, and changes in mental status are reported. *(American Academy of Pediatrics, 579–580; Long, 815)*

18. **(E)** The defect in chronic granulomatous disease (CGD) is the inability of polymorphonuclear and mononuclear leukocytes to effect intracellular killing of catalase positive phagocytosed bacteria. The neutrophils can ingest bacteria normally, but cannot produce the intracellular hydrogen peroxide needed to kill the organisms. Common manifestations include recurrent skin and sinopulmonary infections as well as candidal infections. Hepatic abscesses are a common cause of fever and abdominal pain in these patients. CGD is inherited primarily as a sex-linked recessive trait, although some females with the disorder have been reported. Leukocyte adhesion deficiency represents an impairment of leukocyte migration. Children with Ehlers-Danlos syndrome have a defect in collagen synthesis. Increased capillary permeability and impaired wound healing have a variety of causes, including DIC and sepsis, as well as hepatic and renal dysfunction. *(Long, 618–619, 621; Berhman, 715–716)*

19. **(E)** The clinical feature of scabies infestation that is typical for the infant is an intensely pruritic rash with involvement of the entire skin surface including the scalp, palms, and soles with lesions that are often pustulovesicular. In contrast, older children and adults are generally infested between fingers and toes. The eruption is caused by a hypersensitivity reaction to the proteins of the scabies mite, *Sarcoptes scabiei*. Diagnosis is made by microscopic evaluation of skin scraping. *(American Academy of Pediatrics, 584–585)*

20. **(B)** Formerly known as enterohemorrhagic *E coli*, Shiga-toxin-producing strains of *E coli* (STEC) are associated with a range of gastrointestinal symptoms from self-limited nonbloody diarrhea to hemorrhagic colitis. A triad of microangiopathic hemolytic anemia, thrombocytopenia, and acute renal dysfunction is termed hemolytic-uremic syndrome and may follow the diarrheal illness within a week in 2%–20% of infected children. *E coli* is one of the most common causes of meningitis in the neonate. Chronic diarrhea, pneumonia, and

endocarditis are unlikely manifestations of diarrheal illness related to *E coli*. *(Long, 796–798; American Academy of Pediatrics, 291–293)*

21. **(E)** In general, *T pallidum* can be demonstrated in any mucous membrane or cutaneous lesion of congenital syphilis, especially a moist one. All of these lesions are capable of spreading the organism and are highly infectious. The classical cutaneous manifestations of congenital syphilis are a copper-colored maculopapular rash and vesiculobullous lesions of the palms and soles, often referred to as pemphigus syphiliticus. *(Long, 932)*

22. **(A)** Infants less than 2 months of age who present with undifferentiated fever are at high risk for serious bacterial infection. The standard of care for such infants is a meticulous history and physical examination with laboratory evaluation to detect urinary tract, bloodstream, or CNS infection. The most common serious bacterial infection encountered in this young infant population is urinary tract infection with 90% of infections caused by *E coli*. While seen sporadically, *H influenzae* type B meningitis has largely been eradicated due to widespread use of HIB vaccine. Salmonella enteritis, group A streptococcal bacteremia, and meningococcemia are unlikely in an infant. *(Long, 124, 533)*

23. **(E)** Vaginitis is the most common form of gonococcal infection in the prepubertal female. The unestrogenized, alkaline vaginal mucosa of the prepubertal girl is especially vulnerable to colonization and infection with *N gonorrhoeae*. One study confirmed the diagnosis of gonorrhea in 9% of prepubertal children presenting with a chief complaint of vaginal discharge; sexual abuse must be considered in such patients. Ascending infection (salpingitis, peritonitis) occurs, but only rarely in prepubertal children. Arthritis is uncommon, and conjunctivitis is essentially restricted to the newborn period. *(Long, 361; American Academy of Pediatrics, 302)*

24. **(B)** Gonococcal infection in the female adolescent is often asymptomatic; clinical infection usually manifests as cervicitis, urethritis, and salpingitis. The incubation period is 2–10 days.

Complications can include bartholinitis, PID, and perihepatitis (Fitz-Hugh-Curtis syndrome). Hematogenous spread can involve skin and joints (arthritis-dermatitis syndrome) and can occur in approximately 3% of untreated people. This is most common when infected within 1 week of menstruation. Hematuria can occur, but is not the most common manifestation. Fever and shaking chills would be associated with PID, a secondary complication. Chancres are not associated with gonococcal infections. *(American Academy of Pediatrics, 302; Long, 367)*

25. **(D)** Staphylococcal food poisoning is caused by a toxin elaborated in spoiled food before ingestion. Bacteremia does not occur, since this is not an infection. Fever is uncommon. Symptoms—vomiting, abdominal cramps, and diarrhea—usually begin within 2–4 hours of ingestion of the toxin and are generally limited to the gastrointestinal system. Rash, high fever, and bacteremia are features of staphylococcal toxic shock syndrome. *(American Academy of Pediatrics, 597; Long, 111)*

26. **(E)** Group A streptococcal infection in young children is commonly manifested by persistent fever and mucoserous nasal discharge. This syndrome has been referred to as "streptococcosis." Localized pharyngeal involvement is uncommon in the first year of life. Meningitis caused by this organism is very uncommon at all ages and is generally associated with foreign body. The clinical picture of scarlet fever is rarely seen in the first 3 years of life and acute rheumatic fever is rare before 4 or 5 years of age. *(Long, 172)*

27. **(C)** In temperate climates, summer and late fall outbreaks of enteroviral infection are common with many thousands of cases of meningitis reported each year, the vast majority caused by enteroviruses. Fever, headache, and photophobia are commonly reported in children with enteroviral meningitis. CSF pleocytosis is usually noted with white blood cell counts typically between 100–1000. While neutrophil (PMN) predominance can be seen early on, lymphocytes become predominant between 8 and 48 hours of onset. Definitive diagnosis is made by culture;

although PCR detection is faster, more sensitive, and 100% specific. *(Long, 306)*

28. **(B)** Pharyngotonsillitis is the typical clinical manifestation of group A streptococcal infection. Scarlet fever is a syndrome of tonsillitis, fever, and rash caused by an erythrogenic toxin-producing streptococcus in a patient lacking antitoxin immunity. Streptococcal respiratory tract infections generally peak in children aged 5–11 years and winter predominance is generally noted. Patients younger than 3 years of age with exudative pharyngitis are more likely to have viral disease, as are older children who present with sore throat, cough, and/or rhinorrhea. Slapped cheek appearance is characteristic of parvovirus infection. *(American Academy of Pediatrics, 610; Long, 442)*

29. **(D)** Pneumococcal pneumonia is the most common acute bacterial pneumonia of infants (excluding the neonate) and children. It usually occurs in association with, or as a complication of, a viral upper respiratory illness. The onset of clinical manifestations is usually rapid and abrupt, and although fever is a prominent feature, respiratory signs and symptoms are common and usually are present early. *Staphylococcus epidermidis* is a known cause of bacteremia in the immunocompromised host or those with indwelling central catheter. *Mycoplasma pneumoniae* and *Chlamydophil pneumoniae* typically cause patchy infiltrates seen on chest x-ray in the older age child. *Streptococcus pyogenes* is a less likely cause of pneumonia, but can cause invasive infection with bacteremia, multiple organ involvement, and pneumonia. *(Long, 247, 249, 693, 876, 983)*

30. **(A)** Staphylococcal scalded skin syndrome is mediated by exfoliative toxins A and B. Infants are most commonly affected and clinically present with tender, generalized erythroderma followed by generalized appearance of flaccid bullae, which rupture. Lipopolysaccharide is an endotoxin in the cell wall of gram-negative bacteria. Enterotoxin A and toxic shock syndrome toxin-1 are produced by *S aureus*, the former is associated with food poisoning and the latter is associated with toxic shock syndrome. Shiga toxin may be produced by shigella and

various strains of E *coli*. It is associated with diarrheal illness and HUS. *(Long, 102, 688–689; American Academy of Pediatrics,:291, 597–599)*

31. **(B)** Rotaviruses are recognized as the major cause of severe gastroenteritis in children. Most cases in the United States occur during the winter months. The clinical manifestations of rotavirus infection include nonbloody diarrhea often preceded by fever and vomiting. Approximately 10% of infected infants are hospitalized to correct dehydration. Adenovirus and enterovirus are not typical causes of diarrheal infection in the winter months. While salmonella and shigella cause diarrheal illness, there is no predilection for winter months. Shigella outbreaks have been documented in day care settings. *(Long, 1079–1080; American Academy of Pediatrics, 202–203, 590, 284–285)*

32. **(D)** Rocky Mountain spotted fever (*Rickettsia rickettsii*) infection causes a vasculitis. Electrolyte and hematologic abnormalities seen with this disease include: hyponatremia, thrombocytopenia, leucopenia, and anemia. *(American Academy of Pediatrics, 570; Long, 916–917)*

33. **(D)** Pertussis classically begins with a catarrhal stage indistinguishable from a common cold and lasts up to a week. This is followed by gradual worsening of the cough, finally reaching the paroxysmal stage, characterized by thick, tenacious secretions and fits of forceful coughing that often end in a whoop as the child is finally able to take a full breath. Fever is usually mild or absent. *(American Academy of Pediatrics, 498; Long, 861–862)*

34. **(B)** Pertussis usually is associated with a marked absolute lymphocytosis. Peripheral white blood cell counts in the range of 20,000–30,000/mm^3 with a majority of lymphocytes are characteristic of this infection. This is a useful and important diagnostic feature. *(Long, 863)*

35. **(B)** Typhoid fever (infection with *S typhi*) is characterized by an incubation period of 6–21 days, followed by fever, malaise, and, in some cases, rose spots. These are small, palpable erythematous lesions on the trunk. (Petechiae are smaller and not palpable, see Figure 7-3.)

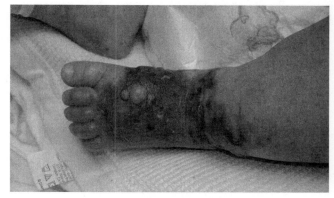

Figure 7-3
(Courtesy of Mary Anne Jackson, MD)

Diarrhea, if present, usually clears and often is followed by constipation. Measles is characterized by cough, conjunctivitis, coryza, and an erythematous maculopapular rash. *Neisseria meningitidis* infection causes meningitis and/or meningococcemia, the latter of which is an acute febrile illness manifested by malaise, prostration, and rash that can evolve into septic shock with DIC and death. Rat bite fever and leptospirosis do not have diarrhea as a part of their constellation of symptoms. *(Long, 815; American Academy of Pediatrics, 424, 441, 452, 559, 579–580)*

36. **(D)** Mumps causes subclinical infection in one-third of cases. The most common manifestation is unilateral parotid swelling that becomes bilateral with a prodrome of headache, fever, abdominal pain, and anorexia. EBV infection typically manifests as exudative pharyngitis and cervical chain adenopathy. Brucellosis is a systemic illness that typically causes fever, joint pain, malaise, and anorexia. Leukemia may vary in presentation, but often presents with fever, hematologic abnormality, petechial rash, and nonspecific complaints. The initial sign of cysticercosis in children is oftentimes a seizure in an otherwise healthy child. *(Long, 856, 1038, 1109–1110; Behrman, 1694–1695)*

37. **(D)** In this patient, the acute onset in association with fever, headache, and stiff neck favor the diagnosis of meningitis. Brain tumor is unlikely to cause fever, and typically either

presents with signs/symptoms of increased ICP or focal neurologic signs. Subarachnoid hemorrhage does not have fever or respiratory symptoms as part of the clinical findings. Bacterial sepsis, without meningitis, should not cause stiff neck. Optic neuritis is characterized by inflammation, degeneration, or demyelination of the optic nerve. Meningitis is confirmed by examination of the cerebrospinal fluid and the accompanying Figure 7-4 shows the typical findings of bacteria seen on Gram-stained smear. *(Long, 285–286, 307–308; Behrman, 849, 1703, 2041, 2121)*

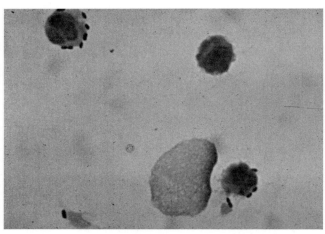

Figure 7-4
(Courtesy of Mary Anne Jackson, MD)

38. **(E)** Subdural fluid collections (effusions) develop in 10%–30% of patients, and are especially common in infants. The exact pathogenesis is unknown, but they are usually sterile and not related either to inadequate therapy or to a bleeding disorder. They are asymptomatic in 85%–90% of patients, and are rarely fatal. The symptomatology that is associated with effusions is headache, vomiting, seizures, and fever. However, these are also common symptoms of meningitis. *(Behrman, 2043–2044, Snedeker, 86:163–170)*

39. **(A)** Although the combination of fever, hemorrhagic eruption, and shock can be seen with bacteremic infection caused by a wide variety of organisms including *H influenzae, S pneumoniae, S aureus,* and beta-hemolytic streptococcus, this combination of findings is most commonly seen with meningococcal (*N meningitidis*) infection. The hemorrhagic skin lesions (purpura fulminans) suggest disseminated intravascular coagulation, an ominous prognostic sign. *(Long, 738–739)*

40. **(C)** While all of the answers are important in clinical evaluation and treatment of the child with meningococcemia, starting with the ABCs of basic life support still applies. As airway management choices are not available, addressing the circulatory status with intravenous fluids would be the most appropriate initial step. Antibiotic administration should occur rapidly and preferably after blood cultures have been drawn. Initial CSF evaluation including culture is helpful, but is not always feasible depending on the degree of illness of the child. It should be completed prior to antibiotics when possible; however it can still be useful after antibiotic administration to evaluate for pleocytosis. *(Long, 740.)*

41. **(D)** The monospot tests for heterophile antibodies, which are rarely produced by children younger than 4 years. A negative result does not exclude EBV infection. Patients present with a typical clinical picture of lymphadenopathy, splenomegaly, and atypical (reactive) lymphocytes on peripheral blood smear. Respiratory syncytial virus, herpes infection, and rubella infection are unlikely to cause atypical lymphocytosis or splenomegaly. Although both HSV and noncongenitally acquired rubella may present with lymphadenopathy, adenovirus typically causes an upper respiratory tract infection and pharyngoconjunctival fever. *(American Academy of Pediatrics, 286–487, 361–362, 560–561, 574)*

42. **(A)** Household contacts of those with meningococcal disease are at 500–1000 times greater risk for acquisition of meningococcal infection than the general population. Although several drug regimens for prophylaxis of contacts of meningococcal disease are acceptable, the primary regimen recommended at this time is rifampin, 10 mg/kg every 12 hours (q12h) for a total of four doses for children and a single dose of ciprofloxacin for those older than 18 years. *(American Academy of Pediatrics, 455–456; Long, 741–742)*

43. **(A)** Group B streptococcus is the leading bacterial cause of neonatal infection in most medical centers in the United States. Two clinical syndromes, early onset and late onset, have been described, although some features do overlap both groups. The early-onset picture is most frequent in high-risk infants (eg, premature, prolonged rupture of membranes) and usually presents as a severe, rapidly progressive illness in the first day or even hours of life. Pneumonia and bacteremia are the most common manifestations, but meningitis occurs in about one-third of cases. Manifestations of late-onset infection are often indolent and include bacteremia and meningitis, as well as other focal infections such as osteomyelitis, septic arthritis, omphalitis, and breast abscess. (*American Academy of Pediatrics, 620–621; Long, 712–713*)

44. **(C)** *Listeria monocytogenes* meningitis is uncommon in childhood except for the newborn period, where in some series it accounts for up to 10% of cases of bacterial meningitis. A few pediatric cases occur in immunodeficient children, and a rare case in the otherwise normal child. Risk factors for the development of listeriosis in a newborn infant is maternal ingestion of unpasteurized dairy products or prepared meats (hotdogs, deli meat) and ingestion of unwashed raw vegetables. Exposure to cat feces increases the risk of toxoplasmosis, which may also be transmitted transplacentally. Exposure to bird droppings is associated with histoplasmosis and *C psittaci* pneumonia. Ingestion of shellfish is not associated with listeriosis or neonatal infection.(*American Academy of Pediatrics, 251, 426, 666, 728; Long, 763–764*)

45. **(C)** Active immunization with live measles vaccine at the time of contact is too late to assure protection. Additionally, children should not receive the vaccine before the age of 6 months to assure an adequate immunologic response. The recommended management of susceptible siblings of a contact case is the use of a preventive dose of gamma globulin (0.25 mg/kg) and later immunization with the live-virus vaccine. In the past, when most women had natural measles infection, maternal IgG levels of measles antibody were very high, and transplacental IgG

afforded the young infant relatively strong protection. Cases of measles infection in this age-group were often milder than in older children. Such is not the case now. Many mothers have low levels of measles antibody (from immunization rather than natural infection), and their infants are susceptible to severe measles infection. (*American Academy of Pediatrics, 443–444*)

46. **(B)** The dog ascarid, *T canis*, cannot complete its life cycle in human beings, therefore eggs or worms are not discharged in the stool. The clinical picture of toxocariasis (often referred to as visceral larva migrans) is characterized by fever, hepatomegaly, and eosinophilia. Less frequently, there may be involvement of the lung, central nervous system, heart, or retina. None of the other parasites listed characteristically causes hepatomegaly. (*American Academy of Pediatrics, 665; Long, 1304–1306*)

47. **(C)** *Ascaris lumbricoides* is the largest intestinal roundworm, and occasionally intestinal obstruction may result from heavy infection. The incidence of this complication has been estimated at 2 per 1,000 infected children per year. Intestinal obstruction has not been observed with any of the other parasites listed. (*American Academy of Pediatrics, 218; Long, 1297-1298*)

48. **(B)** Kawasaki syndrome is a multisystem vasculitis which typically manifests with high, spiking fever for 5 or more days along with conjunctival infection, mucositis, polymorphous rash, changes in peripheral extremities, and single cervical lymph node swelling. Treatment with aspirin and intravenous immune globulin is indicated; without treatment, 20% of children develop coronary artery aneurysms. Fulminant hepatitis, recurrent pericarditis, cerebral edema, and renal failure are not features of Kawasaki syndrome. (*American Academy of Pediatrics, 412–413; Long, 989–991*)

49. **(C)** The clinical manifestations of human parvovirus B-19 include erythema infectiosum (healthy child), polyarthropathy syndrome (adults especially women), chronic anemia/pure red cell aplasia (immunocompromised hosts), transient aplastic crisis (sickle cell patients), and

hydrops fetalis/congenital anemia (fetus). Erythema infectiosum is most commonly diagnosed and easily recognized. A distinctive rash featuring a "slapped cheek" appearance is noted that is often associated with circumoral pallor. Coxsackievirus A16 and enterovirus 71 are causes of hand-foot-and-mouth syndrome. Enterovirus 71 is also associated with encephalitis. Adenovirus is not associated with a characteristic exanthem, however it may cause conjunctivitis. Rubeola virus is the causative agent of measles, and generally presents with a triad of cough, coryza, and conjunctivitis, as well as Koplik spots and rash. *(American Academy of Pediatrics, 202, 284, 484–485)*

50. **(B)** Neonatal herpes simplex virus (HSV) infection is typically transmitted in infants when mothers experience primary infection at the time of delivery and typically manifest in the first 1–4 weeks of life. There are three forms of disease, though clinical overlap is often noted. Disease may be localized to the skin, eyes, and mouth, it may be disseminated with prominent involvement of lungs and liver or localized central nervous system involvement may occur. Perinatally acquired HIV infection is typically asymptomatic initially. Congenital syphilis may present with vesicular rash, but is not associated with sepsis. Group B streptococcal infection does not present with rash. Congenital varicella occurs when maternal infection presents within 5 days before or 2 days after delivery. *(Long, 1016–1017; American Academy of Pediatrics, 361, 637, 711)*

51. **(D)** A full sepsis evaluation should be performed, as well as viral cultures of CSF, lesions, eye, and mucous membranes (NP and rectal). HSV DNA can be detected by polymerase chain reaction assay in the CSF of patients with central nervous system disease and is the diagnostic test of choice for such patients. *(American Academy of Pediatrics, 363–364)*

52. **(C)** Hepatitis A virus infection is generally an acute self-limited illness. Symptoms include fever, malaise, jaundice, anorexia, and nausea. Only 30% of infected children fewer than 6 years of age are symptomatic. Few of these children develop jaundice. *(American Academy of Pediatrics, 326–327)*

53. **(C)** Symptomatology with hepatitis B infection is age dependent, and infants are typically asymptomatic. Between 5% and 15% of children between 1 and 5 years of age develop typical symptoms such as anorexia, nausea, malaise, and jaundice, while 30%–50% of adolescents and adults will develop acute symptoms. *(Long, 1066–1067, American Academy of Pediatrics, 335–336)*

54. **(B)** Chronic infection with hepatitis B virus (HBV) occurs in over 90% of perinatally infected infants, 25%–50% of those infected are between ages 1 and 5 years and between 6% and 10% of older children and adults. Those patients with detectable HBeAg are more likely to transmit infection as they have higher blood concentrations of HBV DNA. *(American Academy of Pediatrics, 336)*

55. **(B)** High fever without other signs and clearing of the fever on appearance of a rash are characteristic of roseola and is the defining clinical expression of primary infection with human herpes virus 6. In measles infection, fever continues for several days after the appearance of the rash. The same is true for the several types of typhus. In infection to echovirus, the rash and fever usually appear together. The rash of scarlet fever often appears at the time of temperature elevation. *(American Academy of Pediatrics, 375–376)*

56. **(B)** Herpangina is a syndrome characterized by small vesicles or punched-out ulcers on the tonsils and fauces, uvula, pharynx, and edge of soft palate. The remainder of the mouth and throat usually appear normal on examination. Infections caused by group A streptococcus and candida do not present with vesicular lesions. The vesicular lesions seen in HSV infection are generally limited to the anterior portion of the mouth in immunocompetent individuals. HHV-6 is the causative agent of roseola, which does not generally cause an enanthem. *(Long, 201, 1151)*

57. **(D)** Hand-foot-and-mouth syndrome is a specific syndrome that can be caused by a variety of viral agents. It was originally described in association with coxsackievirus A16, but enterovirus 71 can cause an identical clinical picture. Group A streptococcus and *Arcanobacterium haemolyticum* cause similar manifestations of exudative pharyngitis. However the latter is a much less common cause of pharyngitis. Adenovirus does not typically cause enanthem. While HSV infection can cause oral as well as digital lesions, this is an atypical presentation with occurrence on both the palms and soles. *(American Academy of Pediatrics, 284; Long, 1152)*

58. **(A)** Meningococcal meningitis is one of the most common causes of bacterial meningitis in children along with *S pneumoniae*. Chemoprophylaxis of all contacts who live in the household is routine as the risk of secondary transmission is 100–1000 times that of the general population. *(American Academy of Pediatrics, 455)*

59. **(C)** Most cases of pharyngitis are caused by viruses, though the finding of an exudative pharyngitis often leads the practitioner to consider the diagnosis of group A streptococcal infection. However, there are a number of pathogens which may produce exudative changes in children with pharyngeal infection, including adenovirus, Epstein-Barr virus, *Corynebacterium diphtheriae*, and *N gonorrhoeae*. Kawasaki syndrome, Behçet syndrome, parainfluenza, and respiratory syncytial virus do not cause exudative pharyngitis. *(American Academy of Pediatrics, 202)*

60. **(D)** The clinical and laboratory findings described are most suggestive of infectious mononucleosis from Epstein-Barr virus. Hepatic involvement evidenced by elevated serum transaminase levels is common. Syphilis, HBV, rubella, and toxoplasmosis do not present with this constellation of symptoms. *(American Academy of Pediatrics, 286)*

61. **(D)** The clinical picture described is typical of herpes simplex keratoconjunctivitis. The associated vesicular lesions on the skin and the dendritic corneal ulcers are almost pathognomonic

of this infection. It is important to diagnose herpes keratitis correctly because infection can be recurrent and lead to loss of vision, and because therapy is available. The other choices do not cause dendritic ulcers. *(Long, 1014–1015)*

62. **(A)** Infants with perinatally acquired HIV infection often present with nonspecific symptoms and signs including lymphadenopathy, hepatosplenomegaly, failure to thrive, oral candidiasis, and recurrent diarrhea. Among the diseases listed, *Pneumocystis jiroveci* pneumonia (PCP) is the most commonly encountered opportunistic infection in infants with perinatally acquired infection. *(American Academy of Pediatrics, 378)*

63. **(B)** Infants with congenitally acquired cytomegalovirus infection are generally asymptomatic though 10% present with a syndrome that includes intrauterine growth retardation, thrombocytopenia, jaundice, hepatosplenomegaly, microcephaly, intracerebral calcifications, and retinitis. EBV infection is not associated with congenital infection. Perinatal coxsackievirus infection may manifest with myocarditis and encephalitis, human parvovirus B-19 as congenital anemia or hydrops fetalis, and perinatally HIV-infected infants are generally asymptomatic at birth. *(American Academy of Pediatrics, 274, 284, 385, 484)*

64. **(C)** Human monocytotrophic ehrlichiosis infection is an acute systemic febrile illness seen most commonly in the south central, southeastern United States with infection caused by *Ehrlichia chaffeensis* and transmitted via the bite of the Lone star tick (*Amblyomma americanum*). *Anaplasma phagocytophilum* causes human granulocytotrophic anaplasmosis (formerly ehrlichiosis) with a similar clinical picture, but predominantly in the north central and northeastern United States and transmitted by the deer tick (*Ixodes scapularis*). The clinical picture is similar to Rocky Mountain spotted fever (though more often without rash) is reported with prominent CNS and gastrointestinal symptoms; hyponatremia, leukopenia, anemia, and elevated liver transaminases are common laboratory manifestations. Doxycycline is the drug of choice and should be used even in young patients as severe and fatal disease has

been noted. *Rickettsia typhi* and *R prowazekii* cause endemic and epidemic typhus respectively. *Coxiella burnetii* is the causative agent of Q fever which generally does not cause these laboratory findings. The organism *B burgdorferi* causes Lyme disease which has the characteristic finding of erythema migrans. *(American Academy of Pediatrics, 281–282, 428, 550, 567, 570; Long, 888–889)*

65. **(B)** In the asplenic patient, there is an increased risk for fulminant life-threatening infection caused by *S pneumoniae*. Infection occurs in those with posttraumatic asplenia, HIV infection, congenital asplenia, polysplenia syndromes, or those who undergo splenectomy in the course of treatment for malignancy as well as patients with sickle cell disease. *(Long, 635–636; American Academy of Pediatrics, 526–527)*

66. **(E)** The rash of varicella follows an incubation period of 10–21 days. There is the onset of a very pruritic rash, with crops of lesions that begin as papules and progress to vesicles and finally crusted scabs. Typically, all three stages of skin lesions are identified on clinical examination. Fever usually is mild to moderate. While a generally self-limited and benign course is noted, severe disease may occur occasionally in the otherwise healthy host, especially adolescents and adults. A progressive and severe disease with visceral dissemination is seen in 30%–50% of children with lymphoproliferative malignancies, solid tumors, or posttransplantation with the development of hepatitis, encephalitis, and pneumonia. Fatal disease has also been reported in those treated with high-dose corticosteroids and in those with other defects of T-cell function. *(Long, 1022–1024)*

67. **(A)** Congenital malformations, stillborns, and abortions all have been reported with rubella infection during pregnancy. The congenital rubella syndrome consists of ophthalmologic, cardiac, auditory, and neurologic abnormalities with rates as high as 85% if infection occurs in the first 4 weeks of gestation, decreasing to 20%–30% during the second month, and 5% during the third or fourth month. These infants may continue to excrete rubella virus for 1 year

or more after birth and pose a risk of infection for susceptible hosts. *(American Academy of Pediatrics, 574)*

68. **(E)** Infectious mononucleosis syndrome generally presents with exudative pharyngitis that may be associated with petechiae or erythematous macules on the palate. A rash occurs occasionally and splenomegaly may be noted. Airway obstruction secondary to markedly enlarged tonsils is an infrequent but important complication. *(Long, 1040)*

69. **(A)** The most common cause of *Pasteurella* infection in children is a dog or cat bite. The organism is present in the oropharyngeal flora of 70%–95% of cats, and 25%–50% of dogs. The infection typically occurs within 24 hours, and can include regional lymphadenopathy, chills, and fever, as well as swelling, erythema, and purulent discharge at the site. *Eikenella corrodens* infections generally occur after human bites. *Streptobacillus moniliformis* is the causative agent of rat bite fever. Infections with Group A streptococcus or *Staphylococcus aureus* are possible, but much less common than *Pasteurella* in patients with animal bites. *(American Academy of Pediatrics, 487)*

70. **(A)** Pharyngitis caused by *A haemolyticum* infection is hard to differentiate from that of streptococcal infection. The rash associated with Arcanobacterium is scarlatiniform, similar to that of group A streptococcus, and infection should be suspected in the adolescent who presents with pharyngeal exudates and rash after streptococcal infection has been excluded. *(American Academy of Pediatrics, 217)*

71. **(A)** Brucellosis is a zoonotic disease in which children are an accidental host, most commonly contracting infection by ingesting unpasteurized milk. Onset of illness can be acute or insidious. Symptoms of disease are usually nonspecific and include fever, malaise, anorexia, joint pains, headache, and night sweats. Physical findings include lymphadenopathy, hepatosplenomegaly, and occasionally arthritis. Meningitis, endocarditis, and osteomyelitis are rare complications of disease. Glaucoma is not reported. *(American Academy of Pediatrics, 235, Long, 856–857)*

72. **(A)** Campylobacter infection is characterized by watery diarrhea possibly followed by blood-streaked stools, fever, abdominal pain, and malaise. It is usually self-limited, but may have immunoreactive complications (Guillain-Barré syndrome, reactive arthritis [monoarticular], Reiter syndrome, and erythema nodosum) occur during convalescence. It is estimated that in 30%–40% of cases of Guillain-Barré syndrome occurred within 2 weeks of *Campylobacter* infection. Anterior uveitis, inguinal lymphadenitis, and encephalitis are not sequelae of *Campylobacter* infection. (*American Academy of Pediatrics, 240–241, Long, 871*)

73. **(C)** Cat-scratch disease (CSD) is caused by *B henselae*. The most common manifestation is unilateral regional lymphadenopathy. Small erythematous papules can occur at the inoculation site and precede the lymphadenopathy by 1–2 weeks. The typical patient lacks constitutional symptoms, but 30% may have mild fever, malaise, headache, and anorexia. Systemic CSD is rare. Infections due to nontuberculous mycobacterium, such as *M avium*, are typically subacute and nontender. *Streptobacillus moniliformis* is the causative agent of rat bite fever. *Coxiella burnetii* is the causative agent of Q fever. *Mycobacterium tuberculosis* infection is less likely in a child with a history of kitten exposure, who is not from a TB-endemic area. (*American Academy of Pediatrics, 246, Long, 851–854*)

74. **(A)** Respiratory syncytial virus (RSV) is the most important cause of bronchiolitis in infants and young children and causes acute respiratory tract illness in patients of all ages. Typical roentgenographic findings include hyperinflation, peribronchial thickening, and atelectasis especially involving the right upper lobe. Infiltrates are typically associated with bacterial pneumonia. Pleural effusions and hilar adenopathy are findings not typically associated with bronchiolitis. (*Long, 1115–1116*)

75. **(B)** *Giardia lamblia* infection can cause a broad spectrum of clinical manifestations. Findings from asymptomatic secretion of organisms to chronic diarrhea and failure to thrive are seen. Most commonly, children either are asymptomatic or have an acute episode of watery diarrhea. Low-grade fever, abdominal pain, nausea, and anorexia may occur with the acute process. Protracted illness is usually associated with passage of foul-smelling stools, abdominal distention, and malabsorption. These can lead to failure to thrive. Bloody diarrhea and cough are not associated with giardiasis. (*American Academy of Pediatrics, 283, Long, 1242–1243*)

76. **(E)** In addition to correcting dehydration and electrolyte abnormalities, metronidazole is the drug of choice. A 5–7-day course of therapy has a cure rate of 85%–90%. Relapse is common in immunocompromised patients, who may require prolonged treatment. Treatment of asymptomatic carriers is generally not recommended. (*American Academy of Pediatrics, 300*)

77. **(D)** Tuberculous meningitis is the most serious complication of tuberculosis in children. It usually occurs within 2–6 months of initial infection. It is difficult to diagnose rapidly as skin testing may be negative and chest films may be normal. Culture results can take anywhere from 1–10 weeks to yield a positive result. CSF findings can give clues of the diagnosis. CSF white cell counts range from 10 to 500 with usual lymphocytic predomination. Glucose is typically 20–40. Protein concentration is elevated, often markedly. Blood-tinged CSF is not associated with tuberculous meningitis. (*Long, 776–777, American Academy of Pediatrics, 678*)

78. **(E)** Children less than 1 year of age are at greatest risk for infection. Patients with increased availability of free iron such as those with sickle cell anemia, B-thalassemia, G6PD, and other hemoglobinopathies, are also at increased risk of infection with *Y. enterocolitica* bacteremia. This is thought to be the result of bacterial iron scavenging systems which increase virulence. The most common manifestation of *Y enterocolitica* is enterocolitis with fever and bloody, mucous-filled diarrhea, not bacteremia. Patients with sickle cell anemia also have functional asplenia and are more susceptible to infections caused by encapsulated organisms. (*American Academy of Pediatrics, 821; Long, 732*)

79. **(A)** Lymphogranuloma venereum is an invasive lymphatic infection caused by *Chlamydia trachomatis*. It starts as an ulcerative lesion on the genitalia along with tender suppurative inguinal and/or femoral adenopathy. It is most often unilateral. HSV can cause a painful ulcer and nonfluctuant adenopathy. Syphilis produces a nontender chancre. Chancroid is caused by *Haemophilus ducreyi* and has an identical presentation to LGV. However, the diagnosis of chancroid is strongly suggested if gram-negative coccobacilli are seen. *(American Academy of Pediatrics, 248, 252)*

80. **(D)** The recommended age range of children for annual influenza immunization has been expanded to include all children 6 months through 18 years of age. This targets all school-aged children and will in turn reduce transmission of influenza to household contacts and community members. The recommendation also includes anyone who wants avoid influenza infection, and caregivers of infants under 6 months of age. Additionally, All healthcare professionals, pregnant women, people over age 50, and people with a chronic illness should also receive annual vaccine. *(MMWR. 2008:57(RR-07):1–60)*

81. **(D)** Topical nystatin is traditionally used to treat thrush and candidal diaper dermatitis. For uncomplicated infections, topical therapy is recommended. However, candidal esophagitis and systemic candidiasis may be treated with systemic therapy, with fluconazole being a reasonable option in infections with known susceptibility to that therapy. Amphotericin B and itraconazole are effective therapies, but more broad spectrum, and not necessary for this patient. Metronidazole and mebendazole are not antifungal agents. *(American Academy of Pediatrics, 244)*

82. **(C)** Cryptosporidiosis usually causes self-limited infection in the immunocompetent host. In immunocompromised hosts, such as those with HIV, it can cause severe, debilitating disease. Transmission is generally from infected animals, person to person, or contaminated water. Outbreaks have been associated with petting zoos, day care centers, and local swimming pools. Diagnosis is made by identifying oocysts that are 4–6 μm in diameter on stool examination. The presentations of giardiasis, entamebiasis, and isosporiasis can be similar. The oocysts of *E histolytica* and *G lamblia* are generally 10–15 μm in diameter and those of *Isospora belli* are 23–33 μm. Giardiasis is generally recognized by visualization of the flagellated trophozoites in stool. *Cryptococcus neoformans* is a fungi not a protozoan and does not cause gastrointestinal disease. *(American Academy of Pediatrics, 271, Long, 1236, 1241, 1245–1246)*.

83. **(B)** Pneumococcus is the most common cause of acute otitis media and of invasive bacterial infections in children. Nontypeable *H influenzae* is also a common cause, but since the advent of Hib vaccine *H influenzae* type B is rarely seen. *Staphylococcus aureus* and *P aeruginosa* cause complicated otitis media in patients with tympanostomy tubes. *Pseudomonas aeruginosa* is the most common cause of otitis externa. *Streptococcus pyogenes* can cause otitis media, however less frequently. *(American Academy of Pediatrics, 525–526; Block, 57)*

84. **(D)** Amoxicillin is the first-line therapy for otitis media and acute sinusitis in children without penicillin allergy. Initial therapy for acute sinusitis should be with an agent of the narrowest spectrum that is active against the likely pathogens, including *M catarrhalis*, *H influenzae*, and *S pneumoniae*. *(American Academy of Pediatrics, 531)*

85. **(A)** The most common presentation of tularemia is ulceroglandular syndrome, which is characterized by a painful maculopapular lesion at the portal of bacterial entry that subsequently ulcerates. Painful, regional lymphadenopathy is associated, that may eventually drain. Wild mammals, including rabbits, are the hosts. Infection can be spread by arthropods, or water and soil that are contaminated by infected animals. Ingestion of inadequately cooked meat or inhalation of organisms while preparing hides can also cause infection. Lyme disease, RMSF, ehrlichiosis, and Q fever are tick-borne illnesses that do not cause ulceroglandular syndrome. *(American Academy of Pediatrics, 704; Long, 148, 891)*

86. **(E)** A dog, cat, or ferret suspected of having rabies should be captured, confined, and observed for 10 days by a veterinarian. If signs of rabies develop, the animal should be euthanized and the brain should be examined for rabies by a qualified laboratory. If wild mammals can be captured after an unprovoked bite they should be euthanized and examined, as clinical manifestations in wild animals can not be interpreted reliably. *(American Academy of Pediatrics, 554–555)*

87. **(D)** If a child is unimmunized, or immunization is incomplete for tetanus, a dose of the appropriate vaccine for age should be given, along with tetanus immune globulin (TIG) if the wound is considered dirty. As this child is 5 years old, DTaP would be the best choice according to the childhood immunization schedule. *(American Academy of Pediatrics, 650–651)*

88. **(B)** Rash is the first clinical manifestation of Lyme disease and is characteristic of early localized disease. It occurs at the site of the tick bite and first appears 7–14 days later. The rash gradually expands without treatment and can appear as a target lesion with central clearing. The rash associated with RMSF and ehrlichiosis is generally petechial and widespread. The rash that accompanies *R typhi* (endemic typhus) is maculopapular and can occur over any area, typically in more than one area. *Rickettsia prowazekii* (epidemic typhus) confers a rash that begins on the trunk and spreads to the limbs with concentration in the axillae. *(Long, 941; American Academy of Pediatrics, 428–429)*

89. **(C)** The rash of Lyme disease is termed erythema migrans. Erythema nodosum is most commonly associated with group A streptococcal pharyngitis and is represented by painful nodules on the shins. It is also associated with many other organisms. Erythema marginatum is associated with acute rheumatic fever, which occurs in fewer than 3% of patients with rheumatic fever. Erythema toxicum is a common newborn rash with eosinophilic pustules. Erythema multiforme has numerous manifestations; from macular to vesicular to urticarial. Diagnosis is established by finding donut-shaped lesions with an erythematous border and central clearing. It is typically associated with viral infection or drug reaction. *(Long, 451, 707, 941–942)*

90. **(B)** *Trichophyton tonsurans* is the causative agent in greater than 90% of cases in the United States. It is common in school-age children, and can be associated with scaling, hair loss, or kerion, which is a boggy inflammatory mass. Local lymphadenopathy occurs with kerion formation. Topical antifungal medications are not effective. Griseofulvin is the drug of choice, and 4–6 weeks of treatment is generally required. Treatment with oral itraconazole or fluconazole is effective, but licensed in the United States for this indication. *(American Academy of Pediatrics, 655)*

91. **(D)** Detecting HIV in an infant or child less than 18 months of age is complicated as these children can carry maternal antibody to HIV, found on ELISA testing, and not be infected. DNA PCR assay is the preferred diagnostic test. Infants born to HIV-infected mothers should be tested by HIV DNA PCR in the first 48 hours of life. These infants need follow-up tests at 1–2 months of age and again at 2–4 months of age. Infection is confirmed with two separate positive tests. Infection is excluded if two PCR tests performed within the first few months of age and a third performed at 4 months of age or greater are all negative. RNA PCR is utilized in HIV-infected patients to monitor viral load. Western blot is used as a confirmatory test in patients who are older than 18 months. HIV p24 antigen is known to give false-positive results in the first month of life. *(American Academy of Pediatrics, 385–386)*

92. **(B)** Adenosine deaminase deficiency is an autosomal recessive form of severe combined immune deficiency (SCID). It causes increased thymocyte and immature B-cell death from accumulation of purine metabolites. Severe combined immune deficiency (SCID) is an inherited deficiency of T- and B-lymphocyte function that occurs in about 1/50,000 live births. Fungal infections, such as *P jiroveci* pneumonia (PCP), are suggestive of severe CD4 lymphocyte (T cell) deficiency. PCP is a common pathogen associated with SCID. Bruton agammaglobulinemia, common variable

immunodeficiency, Job syndrome, and asplenia are not associated with T-cell defects. *(Long, 603, 627–628)*

93. (E) Patients with terminal compliment deficiencies (C5–C9) are incapable of forming the membrane attack complex, which is responsible for bactericidal activity of neisserial infections. These patients are therefore predisposed to disseminated meningococcal and gonococcal infections. X-linked agammaglobulinemia is a B-cell defect. Patients with Chediak-Higashi syndrome have a defect in phagocytosis. Patients with HIV have poor T-cell function, and patients with Wiskott-Aldrich syndrome have defects in both T- and B-cell function. *(Long, 301, 605)*

94. (A) DTaP vaccine should be given as a primary series at 2, 4, and 6 months of age, followed by a dose at 12–15 months and 4–6 years. MMR vaccine should be given at 12–15 months of age followed by a dose at 4–6 years. Primary varicella vaccine should be given at 12–15 months of age, with a second dose at 4–6 years of age. Pneumococcal conjugate vaccine (PCV) should be given as a primary series at 2, 4, and 6 months of age followed by a fourth dose at 12–15 months. Hepatitis A vaccine series should be given at age 12 months, followed by a second dose in 6 months. The primary series for polio vaccine (IPV) should be performed at 2 and 4 months, followed by a third dose at 6–18 months, and a booster at 4–6 years. *Haemophilus influenzae* (Hib) vaccine should be administered at 2, 4, and 6 months, followed by a dose at 12–15 months. Hepatitis B vaccine should be given at birth followed by two more immunizations with the second being at least 1 month after first, and the third 6 months after the first. *(American Academy of Pediatrics, 26)*

95. (C) Definitive diagnosis of malaria relies on parasite identification on stained blood films. Both thick and thin films should be examined, as small numbers may be seen on the thick film. The thin film is useful for species identification as well. Parasites will not grow on culture. Serologic testing is generally not helpful. PCR is currently being developed, but is not commercially available. Liver biopsy is unnecessary. *(American Academy of Pediatrics, 437)*

96. (B) Children with streptococcal pharyngitis should not return to school for 24 hours after beginning appropriate therapy. *(American Academy of Pediatrics, 617)*

97. (B) Secondary syphilis is a systemic multiorgan disease that begins 6–12 weeks after infection. Mucocutaneous lesions are common. Skin lesions begin on the trunk and eventually involve most of the body, including the palms and soles. Generalized lymphadenopathy is found in 85% of patients. Arthritis, osteitis, gastritis, hepatitis, splenomegaly, and nephritic syndrome can occur. Systemic symptoms do not occur in primary syphilis, which begins as a primary chancre. Chancroid, caused by *H ducreyi,* and lymphogranuloma venereum (LGV) have an identical presentation of a painful chancre with suppurative enlargement of local lymph nodes. Gonococcal infection does not manifest as rash on the palms and soles, or splenomegaly. *(Long, 931; American Academy of Pediatrics, 631)*

98. (A) Syphilis has been successfully treated with penicillin for more than 45 years. Parenteral penicillin remains the preferred treatment. Recommendations for duration of therapy vary depending on clinical manifestations. Desensitization in a hospitalized setting should be undertaken in the penicillin-allergic patient. *(American Academy of Pediatrics, 636–637)*

99. (E) The resistance of *S pneumoniae* to penicillins is due to resistant novel penicillin-binding proteins. *S pneumoniae* lacks beta-lactamases. As the name implies, the presence of the *erm* gene leads to macrolide resistance. Presence of the *mef* gene produces a membrane efflux pump which causes macrolides to actively be pumped from the cell. *S pneumoniae* does not have presence of the *mef* gene. Increasing the antibiotic dose of amoxicillin from standard dose to high dose overwhelms the penicillin-binding protein sites. *(Long, 728–729)*

100. (B) Clindamycin is a lincosamide which are not structurally related to macrolides, but have similar mechanism of action. They inhibit RNA-dependent protein synthesis by binding to the 50S ribosomal subunits, inhibiting peptide bond formation in susceptible organisms. Clindamycin is most active against gram-positive organisms and anaerobes. The other choices available are mechanisms of other classes of antibiotics. *(Long, 690)*

101. (C) Kingella infections generally occur in children under 5 years of age, with the most common manifestations being suppurative arthritis and osteomyelitis. The knee is the most commonly involved joint. Kingella organisms are fastidious, gram-negative coccobacilli, which are difficult to isolate in culture. It is best grown in anaerobic conditions with higher recovery when joint fluid is inoculated into a blood culture bottle, and held for at least 7 days. *S aureus* and *S pyogenes* more commonly cause septic arthritis, however they are both gram-positive cocci. Salmonella is a common cause of osteomyelitis in sickle cell patients. Fusobacterium is a rare cause of osteomyelitis. *(American Academy of Pediatrics, 416)*

SELECTED READINGS

Esper F, Boucher D, Weibel C, Martinello RA, Kahn JS. Human metapneumovirus infection in the United States: Clinical manifestations associated with a newly emerging respiratory infection in children. *Pediatrics.* 2003 Jun;111(6 Pt 1):1407–1410.

CHAPTER 8

Injuries, Poisoning, and Substance Abuse

Gary S. Wasserman, DO

Jennifer A. Lowry, MD

Richard J. Mazzaccaro, PhD, MD

Unintentional injuries are the leading cause of death for children aged 1–19 years. Among unintentional injuries, motor vehicle accidents account for nearly two-thirds of deaths. In addition, drownings and poisonings remain common causes of morbidity and mortality in the pediatric population. The rates of firearm-related injuries and deaths are manyfold higher in the United States than in other developed countries. Poisonings, substance abuse, and child abuse often lead to lifelong medical and social consequences. Pediatricians are trained to provide anticipatory guidance to prevent injuries, poisonings, and substance abuse and in practice, age-based advice is well outlined.

Questions

DIRECTIONS (Questions 1 through 42): For each of the multiple choice questions in this section select the one lettered answer that is the best response in each case.

1. A 15-year-old girl was at an overnight rave 24 hours ago and was given Ecstasy by a friend. This morning, she is found comatose and resuscitation is unsuccessful. Most deaths related to Ecstasy have been linked to which of the following?

   (A) cerebrovascular accident
   (B) myocardial infarction
   (C) hyponatremia or hyperthermia
   (D) metabolic alkalosis with compensatory respiratory acidosis
   (E) hyperkalemia or hypothermia

2. A 2-year-old is found with an opened empty bottle of acetaminophen tablets and has pill fragments in his mouth. The major cause of morbidity and mortality in acute poisoning with acetaminophen is which of the following?

   (A) hepatic injury
   (B) gastric bleeding
   (C) metabolic acidosis
   (D) methemoglobinemia
   (E) hypoglycemia

3. A 4-year-old boy has just fallen off the top rung of the ladder while climbing up to the 3-m diving board at the local swimming pool. He lands on the pavement and is motionless when the lifeguard arrives there in less than a minute. Following closed head injury, which of the following would be most ominous?

   (A) irritability
   (B) vomiting
   (C) dilated, fixed pupils
   (D) amnesia for the event
   (E) drowsiness

4. Yearly, over 20,000 individuals younger than 21 years sustain traumatic head injuries while bicycling. Helmet use while bicycling prevents what percent of serious brain injury?

   (A) less than 10%
   (B) 20%–25%
   (C) 50%
   (D) 80%–90%
   (E) 99%

5. An 18-month-old presents to the emergency department with a 2-day history of lethargy. Blue and yellow bruising over the buttocks and thighs are noted and retinal hemmorhages are seen on fundoscopic examination. Parents deny any history of bleeding or bruising other than what you see. Laboratory studies including a urine analysis, platelet count, bleeding time, and PT/PTT reveal normal values. Which of the following is the most likely diagnosis to explain this child's findings?

   (A) von Willebrand disease
   (B) acute lymphoblastic leukemia
   (C) Henoch-Schöenlein purpura
   (D) idiopathic thrombocytopenic purpura.
   (E) child abuse

6. Most cases of serious physical child abuse involving children occur at what age?

(A) less than 1-month old

(B) between 1 month and 4 years old

(C) between 5 and 12 years old

(D) between 13 and 16 years old

(E) who are neurologically impaired

7. A 24-month-old is seen for a well-child visit. The family resides in a 45-year-old home and the parent notes that the child has developed a habit of eating paint which has chipped off of the window sills. You are concerned that the child could be at risk for lead toxicity. In the United States, the appropriate recommendations for routine lead screening is at which of the following ages?

(A) at the 6 months check up

(B) at the 6 and 9 months check up

(C) at the 1- and 2-year check up

(D) at 3- and 5-year check up

(E) at the 12–15-year check up

8. Which of the following combinations of signs and symptoms is most suggestive of chronic lead poisoning?

(A) ataxia, fever, diarrhea, and polycythemia

(B) lethargy, vomiting, hallucinations, and vesicular rash

(C) anemia, leukopenia, thrombocytopenia, and hepatomegaly

(D) lethargy, abdominal cramps, constipation, and anemia

(E) hypertension, rash, cough, and leukocytosis

9. A 3-year-old child is brought to the emergency room 3 hours after he was found playing with an open kerosene bottle. The parents state the child initially had some gagging and coughing and within an hour developed labored breathing. At the time of your evaluation though, the child's examination is completely normal. What is the most appropriate action at this time?

(A) discharge to home, advise parents to return if they note any problems

(B) obtain a chest x-ray

(C) observe child in emergency room for 1 hour

(D) induce emesis with syrup of ipecac

(E) admit to the hospital for 24 hours of observation

10. A 4-year-old child is brought to the urgent care by parents who were concerned because the child suddenly developed unusual posture and movements. Examination reveals an alert child who holds the head in a tilted position and has uncontrolled, writhing movements of the hands and arms. The examination is otherwise normal. When questioned regarding medications at home, parents state they do have routine cold medicine, acetaminophen, and some kind of antiemetic medication in an unlocked medicine cabinet. At this time you should do which of the following?

(A) perform a head computerized tomography (CT) scan

(B) perform a lumbar puncture

(C) obtain an electroencephalogram

(D) administer naloxone intravenously

(E) administer diphenhydramine intravenously

11. A 4-year-old boy was found playing with an open bottle of drain cleaner about 1 hour ago. His mother reports that he now refuses to drink and talk but appears alert though anxious. You should advise the mother to do which of the following?

(A) administer syrup of ipecac

(B) closely observe the child and bring to the emergency room if condition worsens

(C) administer milk of magnesia

(D) give the child cold frozen fruit popsicles

(E) immediately bring the child to the emergency room for evaluation

12. Shellfish poisoning, which is caused by eating shellfish that have ingested toxic dinoflagellates (red tide), is characterized by which of the following?

    (A) blindness
    (B) vomiting and diarrhea
    (C) seizures and coma
    (D) weakness and paralysis
    (E) rash and fever

13. A toddler presents with a known ingestion of iron tablets. By parental count of pills remaining in the bottle it appears he ingested more than 60 mg/kg of elemental iron. Upon admission to the pediatric intensive care unit, he is vomiting. Which of the following chelating agents should be administered?

    (A) deferoxamine mesylate
    (B) ethylene diamine tetraacetic acid (EDTA)
    (C) British anti-Lewisite (BAL)
    (D) hemoglobin
    (E) penicillamine

14. A 3-year-old child who is unresponsive presents with weakness, excessive salivation, bradycardia, and constricted pupils. The parents are so distraught, it is difficult to get information. However, an astute emergency room physician realizes the most likely drug or toxin to cause these signs is which of the following?

    (A) diphenhydramine
    (B) phenobarbital
    (C) ethyl alcohol
    (D) a hydrocarbon
    (E) an organophosphate

15. Following stabilization of the patient in the above question, the emergency room physician administers a test dose of a drug and the patient clinically improves. What drug did this physician most likely administer?

    (A) naloxone
    (B) diphenhydramine
    (C) atropine
    (D) N-acetylcysteine
    (E) phenobarbital

16. The mother of a high school senior varsity football player is concerned that her son may be taking some type of performance-enhancing drug. Among 18-year-old males, approximately what percent have used anabolic steroids as performance enhancers?

    (A) 1%
    (B) 5%–10%
    (C) 15%–20%
    (D) 30%–40%
    (E) 60%

17. Three symptomatic adolescents with a history of ingesting seeds of jimsonweed are arriving via ambulance from a referring hospital emergency room. Which of the following best describes the expected signs and symptoms of jimsonweed poisoning?

    (A) agitation/hallucinations, dilated pupils
    (B) coma, pinpoint pupils
    (C) hallucinations, bradycardia
    (D) coma, bradycardia
    (E) pallor, pinpoint pupil

18. Ingestion of LSD will most likely result in which of the following?

    (A) convulsions
    (B) euphoria
    (C) hallucinations
    (D) sedation
    (E) tremors

19. A teenager who sniffs spot remover and then engages in stressful physical activity is at risk for

    (A) convulsions
    (B) hypertension
    (C) rhabdomyolysis
    (D) severe headache
    (E) sudden death

20. Which of the following are the most commonly used "date-rape" drug?

    (A) amphetamines and LSD
    (B) gamma-hydroxybutyrate and flunitrazepam

(C)   cocaine and phenobarbital

(D)   ephedra and codeine

(E)   phenobarbital and gamma-
       hydroxybutryate

21.   After being lifted up by one hand, a young tod-
       dler refuses to use that arm and holds it against
       her trunk flexed at the elbow with the forearm
       midway between pronation and supination.
       The child most likely has which of the following?

(A)   a shoulder dislocation

(B)   a radial head subluxation

(C)   a fracture of a carpal bone

(D)   avulsion of the ulnar nerve

(E)   a fracture of the radius

22.   A 4-year-old child falls on an outstretched
       arm. The child is likely to sustain which of the
       following?

(A)   fracture displacement of the radial
       epiphysis

(B)   Colles fracture

(C)   comminuted radial and ulnar fracture

(D)   shoulder dislocation

(E)   humeral fracture

23.   Which of the following sets of blood gas values
       is most compatible with acute aspirin poison-
       ing in a 16-month-old child?

(A)   pH 7.60, PCO_2 40, HCO_3 40

(B)   pH 7.5, PCO_2 40, HCO_3 30

(C)   pH 7.25, PCO_2 20, HCO_3 8

(D)   pH 7.20, PCO_2 45, HCO_3 20

(E)   pH 7.00, PCO_2 35, HCO_3 8

24.   Hyperventilation due to salicylate poisoning

(A)   is apparent on physical examination
       within minutes of ingestion

(B)   is characterized by an increase in rate
       and depth of ventilation

(C)   is characterized by an increase in depth
       of ventilation only

(D)   is characterized by an increase in rate of
       ventilation only

(E)   does not occur in young children

25.   Which of the following findings would be most
       suggestive of the form of child abuse referred
       to as the abusive head trauma syndrome
       (formally called shaken babt syndrome)

(A)   ecchymosis over the mastoid area

(B)   retinal hemorrhages

(C)   ecchymoses and petechiae over the
       upper arms and upper trunk

(D)   circumferential ecchymosis on extremities

(E)   cervical spine dislocation

26.   A 9-year-old is injured while sledding. On
       admission, the child appears in shock and is
       complaining of pain in the left shoulder. Of
       immediate concern is the likely diagnosis
       of

(A)   rupture of the descending aorta

(B)   dislocation of the left shoulder

(C)   rupture of the spleen

(D)   rupture of the left diaphragm

(E)   fracture of the humerus

27.   Which of the following is the most common
       unintentional fatal injury to children 1–19 years
       of age

(A)   motor vehicles

(B)   swimming pools

(C)   firearms

(D)   bicycles

(E)   fireworks

28. A 1-year-old child is brought to the emergency room because of a swollen left thigh. The parents, who appear very concerned, state they left the child in the care of a newly hired housekeeper early that morning, and when they returned home in the evening they noted the swelling. Other than tender swelling of the thigh, physical examination is entirely normal. X-ray examination discloses a displaced fracture of the shaft of the femur; skeletal survey reveals no other fractures or abnormalities. The grandparents, who live with the parents and who had accompanied them on their trip, corroborate the parents' story. After first admitting the child for treatment of the fracture, what is the most appropriate next step?

   (A) order a computerized tomography (CT) scan of the head
   (B) order a complete coagulation profile
   (C) order magnetic resonance imaging (MRI) of the leg
   (D) order calcium, phosphate, and uric acid laboratory tests
   (E) report the incident to a child protection agency

29. Syrup of ipecac should be administered in the home to which of the following children?

   (A) 3-year-old child who ingested lye (sodium hydroxide) 5 minutes prior
   (B) 4-year-old child found obtunded, suspected of narcotic poisoning
   (C) 2-year-old child who is having brief seizures, suspected of ingesting sibling's phenytoin
   (D) 2-year-old child who ingested toilet bowl cleaner
   (E) none of the above

30. A 4-year-old child is playing in the basement. The child suddenly comes upstairs, screaming of being bitten by a spider. There is an erythematous 2 cm macule on the child's face which appears to have a central tiny puncture site. Over the next few hours the lesion becomes larger, more painful, and in 24 hours it appears darker. The most likely complication in this child would be which of the following?

   (A) necrosis at the site of the bite
   (B) renal failure
   (C) hepatic failure
   (D) muscle cramps and seizures
   (E) convulsions

31. Management with multiple-dose activated charcoal may be indicated in the overdose of which of the following?

   (A) iron
   (B) cyanide
   (C) carbamazepine
   (D) tricyclic antidepressants
   (E) methanol

32. A 2-year-old child is retrieved from a near-drowning episode in a pool. The child is apneic on retrieval, but is quickly and successfully resuscitated. On arrival in the emergency room, abnormalities which of the following are most likely to be present and require immediate attention?

   (A) hyponatremia and hypokalemia
   (B) hyponatremia and hyperkalemia
   (C) hyperkalemia and acidosis
   (D) acidosis and hypoxemia
   (E) hypoxemia and hemolysis

33. Manifestations of the first stage of severe acute iron poisoning include

   (A) lethargy and gastrointestinal irritation
   (B) metabolic alkalosis and hypertension
   (C) hemolysis and neutropenia
   (D) renal, hepatic, and cardiac failure
   (E) hypoglycemia and hepatic injury

34. Which of the following statements regarding automobile safety for children is correct?

   (A) Children, beyond the age of 1 year, or 20 lb, may ride either facing the front or rear of the car.
   (B) Children over 25 lb may use adult-type restraints.
   (C) A 1-year-old child held in the lap of a seat-belted adult is almost as safe as in an infant restraint device.

(D) Safety restraints are not needed for infants less than 3 months of age or 10 lb of body weight.

(E) Infants under the age of 1 year should ride in restraint devices facing the rear of the car.

35. Which of the following statements regarding drowning and near-drowning is correct?

(A) Four-sided fencing around pools has not decreased the incidence of drownings.

(B) Children under the age of 5 years who drown in home pools most often enter the pool by climbing over a fence.

(C) The incidence of drowning peaks in elementary school-age children.

(D) Approximately 50% of those who die are declared dead at the scene.

(E) Among children who survive, neurologic impairment is generally uncommon.

36. Concerning child sexual abuse, which of the following is correct?

(A) Boys and girls are at equal risk.

(B) In the majority of cases, the abuser is well known to the child.

(C) Physical contact is necessary to fulfill diagnostic criteria for child sexual abuse.

(D) An estimated 10% of children are sexually abused each year in the United States.

(E) There must be evidence of sexual intercourse for successful prosecution.

37. Which of the following statements regarding firearm-related injuries in children less than 19 years of age is correct?

(A) Intentional firearm-related injuries far outnumber unintentional firearm-related injuries.

(B) Half of firearm-related deaths are the result of suicide.

(C) Firearms account for the majority of all injury deaths in this age group.

(D) Firearm-related injuries result in more deaths than do motor vehicle accidents each year.

(E) Most firearm-related deaths occur after prolonged hospital course.

38. Which of the following is most suggestive of unintentional (nonabuse) injuries in children?

(A) hand print bruise on the face of a child

(B) belt marks on the buttocks of a 3-year-old child

(C) bruises on upper thighs reported to result from "spanking"

(D) fractured femur of a 1-month-old baby from rolling off the bed

(E) multicolored bruises along the shins of a 4-year-old child

39. Injuries remain the leading cause of death among all children of age 1–19 years. For those 15–19 years of age, which of the following lists the categories of injuries from most common to least common?

(A) suicide, homicide, motor vehicle accidents (MVA)

(B) homicide, suicide, MVA

(C) MVA, suicide, homicide

(D) MVA, homicide, suicide

(E) homicide, MVA, suicide

40. Overdose of which of the following is most likely to be complicated by hypoglycemia?

(A) salicylates

(B) lead

(C) tricyclic antidepressants

(D) opioids

(E) organophosphates

41. Last week, a 14 year old boy is caught smoking a cigarette by his mother and the teen is now being seen in your pediatric clinic. His mother is concerned about short- and long-term effects of smoking tobacco at such a young age. Which of the following statements concerning tobacco/cigarette smoking in preadolescent and adolescent years is most accurate?

   (A) The average smoker in the United States starts at age 16 years.
   (B) 50% of adolescent smokers become adult smokers.
   (C) Adolescent smokers become nicotine dependent after smoking fewer cigarettes than the adult smoker.
   (D) The use of cigars and smokeless tobacco is rare in adolescence.
   (E) Cigarette use cannot be detected by evaluating a urine drug screen.

42. A 12-month-old infant who has been walking well for 3–4 weeks, now limps on the right leg. No specific injury can be recalled by the parents. The child is afebrile. Examination reveals tenderness with gentle twisting of the lower right leg. An x-ray reveals an oblique nondisplaced fracture of the distal tibia. This condition is referred to as which of the following?

   (A) toddler fracture
   (B) Monteggia fracture
   (C) nursemaid ankle
   (D) Cozen fracture
   (E) Osgood-Schlatter disease

DIRECTIONS (Questions 43 through 52): The following group of questions is preceded by a list of lettered answer options. For each question, match the one lettered option that is most closely associated with the question. Each lettered option may be selected once, multiple times, or not at all.

Questions 43 through 52

   (A) naloxone
   (B) flumazenil
   (C) oxygen
   (D) ethanol or 4-methylpyrazole
   (E) deferoxamine
   (F) sodium bicarbonate
   (G) atropine
   (H) sodium nitrite/sodium thiosulfate or hydroxocobalamin
   (I) methylene blue

43. organophosphates

44. cyanide

45. tricyclic antidepressants

46. benzodiazepines

47. ethylene glycol

48. carbon monoxide

49. methemoglobinemic agents

50. opioids

51. methanol

52. iron

Answers and Explanations

1. **(C)** Raves, or underground all-night parties, typically are attended by adolescents and young adults. Probably the most popular club drug used at raves is Ecstasy, or methlyenedioxymethamphetamine (MDMA). The use of Ecstasy, an amphetamine with hallucinogenic and stimulant properties, results in CNS agitation, tachycardia, hypertension, and diaphoresis. Serotonergic effects of Ecstasy also include enhanced sensual perceptions and blunted perceptions of hunger and thirst. Most Ecstasy-related deaths have been linked to hyperthermia (increased physical activity in enclosed space) or hyponatremia (water intoxication or SIADH). *(Poirier, 2002;18:216–218, www.usdoj.gov/ndic)*

2. **(A)** Ingestion of acetaminophen in therapeutic doses typically does not result in side effects. However, ingestion of potentially toxic doses (> 10 g in adults and > 200 mg/kg in children) may result in hepatotoxicity. When present, hepatotoxicity peaks 48–96 hours after ingestion. The use of antidotal therapy with *N*-acetylcysteine is guided by the serum acetaminophen level drawn no less than 4 hours following ingestion. *(Acetaminophen: Consensus Guideline for out of hospital management; Rudolph, 2002;409–411)*

3. **(C)** Following head trauma, eye changes such as fixed, dilated pupils usually are indicative of increasing intracranial pressure or focal neurologic damage. A history of unconsciousness, irritability and lethargy, amnesia for the event, and/or vomiting are seen commonly in the absence of major intracranial injury. *(Rudolph, 348, 2244; Singer, 62:819, 1978)*

4. **(D)** An astounding 88% of serious brain injury sustained while bicycling is prevented with helmet use. Additionally, helmet use prevents an estimated 65% of injuries to the mid and upper face. Two factors have been identified as having a strong association with bicycle helmet use by young children. These are helmet use by an accompanying parent and a state mandatory helmet use law or local ordinance. Communities have successfully raised the rate of helmet use with a variety of programs. *(AAP Committee on Injury and Poison Prevention 2001;108:1030–1032)*

5. **(E)** Physical abuse is the leading cause of serious head injury among infants, and studies suggest 95% of serious head injuries in infants under 1 year of age are related to child abuse. The entity "abusive head trauma syndrome (formally referred to as shaken baby syndrome)" typically occurs in infants less than 2 years and was first described as a constellation of findings which included retinal hemorrhages, subdural and/or subarachnoid hemorrhages, and little or no evidence of external cranial trauma caused by "extreme rotational cranial acceleration induced by violent shaking." Evidence of other injuries, such as bruises, rib fractures, long-bone fractures, and abdominal injuries are often not present. In up to 90% of cases, unilateral or bilateral retinal hemorrhages are present. In cases of leukemia and idiopathic thrombocytopenic purpura, hematologic abnormalities generally are present and suggestive of the diagnosis. Henoch-Schöenlein purpura is a systemic vasculitis typically manifest by a triad of arthritis, abdominal pain (related to small bowel edema and inflammation and occasionally to

intussusception), and a classic purpuric rash which appears on the buttocks and legs of the child; neurologic manifestations may occur but are not characterized by retinal hemorrhage. *(AAP Committee on Injury and Poison Prevention, July 2001;108(1):206–210; Kliegman, 2007)*

6. **(B)** Most cases of physical child abuse and almost all deaths from abuse occur in the age group less than 4 years, especially less than 2 or 3 years, before the child can communicate effectively with others. In approximately 10% of all emergency room visits for injuries in children younger than 5 years, abuse is the etiology of those injuries. Although neurologically impaired children are at increased risk for abuse, most victims are previously healthy and have no pre-existing neurologic deficits. *(Behrman, 111)*

7. **(C)** Cases of lead poisoning in the United States are seen chiefly in the toddler age group. This is understandable, considering the mechanism of poisoning. The major source of lead poisoning in children living in urban areas is old, flaking lead paint, found in pre-1950 buildings; it is estimated that 25% of US children reside in buildings with lead-based paint. Some children will chronically ingest the paint flakes. Although it is no longer legal to use lead paints indoors, old buildings still may have layers of paint with high lead content beneath the more recent coats of "lead-free" paint. Children become exposed to lead as older homes are renovated. As severe, overt lead poisoning has become less common, there has been an increased concern about the long-term neurodevelopmental effects of subclinical lead poisoning, and guidelines for lead screening are issued by the CDC. Current guidelines from the American Academy of Pediatrics state that routine screening should occur at 1 and 2 years of age. *(McMillan, 599–632; AAP Committee on Environmental Health, October 2005;116(4):1036–1046 [doi:10.1542/peds.2005-1947])*

8. **(D)** Common signs of lead poisoning include lethargy, abdominal cramps, constipation, and anemia. Vomiting also is common. Ataxia is seen occasionally. The other items listed—fever, diarrhea, rash, hallucinations, hypertension, thrombocytopenia, and cough—are not associated with lead poisoning. *(McMillan, 632; AAP Committee on Environmental Health, October 2005;116(4):1036–1046 [doi:10.1542/peds.2005-1947])*

9. **(B)** Up to 28,000 children (usually < 5 years of age) ingest hydrocarbons each year. Most children will remain asymptomatic. Those who develop respiratory symptoms, even if transient, should be evaluated by a physician. A chest radiograph should be part of the initial evaluation of all those children who developed respiratory symptoms, such as wheezing, coughing, gagging, or dyspnea, even if symptoms were transient. Pneumonitis is most commonly encountered in children with respiratory symptoms; radiographs can be normal initially. The decision to hospitalize a child is not based on chest radiograph alone but based on clinical symptoms and need for oxygen or other supportive care. Syrup of ipecac should never be given as vomiting is associated with an increase risk for aspiration and subsequent respiratory complications. *(Fleisher, 914–915; Flomenbaum, 1435–1442)*

10. **(E)** The child described has developed extrapyramidal symptoms typical of phenothiazine toxicity. These findings may occur with therapeutic as well as excessive dosage and are common in children. Akinesia, trismus, opisthotonos, torticollis, chorea, dystonia, and oculogyric crises may be seen. These symptoms usually respond dramatically to intravenous diphenhydramine (Benadryl) or benztropine mesylate (Cogentin), although relapses are frequent. The clinical picture is so classic that it can be suspected even in the absence of a history of ingestion. Aside from managing this ingestion and screening for other medications this child may have ingested, you must work with these parents to prevent future episodes of ingestion. *(Flomenbaum, 1043–1044)*

11. **(E)** This child should be evaluated immediately by a physician. Ingestion of caustic agents, alkaline or acidic, results in dermal and mucosal injury from contact. Refusal to drink may indicate tissue damage and an assessment should be performed to determine the extent of this damage. The physical examination should include close examination of the oropharynx. Clinical or

radiographic evaluation can demonstrate signs of esophageal or tracheal perforation. This includes subcutaneous air and crepitus, pneumothorax, pneumomediastinum, or pneumoperitoneum. If endoscopic evaluation is indicated, it should be performed within the first 24 hours because of increased risk of iatrogenic perforation with this procedure after 48 hours following ingestion. Long-term effects of caustic ingestions include esophageal stricture formation. *(Flomenbaum, 1410–1413)*

12. **(D)** Shellfish poisoning is characterized by paresthesia and numbness of the mouth and face, generalized weakness, and paralysis. The incubation period is brief, lasting from minutes to hours. Treatment is supportive; in severe cases, mechanical ventilatory assistance may be required. Presumably the flagellates ingested by the shellfish produce a neurotoxin, which is, in turn, ingested when the shellfish are eaten (typically oysters, clams, mussels, or scallops), accounting for the symptoms. Larger numbers of dinoflagellates in the water where the shellfish are harvested can impart a red or reddish-brown color to the water, the so-called red tide. *(Flomenbaum, 703–704)*

13. **(A)** Iron poisoning in children generally does not occur with ingestion of multivitamins, but more commonly it is associated with prenatal vitamins or stand-alone iron-containing tablets. Deferoxamine it is the chelating agent of choice for iron poisoning. It combines with iron to form ferrioxamine, which is excreted in the urine. Parenteral administration (intravenous) is given for children with severe poisoning (typically defined by clinical symptoms/toxicity and/or a measurement of iron greater than 500 mg/dL). *(Flomenbaum, 634)*

14. **(E)** The signs described—coma, weakness, excessive salivation, bradycardia, and constricted pupils—are classic for organophosphate poisoning. Organophosphates are potent and irreversible inhibitors of acetylcholinesterase and can bind to muscarinic and nicotinic receptors. Excessive salivation is not seen in phenobarbital, diphenhydramine, ethyl alcohol, or hydrocarbon poisoning. *(Flomenbaum, 1500–1502)*

15. **(C)** Atropine is the major antidote in the treatment of organophosphate poisoning. Administered intravenously, it can result in rapid improvement in signs and symptoms. This improvement, however, typically is short-lived, necessitating repeat dosing. *(Flomenbaum, 1505–1506)*

16. **(B)** It is estimated that 6.6% of high school seniors have used anabolic steroids and one-third of them were not even participating in organized high school sports. Other performance-enhancing drugs include substances classified as supplements (such as caffeine, creatine, or androstenedione), or prescription drugs (such as beta-blockers, or diuretics). Some have been banned by governing boards or made illegal by law. These are classified as illicit or banned substances and include, among others, narcotics, human growth hormone, anabolic steroids, and gamma-hydroxybutyrate. A common triad consisting of acne, striae, and gynecomastia is reported in men. Multiorgan toxicity is possible and involvement of the heart (myocardial infarction), liver (hematomas, hepatitis), skin (acne, hirsutism in women), endocrine (gynecomastia, testicular atrophy, amenorrhea, and breast atrophy in women), and neurologic (depression, mania, mood lability, and aggressiveness) systems may be seen. *(Flomenbaum, 1688)*

17. **(A)** Jimsonweed seeds are abused because of their profound hallucinogenic effect. This, as named, is a weed with widespread growth through the continental United States and many other countries. Though some data suggest the use of this substance by adolescents is declining, fatalities associated with ingestion of jimsonweed continue to be reported. Typically patients present as agitated adolescents with signs of anticholinergic toxicity such as tachycardia, dilated pupils, and flushed skin. Convulsions are infrequent, but can be severe and difficult to control. *(Flomenbaum, 220)*

18. **(C)** Hallucinations, especially visual, are the most common and most striking effect of LSD. Sensations are magnified and distorted. The patient may imagine seeing odors or hearing colors. The emotional response can be either positive and pleasurable or negative and frightening. *(Fleisher, 934)*

19. **(E)** Sudden death is not infrequent in those who sniff organic solvents. The risk appears to be especially great if the inhalation involves a halogenated hydrocarbon (frequently used as solvents or spot removers) and is followed by exercise or other vigorous physical activity. It has been postulated that this may be related to sensitization of the myocardium by the volatile hydrocarbons. A lethal arrhythmia then is precipitated by the catecholamine release occasioned by the exercise. *(Knight, 1987;34:335,337)*

20. **(B)** Both flunitrazepam (Rophynol®; street names: roachies, roofies, the forget pill, roofenol) and gamma-hydroxybutyrate (GHB; street names: easy lay, grievous body harm) are used as agents in date-rape. Flunitrazepam, a benzodiazepine not licensed for use in the United States but readily available from dealers for less than $5 per tablet, quickly dissolves in liquids as a colorless and odorless sedative/hypnotic agent. Symptoms of dizziness, disorientation, and/or nausea begin within 15–20 minutes following ingestion, and peak with unconsciousness within 1–2 hours. These, along with the amnestic properties of flunitrazepam, have enabled sexual predators to render their victims helpless, and have made prosecution for sexual assault crimes even more challenging. GHB, commonly used as a euphoriant or aphrodisiac at parties or raves, also can be unknowingly ingested by a victim who is subsequently sexually assaulted or raped. This compound can be obtained in small quantities at large parties or in liter bottles from Canadian web sites. GHB also is popular among body builders because it is reputed to increase the production of growth hormone which increases muscle mass. *(Fleisher, 939, www.rapecrisiscenter.com; Poirier, 2002;18:53–59)*

21. **(B)** When a young child is lifted off the ground, dragged, or swung by one arm, the radius may partially escape from the annular ligament at the elbow. This subluxation of the radial head is a common injury, also commonly called nursemaid injury or nursemaid elbow. The child holds the injured arm flexed at the elbow and refuses to move it. The subluxation usually is easily reduced by supination of the arm. Recurrent radial head subluxations are seen in 33% of patients. Therefore,

caretakers should be informed of this risk and of preventive measures. *(Fleisher, 1945)*

22. **(A)** Epiphyseal separations are common childhood injuries. The growth plate or epiphysis is generally the weakest part of a child's bone, weaker even than surrounding ligaments. Trauma which would result in a tear of the ligament in an adult, often results in an epiphyseal fracture in a child. A fall onto an outstretched arm, which might result in a Colles fracture in an adult, is likely to cause a separation fracture of the distal radial epiphysis in a child. *(Rudolph, 1436)*

23. **(C)** Aspirin poisoning results in a mixed disturbance of metabolic acidosis and respiratory alkalosis. In adolescents and adults, the predominant early abnormality usually is the respiratory alkalosis. Before the age of 2 years, however, metabolic acidosis is the predominant process and the net change in arterial pH generally is a decrease. *(Rudolph, 375–376; Gaudreault,1982;70:566)*

24. **(B)** Salicylate poisoning results in an increase in both rate and depth of ventilation. The latter usually is especially striking. Generally, neither tachypnea nor deep respirations are clinically apparent until several hours after ingestion. Even young infants show this response. *(Rudolph, 375–376; Gaudreault, 1982;70:566)*

25. **(B)** Retinal hemorrhages and cerebral hemorrhages are characteristic of the abusive head trauma syndrome. Often, there are no external signs of trauma. This type of child abuse occurs most commonly in children less than 1 year of age and is associated with high morbidity and mortality. Of children who survive this injury, 35% will be blind or visually impaired. Increasingly, this syndrome is referred to by other names such as shaken baby/impact syndrome, nonaccidental head trauma, and abusive head trauma. *(Fleisher, 1677; Rudolph, 2415; Caffey, 1974;54:396)*

26. **(C)** The child described most likely has sustained an injury to the spleen. Splenic trauma, with or without rupture, is a common sledding injury. Shock can occur rapidly, or some time later. Pain in the left shoulder is common and

reflects irritation to the left diaphragm by sub-phrenic blood. Hospitalization with careful monitoring is the current approach to management, with every attempt to salvage, rather than remove, the spleen. *(Fleisher, 1365)*

27. **(A)** Unintentional injuries remain the leading cause of death among children aged 1–19 years. Of these fatal unintentional injuries, two-thirds involve motor vehicles. *(McMillan, 9; MacDorman, 2002;110:1037–1052)*

28. **(E)** All states have laws requiring any person having reason to suspect child abuse or neglect to report the case to the proper child protective authority. Proof is not a prerequisite for reporting. In a case of suspected abuse, physicians must identify and treat physical injuries and must ensure the child's immediate safety. Detailed recording of exact history given, including history in the child's own words if he/she is old enough to speak, and physical findings (photographs or videos) can be extremely useful to the child protective team. In this case, further evaluation by scanning, or blood tests are not necessary since the fracture is clearly seen on plain films. *(Rudolph, 2002;415–418)*

29. **(E)** In November 2003, the American Academy of Pediatrics (AAP) issued a policy statement, Poison Treatment in the Home, which stated syrup of ipecac should no longer be used routinely as a home treatment strategy. Further, it recommends safe disposal of all ipecac from homes. The policy identifies the incidence of significant vomiting often with prolonged duration (potentially impacting the efficiency of activated charcoal therapy), lack of efficacy for the vast majority of children, and potential for abuse (eg, eating disorders and Munchausen by proxy ie, Pediatric Falsification Condition). Caregivers of a child who may have ingested a toxic substance should consult with local poison control centers by telephoning 800-222-1222. *(AAP Committee on Injury, Violence and Poison Prevention, 2003;112:1182–1185)*

30. **(A)** The most likely villain in this case is the brown recluse spider (fiddler spider, *Loxoseles reclusa*). Envenomation is characterized by severe local reaction, often a blister at the bite site

which often progresses to local tissue necrosis, particularly in bites that occur over fatty areas of the body. An associated rash is often noted. Severe systemic symptoms and painful muscle cramps are characteristic of black widow spider (*Latrodectus mactans*) bite, in which case there is little local reaction, although local pain is common. *(Fleisher, 1049–1050)*

31. **(C)** Activated charcoal administered orally or via nasogastric tube adsorbs certain substances onto its surface, thereby decreasing the amount available for absorption from the gastrointestinal tract. Multiple-dose activated charcoal (MDAC) is defined as the administration of more than two doses of activated charcoal in the treatment of a given poisoning. It is believed that drugs with a prolonged elimination half-life, low plasma protein binding, and a small apparent volume of distribution (eg, ≤ 0.6 L/kg) may be more quickly eliminated by use of multiple doses of activated charcoal and as a result, the clinical course of the patient improved. In addition, some drugs undergo enterohepatic or enteroenteric recirculation which, in the case of an overdose, may be enhanced by such therapy. Multiple-dose activated charcoal should be considered for life-threatening ingestions of carbamazepine, dapsone, phenobarbital, quinine, and theophylline. The decision to use multiple-dose activated charcoal should be based on the physician's clinical judgment, lack of contraindications to its use, and the potential of other alternative therapies. *(Lowry, 2008; Flomenbaum, 115–116, 130–131)*

32. **(D)** The most immediate concern in patients successfully resuscitated from a near-drowning episode is correction of hypoxemia and acidosis. The consequences of cerebral hypoxia with acute brain swelling are the major causes of morbidity and mortality. Aspiration pneumonia is common. Life-threatening electrolyte disturbances are quite rare in patients who survive to the emergency room. Most victims of near-drowning aspirate relatively late in the immersion episode, after they have become severely hypoxic secondary to apnea. Aspiration of large quantities of fluid, therefore, is rare. (Note: A key to answering this question correctly is

attention to the phrase "require immediate attention.") *(Fleisher, 1009–1012)*

33. **(A)** The clinical manifestations of iron poisoning have been organized into four stages. The first stage is characterized by gastrointestinal (vomiting, diarrhea, abdominal pain, and gastrointestinal bleeding) and neurologic (lethargy or coma) signs. This is followed by a second stage of deceptive quiescence, of up to 48 hours, and then a third stage characterized by shock and metabolic acidosis, with or without evidence of hepatic injury. Leukocytosis is common. Late sequelae (stage four) include pyloric or antral stenosis and hepatic cirrhosis. *(Fleisher, 979–982, Behrman, 350–351)*

34. **(E)** The head of an infant is relatively larger (compared to total body size or weight) than the older child or adult. For this reason, the neck is subjected to proportionally increased force during a crash. Having the infant face backward diffuses the blow (deceleration) over the entire back. Infants under the age of 1 year should ride facing the rear of the car. All older children should ride properly restrained, facing forward. It has been shown that the force generated by a 1-year-old infant in a front-end crash far exceeds the ability of an adult to hold a child in the lap. The child will be propelled against the interior of the automobile or outside the automobile. *(McMillan, 139–141)*

35. **(D)** Drowning is defined as death from suffocation within 24 hours of submersion in water. Near-drowning victims survive at least 24 hours. Therefore, near-drowning victims may survive or die from complications of the submersion. As with many injuries and poisonings, there are peaks in occurrence of drownings in toddlers and in teenagers. In the United States, almost one-half of those who die of drowning are declared dead at the scene and never present to a medical facility for care. Of children and adolescents who survive near-drowning, an estimated 35% will have significant neurologic impairment. Prevention is of utmost importance. Installation of four-sided fences around pools decreases the number of pool immersion injuries by more than 50% in children aged 1–4 years.

As with all injuries, brief lapses in appropriate supervision may result in tragedies. *(Fleisher, 1011–1012; Behrman, 438–449)*

36. **(B)** Childhood sexual abuse is defined as "the engaging of dependent, developmentally immature children in sexual activities that they do not fully comprehend and to which they cannot give consent or activities that violate the laws and taboos of a society." The abusers frequently are relatives or others well known to the child. Impotence and low self-esteem are often seen in abusers. It is estimated that about 1% of children are sexually abused each year in the United States. Girls are six times more likely than boys to be victims of sexual abuse. *(Fleisher, 1780, Behrman, 178–182)*

37. **(A)** Firearm-related deaths in children aged 1–19 years are overwhelmingly intentional, with fewer than 8% unintentional. Most of these deaths occur prior to arrival at the hospital. Firearms remain the most common means of suicide in males of all ages. Though the rates of motor vehicle accident deaths have declined over the past two decades, they remain the leading cause of injury-related deaths in this age group. *(McMillan, 135–144, Behrman, 373)*

38. **(E)** It is extremely important to recognize patterns of abuse to prevent escalating abuse or additional injury and also to prevent unnecessary family anxiety with unwarranted referrals to child protective authorities. Trends found in cases of child abuse include a history not consistent with the injury or the developmental stage of the child (he rolled off the bed and broke his leg, said by the parent of the 1-month-old baby), the presence of a pattern of injuries known not to occur except with abuse (handprint bruise on the face), a pattern of injury that reflects injury with an instrument in a manner that would not occur in play or natural injury (hanger or loop cord marks on buttocks), delay in seeking medical attention, a history that changes during the course of the evaluation, and a history of recurrent injuries. On the other hand, bruises along the anterior lower leg, where children often bump into objects and where the bone is close to the skin, are characteristic of active preschoolers.

Figure 8-1 demonstrates a burn injury incurred when a child was placed in scalding water. The story the parents gave that the child fell forward into the water in a pot on the stove is inconsistent with the pattern of burn. *(Behrman, 171–178)*

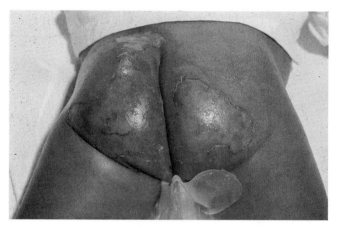

Figure 8-1
(Courtesy of Mary Anne Jackson, MD)

39. **(D)** Motor vehicle accidents, homicide, and suicide account for approximately 70% of all deaths in this age group. Motor vehicle injuries lead the list of injury deaths at all ages during childhood and adolscence, even in children younger than 1 year of age. Homicide is the third leading cause of injury death in children ages 1–4 years and second for the 15–19-year-old group. Suicide is the third leading cause of death for 15–19-year olds. *(McMillan, 9; MacDorman, 2002(110):1037–1052, Behrman, 366–375)*

40. **(A)** Ingestion of an overdose of salicylates, ethanol, or an oral hypoglycemic agent may result in symptomatic hypoglycemia. Close monitoring and aggressive therapy with dextrose is appropriate. *(Fleisher, 968–970, 1174; Flomenbaum, 750,764–767)*

41. **(C)** Compared to all other substances and firearms, tobacco kills more individuals in the United States each year than all other causes combined. Among adults aged >25 years, 59% of all deaths in the United States result from cardiovascular disease (36%) and cancer (23%). The leading causes of morbidity and mortality among youth and adults in the United States are related to six categories of health-risk behaviors: violence, tobacco use; alcohol and other drug use; sexual activity that contribute to unintended pregnancy and STDs, including HIV infection; unhealthy dietary behaviors; and physical inactivity. These behaviors frequently are interrelated and are established during childhood and adolescence and extend into adulthood. The average smoker in the United States starts at age 12 years and most are regular smokers by age 14 years. Adolsecent smokers may become nicotine dependent after smoking fewer cigarettes than adults. Nicotine's effect in the brain takes less than 20 seconds. While cigarettes are the most common tobacco products used by adolescents, cigars and smokeless tobacco use is common (11% and 6% respectively). Cotinine is the major metabolite of nicotine and can be detected in urine. *(Behrman, 829)*

42. **(A)** This clinical scenario is classic for a toddler fracture, which is seen most often in children aged 9–36 months. History of injury may not be elicited, and physical findings often are subtle. Care and time must be taken in the physical examination. Approximately one-fourth of the time, these fractures are not evident radiographically and must be diagnosed by physical examination or bone scan, with confirmatory x-ray revealing subperiosteal new bone 2–3 weeks later. *(Fleisher, 1561–1562)*

43. **(G), 44. (H), 45. (F), 46. (B), 47. (D), 48. (C), 49. (I), 50. (A), 51. (D), 52. (E)** There are specific antidotes for a number of toxic ingestions. These antidotes should be readily available in emergency room settings, and administered as early as possible in the appropriate dose. Antidote administration should be used in conjunction with meticulous ongoing evaluation, management, and supportive care. *(McMillan, 752, Behrman, 343)*

SELECTED READINGS

Garry Gardner H and the Committee on Injury, Violence, and Poison Prevention. Office-based counseling for unintentional injury prevention. *Pediatrics*. 2007;119:202–206.

Hegenbarth MA and the Committee on Drugs. Preparing for pediatric emergencies: Drugs to consider. *Pediatrics*. 2008; 121:433–443.

Williams JF, Storck M, and the Committee on Substance Abuse, and Committee on Native American Child Health. Inhalant abuse. *Pediatrics*. 2007;119:1009–1017.

Brenner RA and Committee on Injury, Violence, and Poison Prevention., Prevention of drowning in infants, children, and adolescents. *Pediatrics*. 2003;112:440–445.

AAP Committee on Injury and Poison Prevention. Firearm-related injuries affecting the pediatric population (RE9926). *Pediatrics*. 2000;105:888–895.

AAP Committee on Sports Medicine and Fitness. Adolescents and anabolic steroids: A subject review (RE9720). *Pediatrics*. 1997;99:6.

Committee on Sports Medicine and Fitness. Use of performance-enhancing substances. *Pediatrics*. 2005;115: 1103–1106.

CDC. Youth risk behavior surveillance—United States, 2001. *MMWR*. 2002;51:6–7.

Hughes JM, Merson MH. Fish and shellfish poisoning. *N Engl J Med*. 1976;295:1117–1120.

Koch JJ. Performance-enhancing substances and their use among adolescent athletes. *Pediatr Rev*. 2002;23:310–317.

McHugh MJ. The abuse of volatile substances. *Pediatr Clin North Am*. 1987;34:333–339.

Reece RM, Grodin MA. Recognition of nonaccidental injury. *Pediatr Clin North Am*. 1985;32:41–60.

Tobias JD. *Pediatric Critical Care: The Essentials*. Armonk, NY: Futura Publishing Co.; 1999.

Tong T, Boyer EW. Club drugs, smart drugs, raves and circuit parties: An overview of the club scene. *Pediatr Emerg Care*. 2002;18:216–218.

CHAPTER 9

Critical Care and Pediatric Therapeutics

Jason W. Custer, MD

Kristine A. Parbuoni, PharmD, BCPS

R. Blaine Easley, MD

Questions

1. A 5-year-old, 15 kg girl presents to the emergency room 10 hours after ingesting 7.5 g of acetaminophen. Plasma acetaminophen and hepatic enzymes are obtained and oral N-acetylcysteine is started. The patient is admitted and repeat acetaminophen levels and hepatic enzymes are followed. Peak AST levels are 300 U/L, but return to normal. Her hospital course is uneventful. Young children are less prone to develop hepatic injury following acetaminophen overdoses compared to adults due to which of the following?

    (A) Children are healthier with greater renal clearance of acetaminophen.
    (B) Children have an active sulfate conjugation pathway.
    (C) Acetaminophen undergoes glucuronidation only in young pediatric patients.
    (D) Glutathione stores are larger in adults.

2. A 24-month-old, 10 kg boy with a history of epilepsy, develops a tonic-clonic seizure at home. EMTs arrive and are unable to get IV access. He has been seizing for 60 minutes when you are called. The EMTs have a vial of diazepam. Which route will achieve the safest and quickest therapeutic serum diazepam level?

    (A) administering the diazepam via intramuscular route
    (B) administering the diazepam via intranasal

    (C) administering the diazepam via oral/sublingual route
    (D) administering the diazepam via rectal route
    (E) administering the diazepam via transcutaneous route

3. An 8-year-old male with cystic fibrosis is admitted to the hospital with acute decline in pulmonary function and fever. He is started on ceftazidime and tobramycin. This is his second hospitalization this year. The pharmacy recommends tobramycin be dosed at 2.5 mg/kg IV every 8 hours based on his pharmacokinetics from the last admission. Tobramycin levels obtained appropriately after the third dose are: peak of 3 mg/L and trough of 1.8 mg/L. The timing of the draws is double checked and determined to be accurate. What is the most likely cause of the unexpected tobramycin level?

    (A) The tobramycin dose is too low; he needs his tobramycin dose increased.
    (B) The patient has a much larger volume of distribution than expected.
    (C) The IV pump/system caused a delayed delivery of the drug.
    (D) The ceftazidime is interfering with the drug level.

4. A 2-year-old comes into your clinic with a chief complaint of a rash. You see multiple circular areas with a raised boarder and a scaling interior on the upper arms and back. You also note a bald patch with a similar-looking lesion on the scalp. Which of the following medications is the most appropriate treatment for this patient?

(A) griseofulvin

(B) ketoconazole cream

(C) amoxicillin

(D) fluconazole

(E) triamcinolone cream

5. A 6-year-old male with a known history of asthma presents to the emergency department with the most severe asthma attack of his life. When you listen, you hear very little air movement and your patient has a declining level of consciousness. After your initial measures, you see very little improvement and a decision is made to intubate the patient's trachea. Which combination of drugs is most appropriate in this situation to prevent worsening bronchospasm?

(A) phenobarbital, atropine, and succinyl-choline

(B) pancuronium and lidocaine

(C) ketamine, lidocaine, and rocuronium

(D) versed, fentanyl, and pancuronium

(E) perform endotracheal intubation without medication

6. A 3-year-old girl presents to your clinic with 5 days of rhinorrhea, cough, and congestion. Her mother has been using an over-the-counter cough and cold remedy to help control the symptoms. What is the most appropriate counseling to give this mother regarding over-the-counter medication usage in children?

(A) All over-the-counter medications are safe.

(B) All over-the-counter medications labeled pediatric or children's are safe.

(C) Many over-the-counter medications have a combination of medications that can have serious side effects in children, always consult a physician for dosing and safety.

(D) It is very rare that over-the-counter cold medications have acetaminophen as an ingredient.

(E) It is safe to give over-the-counter medications with acetaminophen as well as regular doses of acetaminophen if a child has a fever.

7. A 4-year-old with a history of renal failure, encopresis, and asthma is brought to the emergency room because of lethargy and difficulty breathing. She has been taking her usual breathing treatment and has not had any respiratory symptoms or fevers. She had recently been severely constipated and her parents have been administering multiple enemas to try to help her stool with no result. Which of the following is the most likely cause of her lethargy and respiratory distress?

(A) hyperphosphatemia secondary to enemas

(B) albuterol overdose

(C) sepsis

(D) asthma exacerbation

(E) anaphylaxis

8. An 11-year-old boy presents to the clinic complaining of itchy, watering eyes; stuffy nose; and a "tickle" in the back of his throat. He had similar symptoms at this time last year. His mother is concerned that he may be developing allergies. Which of the following allergy medications can cause tachycardia and hypertension?

(A) intranasal pseudoephedrine spray

(B) diphenhydramine

(C) intranasal steroid spray

(D) oral decongestants (pseudoephedrine)

(E) cromolyn sodium

9. You are in the delivery room for the birth of a full-term infant who is delivered by c-section for fetal distress. The baby is limp, cyanotic, and not making respiratory effort when placed under the warmer. The heart rate is found to be less than 60 beats per minute. The decision is made to place an endotracheal tube and mechanically ventilate the newborn. Which of the following medications can be safely administered via endotracheal tube?

(A) calcium chloride

(B) atropine

(C) amiodarone

(D) dopamine

(E) phenobarbital

10. A 1-year-old presents to the emergency department with the chief complaint of teething. You noticed in physical examination that the patient has peri-oral cyanosis with an oxygen saturation of 98% on room air. There is no significant past medical history. What is the most likely medication that causes this condition?

   (A) acetaminophen
   (B) ibuprofen
   (C) pseudoephedrine
   (D) orajel (topical benzocaine)
   (E) aspirin

11. A 4-year-old boy presents to the primary care clinic with a complaint of cough. The patient has a history of wheezing with colds, but has recently had a persistent cough and has been taking an albuterol MDI with some relief. The patient's mother says that he has symptoms at least 1 night out of the week and almost every day. What is the most appropriate medication regimen for this patient?

   (A) albuterol as needed
   (B) over-the-counter cough medication
   (C) albuterol twice daily
   (D) inhaled corticosteroid twice daily plus albuterol as needed
   (E) daily systemic corticosteroids

12. A 5-year-old presents to the emergency department with 6 days of fever, conjunctivitis, a "strawberry tongue," swelling of the hands, a diffuse rash, and a large swelling that appears to be a lymph node in the cervical area. Which medication should be included in the initial treatment regimen for this disorder to lessen the risk of complications?

   (A) acetaminophen
   (B) IV antibiotics
   (C) intravenous immunoglobin (IVIG)
   (D) ibuprofen
   (E) corticosteroids

13. A 14-year-old presents to the emergency department after being involved in a car accident. He has a GCS of 15; however he has multiple lacerations which require suturing. In which of the following locations is the use of a local anesthetic with epinephrine contraindicated?

   (A) shoulder
   (B) cheek
   (C) ear
   (D) neck
   (E) forehead

14. A 10-year-old with a history of asthma presents to the emergency department in respiratory distress. You auscultate diffuse wheezing and the patient has increased work of breathing. You initiate albuterol via nebulizer, oral steroids, and establish IV access. The patient is showing signs of worsening work of breathing, which one of the following medications can act as an acute bronchodilator?

   (A) magnesium sulfate
   (B) calcium chloride
   (C) sodium phosphate
   (D) potassium chloride
   (E) sodium bicarbonate

15. A 4-year-old with a seizure disorder presents to the emergency department with increased seizure frequency. Her medication regimen is currently phenytoin twice daily. She has been compliant with her medication and has been on the same dose for over 2 years. What is the next best step in her management?

   (A) add Tegretol (carbamazepine) to her regimen
   (B) add ethosuximide to her regimen
   (C) add phenobarbital to her regimen
   (D) measure a serum phenytoin level
   (E) perform an EEG to be sure that these are seizures

16. A 5-year-old who has just started first grade presents to your clinic with his mother. His mother has a note from his teacher that your patient frequently misbehaves in class, gets up out of his seat, and bothers other children. His mother says that she has a hard time controlling his behavior at home. He is unable to sit

still during your examination and is busy playing with magazines and toys when you try to talk to him. You suspect a diagnosis of ADHD for this patient. Which of the following is the most appropriate medication to offer this patient as a trial?

(A) methylphenidate
(B) imipramine
(C) haloperidol
(D) paroxetine
(E) phenytoin

17. You are caring for a now 5-day-old infant born after 28 weeks of gestation. On physical examination you note bounding pulses and a harsh "washing machine" murmur. The patient has also had an increasing oxygen requirement. You order an echocardiogram and diagnose a patent ductus arteriosus. Which of the following therapies may correct this problem?

(A) opamine infusion
(B) 100% oxygen administration
(C) indomethacin
(D) prostaglandin infusion
(E) corticosteroids

18. A previously healthy 12-year-old presents to the emergency department with nausea and vomiting for 2 days, there are other sick contacts at home. He has no meningeal signs. An IV is placed and he is given IV fluids for rehydration. The vomiting continues and you decide to give him an antiemetic. After the medication is given, the patient begins to slowly turn his head to the right and has extreme arching of his back. He is awake and alert. What is the most likely cause of this reaction?

(A) hypocalcemia
(B) tetanus
(C) seizure disorder
(D) metoclopramide administration
(E) meningitis

19. A 9-year-old boy with Duchenne muscular dystrophy presents to the pediatric emergency room with severe respiratory distress related to pneumonia. The decision is made to intubate the patient for respiratory failure. Which of the following paralytics are contraindicated in this patient?

(A) pancuronium
(B) vecuronium
(C) atracurium
(D) succinylcholine
(E) rocuronium

20. A 6-month-old infant with chronic lung disease (CLD) on home oxygen and high-calorie feeds presents with slow growth. You consider starting a thiazide diuretic to decrease airway resistance and improve lung compliance. Which of the following electrolyte abnormalities may result from the use of thiazide-type diuretics?

(A) hypoglycemia
(B) hyperuricemia
(C) hyperkalemia
(D) hypernatremia
(E) hypocalciuria

21. A 2-year-old child presents from home with a temperature of 39°C and seizure activity. The seizure lasts less than 15 minutes. Despite her mother's aggressive antipyretic administration during the child's febrile illnesses, this is the girl's fourth febrile seizure this year. Which of the following drugs can decrease the rate of recurrence of febrile seizures?

(A) carbamazepine
(B) clonazepam
(C) phenobarbital
(D) phenytoin
(E) felbamate

22. A 6-year-old is brought to your office because of "poor color". At the visit, the child is otherwise appropriate, but slightly less active than normal, and grayish in appearance. He admits to drinking water from a pump-well he found with his older brother. You suspect nitrite poisoning. Which of the following drug should you administer for treatment of acute nitrate poisoning?

(A) hydralazine
(B) morphine
(C) methylene blue
(D) corticosteroids
(E) thiosulfate

23. A 12-year-old child with a surgically corrected pulmonary shunt is to undergo an invasive dental procedure. Which of the following antibiotics would be most appropriate for prophylaxis against bacterial endocarditis?

(A) amoxicillin
(B) clindamycin
(C) erythromycin
(D) oxacillin
(E) vancomycin

24. A 4-year-old child has a history of developing a persistent cough that has endured the past 3 weeks. There are multiple sick contacts in the home with similar respiratory complaints. You suspect atypical pneumonia. Which of the following is most appropriate for the treatment of *Mycoplasma pneumoniae* infection?

(A) cefuroxime
(B) chloramphenicol
(C) erythromycin
(D) penicillin
(E) tetracycline

25. You are caring for a 6-month-old infant following aortic reconstruction in the intensive care unit. You are called with a panic value that cyanohemoglobin levels were detected on the infant. You assess the infant and find her oral-tracheally intubated and mechanically ventilated on numerous vasoactive drips and

sedatives. Cyanide is produced in the metabolism of which of the following?

(A) sodium nitroprusside
(B) nitroglycerin
(C) labetalol
(D) dobutamine
(E) milrinone

26. You have followed a 5-year-old for a series of neurologic and behavioral issues. You refer her to a pediatric neurologist for evaluation. After her evaluation, she returns to your clinic for follow-up and is on ethosuximide. Ethosuximide (Zarontin) is most useful in the treatment of which symptom?

(A) phenobarbital overdosage
(B) absence (petit mal) seizures
(C) akinetic seizures
(D) tonic-clonic seizures
(E) complex partial seizures

27. A 14-month-old male is admitted to the PICU for bleeding from his nose and gums. There is no family history of bleeding tendency. On further history you determine the family has a problem with mice and rats and have rodenticides around the house. Which of the following should be included in initial treatment?

(A) vitamin C
(B) vitamin K
(C) copper sulfate
(D) a phenothiazine
(E) atropine

28. A 14-year-old female presents to the emergency room 20 hours following ingestion of 8.5 g of acetaminophen. Therapy with which of the following should be initiated?

(A) deferoxamine
(B) physostigmine
(C) *N*-acetylcysteine
(D) glutathione
(E) no therapy is indicated

29. A 6-day-old male infant is brought to the emergency center with complaints of poor feeding and lethargy for 2 days. On physical examination, the infant is hypotonic and responds poorly to painful stimuli. The initial Dextrostix is 30 mg/dL. You administer 2 mL/kg of $D_{25}W$ intravenously in addition to 20 mL/kg of normal saline. Initial laboratory evaluation includes sodium 128 meq/L, potassium 8.4 meq/L, bicarbonate 8 meq/L, and chloride 104 meq/L. The next intervention should be which of the following?

(A) obtain plasma for 17-OH progesterone level and administer 10 mg/kg hydrocortisone

(B) start prostaglandin E

(C) administer 3 mL/kg of hypertonic saline

(D) obtain a urine metabolic screen

(E) check serum ammonia and liver function tests

30. An 8-year-old with complex medical history has transferred care to your clinic. The child's current medication list includes: albuterol, carbamazepine, ranitidine, and methylphenidate. Methylphenidate is most commonly prescribed in the management of children with which of the following?

(A) poor appetites

(B) temper tantrums

(C) seizure disorders

(D) breath-holding spells

(E) attention-deficit hyperactivity disorders

31. A 6-month-old infant presents from day care with fever, vomiting, and lethargy. On physical examination, you confirm the lethargy and note a full fontanel despite signs of dehydration. Which of the following would be the initial antibiotic(s) of choice?

(A) cefuroxime and vancomycin

(B) ceftriaxone and vancomycin

(C) clindamycin

(D) vancomycin

(E) amoxicillin

32. A 3-day-old male was born at the hospital and discharged home within 24 hours. The mother relates that he has been a poor breast-feeder. His parents bring him to the emergency room because he has become very pale and listless over a matter of hours. On examination, you note a lethargic newborn in shock with a large liver and a gallop. Chest x-ray reveals increased pulmonary vasculature and cardiomegaly. You begin antibiotic therapy but suspect congenital cardiac disease. Which of the following is the drug of choice?

(A) dobutamine

(B) digoxin

(C) prostaglandin E_1

(D) milrinone

(E) nicardipine

33. A 7-year-old male adopted from Romania presents with hematemesis. He is known to have severe chronic hepatitis. An upper endoscopy reveals esophageal variceal bleeding. Which of the following agents is most likely to be beneficial in controlling the esophageal blood loss?

(A) octreotide

(B) prostaglandin E_1

(C) nitric oxide

(D) prostacyclin

(E) dexamethasone

34. A 15-year-old adolescent comes to spend the summer with her aunt. She has an appointment to be seen in your clinic because of her need for frequent medical care. Prior to seeing the patient you review her records and notice she is on oral pancreatic enzyme replacement therapy. This is most helpful in patients with which of the following?

(A) protein-losing enteropathy

(B) celiac disease

(C) ulcerative colitis

(D) alpha$_1$-antitrypsin deficiency

(E) cystic fibrosis

35. A 2-week-old neonate presents with lethargy, hypothermia, and poor feeding. Evaluation of the cerebrospinal fluid reveals a white blood cell count of 1200 cells/mm³ (95% polymorphonucleocytes) with an elevated protein and decreased glucose. Which of the following is the initial antibiotic regiment of choice?

(A) ampicillin
(B) ceftriaxone
(C) cefotaxime
(D) cefuroxime with ampicillin
(E) gentamicin with ampicillin

36. A 14-year-old undergoing consolidation therapy for high-risk, chronic lymphocytic leukemia develops burning and discomfort with urination. Urine analysis demonstrates large amount of hemoglobin, along with red and white blood cells. Urine culture is negative. You diagnose the child with hemorrhagic cystitis. Hemorrhagic cystitis is associated most closely with large doses of which of the following?

(A) cyclophosphamide
(B) methotrexate
(C) actinomycin D
(D) L-Asparaginase
(E) prednisone

37. A 2-month-old female presents with a 4-day history of coughing spells that last at least 30 seconds. After the coughing spells she vomits. She is otherwise well. Laboratory evaluation reveals a peripheral white blood cell count of 42,000/mm³ with 86% lymphocytes. Which of the following prophylaxis should the family and day-care contacts of this child receive?

(A) rifampin
(B) erythromycin
(C) gentamicin
(D) penicillin
(E) trimethoprim-sulfamethoxazole

38. An 8-year-old male presents to your office with his parents with the chief complaint of wetting the bed. His parents say that he has never had a period longer than 2 weeks in his life when he has not wet the bed in the middle of the night. He does not want to go to sleepovers now because he is embarrassed. He has tried cutting down on nighttime fluids and this has not made a difference. His parents are looking for a solution. What therapy has been shown to have the best success rate?

(A) behavioral conditioning (alarm/arousal system)
(B) DDAVP
(C) imipramine
(D) motivational therapy
(E) furosemide

39. A 4-year-old presents to the emergency department with a chief complaint of swelling around the eyes and ankles. You note the patient to have pitting edema up to the knees bilaterally and peri-orbital edema with no erythema. You astutely send off a urine analysis and find that the patient has 3+ protein in the urine without signs of infection or red blood cells. You make the diagnosis of nephrotic syndrome, likely minimal change disease. What is the next step in this patient's management?

(A) intravenous immunoglobulin (IVIG)
(B) corticosteroids
(C) kidney biopsy
(D) cyclophosphamide
(E) antibiotic therapy

40. A well-appearing, 10-year-old presents to the emergency department with a red rash on his trunk, ankles, elbows, and red lesions on his tongue. You suspect that these look like petechiae and order some laboratory tests including a complete blood count. When the laboratory values come back, you see that the platelet count is read as 5,000/μL. The patient's blood type is A and he is Rh positive. You diagnose the patient with idiopathic thrombocytopenia purpura. What is the next step in your management?

(A) intravenous immunoglobulin (IVIG)
(B) amoxicillin
(C) anti-D immunoglobulin

(D) platelet transfusion

(E) observation

41. A 5-year-old with a history of sickle cell disease presents to the emergency department with a 2-day history of cough and a 1-day history of fever. You order blood work and a chest x-ray and she is found to have an infiltrate that is consistent with pneumonia. What is the next step in your management?

(A) amoxicillin

(B) ceftriaxone

(C) azithromycin

(D) ceftriaxone and azithromycin

(E) no antibiotics needed, likely viral

42. A 12-month-old comes to the emergency department after having 4 days of upper respiratory tract symptoms and fever. Her mother has been giving her acetaminophen every 4 hours and an over-the-counter cold and cough remedy six times daily. She says today that the child has been more sleepy and not as interactive. She shows you the bottle of cough and cold remedy and you notice that it also contains acetaminophen. You suspect acetaminophen toxicity and this is confirmed with a serum acetaminophen level in the toxic range, but liver enzymes are normal. How should you proceed?

(A) contact poison control and administer steroids

(B) administer furosemide and arrange for admission

(C) administer naloxone and monitor for improvement

(D) contact poison control and administer N-acetylcysteine

(E) no therapy needed and observe

43. A 16-year-old presents to your office complaining of abdominal pain and vaginal discharge. She has been sexually active with multiple partners and is concerned that she may be pregnant. You perform a pregnancy test that is negative and during your pelvic examination she is noted to have severe cervical motion tenderness. You suspect a diagnosis

of pelvic inflammatory disease. Which of the following is the most appropriate antibiotic regiment for this patient?

(A) clindamycin

(B) ceftriaxone

(C) doxycycline

(D) ceftriaxone plus doxycycline

(E) metronidazole

44. A 15-year-old comes to your clinic complaining of frequent and heavy menstrual cycles. She had her first period at the age of 12, had some irregularity; however began having regular 28 day cycles at the age of 13. For the last 4 months she has been having bleeding on and off every 1–2 weeks. She is not and has never been sexually active, has not had any vaginal discharge, has no abdominal pain, or other bleeding problems. She is concerned and wants to better predict her menstrual cycle. You tell her that this is likely dysfunctional uterine bleeding. What should you recommend?

(A) testosterone cream

(B) platelet infusion

(C) oral contraceptive pill

(D) nonsteroidal anti-inflammatory drug (NSAID)

(E) careful observation

45. You are called to the newborn nursery to see a 3-day-old that has a rash. The parents are concerned because they did not notice the rash until this morning and are sure that it was not present the first 2 days of life. You find a well-appearing baby who has scattered red papules all over the body and are in clumps on the cheeks and on the trunk, some of them even look like vesicles. You take a scraping of one of the vesicles to examine under the microscope and find that these vesicles contain a large number of eosinophils. What is the recommended treatment for this patient?

(A) acyclovir

(B) topical steroids

(C) antidandruff shampoo

(D) phototherapy

(E) observation

46. A 14-month-old child is brought into the emergency room unresponsive. He is pale, has delayed capillary refill, and minimal respiratory effort. Pulses are barely palpable. You are requested to obtain vascular access. According to current resuscitation guidelines, what should your next step be?

(A) Attempt a central line.
(B) Place an arterial line.
(C) Attempt a peripheral IV catheter, if unsuccessful place an intraosseous needle.
(D) Administer intracardiac medications.
(E) Attempt a central line, if unsuccessful call the surgeon for a vascular cut-down.

47. A 24-month-old returns to your clinic after treatment for Streptococcal pharyngitis. His mother complains that he continues to have an irregular gait after his penicillin shot. You examine the child and find he has a foot drop. The most likely cause of this finding is which of the following?

(A) reaction to penicillin
(B) complication of intramuscular injection into gluteal area
(C) complication of intramuscular injection into anterolateral thigh
(D) complication of the bacterial infection
(E) cerebral vascular accident

48. A 10-year-old boy with Hodgkin lymphoma is undergoing chemotherapy. The oncologist wants to start a new regimen but is worried about cardiac toxicity. Cardiomyopathy is most likely to be caused by which of the following?

(A) bleomycin
(B) doxorubicin
(C) cytarabine
(D) etoposide
(E) cisplatin

49. A 16-year-old girl with acute lymphocytic leukemia nearing the end of induction therapy presents with tingling in her fingers. Peripheral neuropathy is the most common adverse effect of which chemotherapeutic agent?

(A) methotrexate
(B) cyclophosphamide
(C) cytarabine
(D) procarbazine
(E) vincristine

50. A 10-year-old girl with acute myeloid leukemia (AML), now day 75 status post a matched, unrelated bone marrow transplant presents with voluminous diarrhea, nausea, and vomiting. Acute graft-versus-host disease is suspected and high-dose corticosteroids are initiated. Side-effects of corticosteroids most commonly include which of the following?

(A) peripheral obesity
(B) gigantism
(C) cataracts
(D) hypoglycemia
(E) hypotension

51. A 6-year-old girl is brought to the emergency room with head injuries after being hit by a car. Her heart rate is 42 beats per minute, blood pressure is 160/100 mm Hg, respiratory rate is 8 breaths per minute, and she is minimally responsive. The left pupil is larger than the right and minimally reactive to light. The decision is made to perform a rapid sequence intubation since she is unable to protect her airway. Which of the following sedative agents could cause worsening of her condition?

(A) thiopental
(B) propofol
(C) fentanyl
(D) etomidate
(E) ketamine

52. A full-term baby became cyanotic 5 hours after birth. The baby was found to have persistent pulmonary hypertension of the newborn (PPHN) and is now being managed in the NICU on a mechanical ventilator. The baby's condition is worsening, which of the following interventions is indicated?

(A) prostacyclin
(B) arachidonic acid

(C) leukotriene C
(D) nitric oxide
(E) adenosine

53. A 10-year-old boy presents to the emergency department with a 4-day history of fever, runny nose, vomiting, and diarrhea. His mother has been giving him aspirin (325 mg) two tablets every 4–6 hours for the fever and Pepto Bismol (175 mg/15 mL salicylate), one tablespoon every 4–6 hours for the upset stomach. He is lethargic, diaphoretic, and febrile to 102.4°F, BP is 100/60, HR is 120, and RR 40. Arterial blood gas testing shows a pH of 7.44, PCO_2 14 mm Hg, PO_2 93 mm Hg. Giving sodium bicarbonate at this time would have what primary effects?

(A) worsen his acid-base status
(B) prevent cardiac arrhythmias
(C) worsen his hydration status
(D) prevent seizures
(E) prevent absorption of salicylates

54. A 16-year-old male with sickle cell anemia presents to clinic for evaluation of his pain management. He is having acute pain on top of his chronic pain. Which of the following opioids is available as a long-acting and short-acting oral formulation as well as intravenous?

(A) fentanyl
(B) morphine
(C) oxycodone
(D) meperidine
(E) methadone

55. A 3-year-old girl is admitted to the burn unit following an immersion hot water injury with resultant second- and third-degree burns covering 60% of the body surface area. Fluids are started at maintenance plus 4 mL/kg/%BSA burned according to the Parkland formula with half of the fluid administered over the first 8 hours and the remainder over the following 16 hours. A Foley catheter is placed to monitor urine output. Six hours after admission, the urine output has decreased to 0.5 mL/kg/h for the past 2 hours. The most appropriate therapy would be which of the following?

(A) continue to observe the urine output
(B) furosemide 1 mg/kg intravenously
(C) furosemide 2 mg/kg orally
(D) mannitol 0.5 g/kg intravenously
(E) fluid bolus of 20 mL/kg of normal saline

56. A 2-day-old, 1.9-kg boy was delivered to a 19-year-old mother at 36 weeks gestation, with no prenatal care. Upon preparing the infant for discharge, the patient was noted to be tachypneic, with weak peripheral pulses and grayish cyanosis of the lips. Oxygen saturations were noted to be 85% and declining. Chest x-ray shows cardiomegaly and an echocardiogram is ordered which reveals the presence of hypoplastic left heart syndrome (HLHS). Considering the patient's present condition, which one of the following is the best initial intervention that should be taken?

(A) give indomethacin
(B) consult a pediatric cardiologist for surgical options
(C) start prostaglandin E_1
(D) start phenylephrine
(E) give oxygen at 100%

57. A 10-year-old child presents to the emergency department with an erythematous rash on his thigh, fever, and myalgia 2 weeks after hunting with his father in eastern Pennsylvania. The rash appeared about 4 days prior to presentation and has been gradually increasing in size. He thinks he had a bug bite in the same spot of the rash. The initial treatment of choice is which of the following?

(A) streptomycin
(B) azithromycin
(C) clindamycin
(D) vancomycin
(E) doxycycline

58. A 16-year-old male presents with fever, chills, nausea, vomiting, and headache. He was previously healthy, but over the last 24 hours he has felt awful and states he has been unable to concentrate for his exams. He also has a petechial rash on his trunk. Gram stain of CSF fluid shows gram-negative diplococcus. Which of the following is the drug of choice for the treatment of meningococcal meningitis?

(A) cefotaxime
(B) ceftriaxone
(C) vancomycin
(D) chloramphenicol
(E) penicillin

59. A 3-year-old female was found with her mother's prenatal vitamins. The bottle was empty and was estimated to contain 20–25 tablets. At 4 hours postingestion, her serum iron level is 550 mg/dL. Which of the following should be administered?

(A) dimercaprol (BAL)
(B) deferoxamine (desferal)
(C) edetate calcium disodium (EDTA)
(D) ipecac
(E) activated charcoal

60. A 10-year-old male is admitted to the hospital with a 4-day history of nausea, vomiting, and abdominal pain. The pain is located in the epigastrium and radiates to the back. He is currently completing a course of azithromycin for a sinusitis diagnosed 3 days prior. Home medications include acetaminophen, metoclopramide, ranitidine, valproic acid, fluticasone nasal spray, and loratadine. The drug most likely to cause these symptoms is which of the following?

(A) acetaminophen
(B) ranitidine
(C) azithromycin
(D) valproic acid
(E) loratadine

61. An adolescent male presents with a urethral discharge. Gram stain of the exudate reveals intracellular gram-negative diplococci. The initial treatment of choice is which of the following?

(A) azithromycin, 1 g orally once
(B) doxycycline, 100 mg twice a day for 7 days
(C) procaine penicillin G, 1.2 million units IM once
(D) benzathine penicillin G, 2.4 million units IM once
(E) ceftriaxone, 125 mg IM once

62. A 16-year-old girl presents to the emergency department 12 hours after ingesting 30 extra strength Tylenol (acetaminophen) tablets. She is vomiting, diaphoretic, and lethargic. Which of the following statements is true regarding the toxicity of acetaminophen overdose?

(A) primarily involves the liver
(B) primarily involves the central nervous system
(C) is most severe in patients less than 2 years of age
(D) is best treated with sodium bicarbonate to alkalinize the urine
(E) is best treated with dialysis

63. A neonate is receiving intravenous ampicillin and gentamicin for sepsis and possible meningitis. A blood culture reveals group B streptococcus. The antibiotic of choice is which of the following?

(A) clindamycin
(B) penicillin
(C) cefuroxime
(D) vancomycin
(E) tobramycin

Questions 64 and 65

64. A 14-year-old girl is admitted to the emergency department with an acute change in mental status. She recently had a fight with her parents and threatened to kill herself. Her HR is 130, BP is 106/68, and T 37°C. She is placed on a cardiac monitor and an electrocardiogram is obtained which shows prolongation of the QRS interval. Which of the following agents was most likely ingested by this patient?

(A) nortriptyline
(B) phenobarbital
(C) acetaminophen

(D) cocaine

(E) phencyclidine

65. The patient was given activated charcoal and a fluid bolus with normal saline. Minutes later, the QRS complex abruptly widens to 0.16 seconds, BP 86/50, and HR 140. Treatment should include the immediate administration of which of the following?

(A) *N*-acetylcysteine

(B) sodium bicarbonate

(C) sodium nitroprusside

(D) amyl nitrite

(E) lidocaine

66. A 14-year-old patient with acute lymphocytic leukemia presents with fever to 39.6°C. She was most recently discharged 1 week ago after completing a round of chemotherapy. Blood culture reveals a nonlactose fermenting gram-negative rod, which is oxidase positive. Which of the following is the appropriate antibiotic?

(A) levofloxacin

(B) azithromycin

(C) trimethoprim-sulfamethoxazole

(D) piperacillin-tazobactam

(E) ceftriaxone

67. A 2-year-old male presents to the emergency department with fever to 39.1°C, and abnormal mental status for the past 12 hours. Laboratory results show a WBC of 567,000, hemoglobin 3.2, and LDH 1197. Acute lymphoblastic leukemia is suspected and the oncologist asks you to initiate allopurinol therapy. Allopurinol is used most commonly to manage what in acute leukemia of childhood?

(A) to induce remission

(B) to maintain remission

(C) to help alkalinize the urine

(D) to prevent vomiting from chemotherapy

(E) to prevent hyperuricemia associated with tumor lysis syndrome

68. A 4-year-old child presents with profuse watery diarrhea which is positive for occult blood. She complains of abdominal pain and cramping. She is febrile to 38.8°C and her WBC is 19,000. She is currently completing a 7-day course of amoxicillin-clavulanate for an ear infection. Which of the following is the most appropriate therapy at this time would be

(A) IV vancomycin

(B) PO vancomycin

(C) IV metronidazole

(D) PO metronidazole

(E) PO clindamycin

69. A 15-year-old boy with central core disease and a history of malignant hyperthermia crises is undergoing surgery. He would benefit from which agent during a malignant hyperthermia crisis?

(A) ethanol

(B) succinylcholine

(C) halothane

(D) potassium

(E) dantrolene

Questions 70 and 71

Gentamicin and piperacillin-tazobactam is initiated in an 8 year old with acute myeloblastic leukemia for dual coverage of *Pseudomonas aeruginosa* bacteremia. Gentamicin levels will be checked to ensure that the peaks are high enough to kill the bacteria relative to the MIC (peak concentration to MIC or peak/MIC ratio).

70. Which of these drugs is concentration-dependent like the aminoglycosides?

(A) doxycycline

(B) ciprofloxacin

(C) vancomycin

(D) cefdinir

(E) erythromycin

71. For the above patient, the appropriate time to check serum gentamicin levels at steady state would be after how many half-lives?

(A) one

(B) two

(C) three

(D) five

(E) seven

72. A 33-week, 1200 g boy is born to a teenage mother who had poor prenatal care. The baby's head circumference, height, and weight are below average for his age, indicating poor intrauterine growth, likely due to exposure to drugs during pregnancy. Intrauterine growth retardation (IUGR) is a common adverse effect of which drug if taken by the mother during pregnancy?

(A) warfarin
(B) acetaminophen
(C) lithium
(D) lisinopril
(E) phenytoin

73. An 8-year-old girl with uncontrolled asthma is receiving inhaled corticosteroids and beta-agonists (Advair, fluticasone/salmeterol) as well as a leukotriene antagonist (Singulair, montelukast). The decision is made to begin theophylline; however you are worried about the potential toxicities. What side effects should you monitor for that would indicate high levels of theophylline?

(A) nystagmus
(B) myopathy
(C) polyuria
(D) rash
(E) vomiting

DIRECTIONS (Questions 74 through 100): The following group of questions is preceded by a list of lettered answer options. For each question, match the one lettered option that is most closely associated with the question. Each lettered option may be selected once, multiple times, or not at all.

Questions 74 through 78

(A) dopamine
(B) epinephrine
(C) isoproterenol
(D) norepinephrine
(E) dobutamine
(F) milrinone

74. Indicated for septic and spinal shock

75. Has most significant impact on metabolism; possesses β_1 and β_2 effects

76. May lower systemic vascular resistance and pulmonary vascular resistance

77. Increases cardiac output without increasing heart rate or systemic vascular resistance

78. Has greatest effect on increasing heart rate

Questions 79 through 84

(A) albuterol
(B) cromolyn sodium
(C) theophylline
(D) corticosteroids
(E) epinephrine (racemic)
(F) ipratropium bromide
(G) caffeine

79. Reduces airway edema rapidly, with risk of potential recurrence of symptoms

80. Mast cell stabilizer

81. Anticholinergic agent used for airway smooth muscle relaxation

82. Reduces upper and lower airway inflammation

83. Narrow therapeutic window

84. May be given by inhalation, orally, intravenously, and intramuscularly

Questions 85 through 88

(A) μ_1 (mu$_1$)
(B) μ_2 (mu$_2$)
(C) κ (kappa)
(D) δ (delta)
(E) σ (sigma)

85. Sedation, miosis

86. Analgesia

87. Hypertonia, dysphoria

88. Physical dependence

Questions 89 through 91

In a trial evaluating the pharmacology of a new drug in children, the drug is administered in three different fashions and the serum concentration of the drug is measured at different time points. The area in gray represents the minimal effective concentration of the drug in the serum. Match the resulting serum concentration curves (labeled A, B, and C) with the most likely method of administration (see Fig. 9-1).

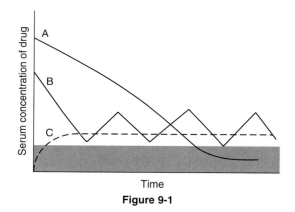

Figure 9-1

89. Continuous intravenous infusion

90. Intermittent intravenous dosing

91. Single intravenous bolus dose

Questions 92 through 93

A 15-year-old male is found unresponsive in his bedroom. The child is intubated but remains minimally responsive. He is admitted directly to the intensive care unit and toxicology screens demonstrate alcohol and benzodiazepines. No other medications are found. If repeat serum tests are performed on these two agents, the illustrated elimination curves would result. Match the agents to their respective elimination kinetics (see Fig. 9-2).

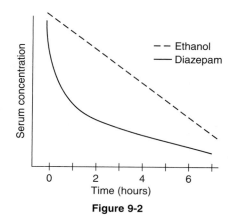

Figure 9-2

(A) first order
(B) zero order

92. Ethanol is eliminated following _____ kinetics.

93. Diazepam is eliminated following _____ kinetics.

Questions 94 through 96

On the following graph, (A) represents the dose-response of a drug acting alone, and (B) depicts the dose-response relationship of the same drug in the presence of a competitive antagonist (see Fig 9-3).

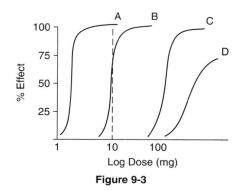

Figure 9-3

94. If the amount of the competitive antagonist is increased, which is the resulting dose-response curve?

95. Which curve illustrates a dose-response curve of lower efficacy than B?

96. Which curve illustrates a dose-response curve of greater potency than B?

Questions 97 through 100

Patients A and B are receiving the same medication at the same dosing interval, and have their serum levels of the drug monitored at the same time intervals. The drug is hepatically metabolized, and then active metabolites are cleared renally. Based on the graph of their serum levels following repetitive dosing of the medication, match the patients with the most likely clinical scenarios (see Fig 9-4).

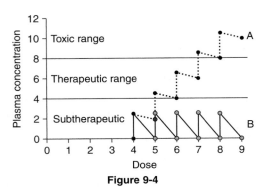

Figure 9-4

97. This patient has renal insufficiency.

98. This patient has elevated cytochrome P-450 activity.

99. This patient demonstrates cumulative drug properties.

100. This patient would benefit in an increase in both the dose amount and frequency of drug administration.

Answers and Explanations

1. **(B)** Children younger than 6 years of age are unlikely to develop significant toxicity after a single ingestion of even relatively large doses of acetaminophen. Although prepubescent children have relatively high hepatic, mixed function oxidase (MFO) activity, they also exhibit a greater capacity than adults to detoxify acetaminophen by phase II metabolic reactions, primarily sulfate conjugation. In addition, children possess higher glutathione turnover which may contribute to protection from hepatotoxicity. Thus, the lower susceptibility of children to acetaminophen poisoning is due to their greater capacity to eliminate the drug by nontoxic pathways. Nevertheless, children with a significant ingestion should have their plasma acetaminophen level measured and receive treatment with N-acetylcysteine (NAC) if the level falls within the toxic range on the nomogram. Notably, adolescents have a higher incidence of toxic plasma levels after ingestion than do younger children. Even if a serious case of hepatotoxicity develops, the mortality rate is less than 0.5%. Children who recover have no sequelae when observed 3–12 months after the acute toxicity; however, severely affected patients may require liver transplantation. *(McMillan, 760–761)*

2. **(D)** Alternative routes for drug administration are required in children more often than adults. Routes to consider are oral, intramuscular (IM), transdermal, and rectal administration. If an IV line cannot be established or the child is some distance from a medical center, rectal diazepam or lorazepam can be used safely. IM midazolam is as effective as IV diazepam initially or refractory. Diazepam diluted in 3 mL 0.9% NaCl is placed into the rectum by a syringe and a flexible tube at a dose of 0.3–0.5 mg/kg. The effective dose of rectal lorazepam is 0.05–0.1 mg/kg. Therapeutic serum levels occur within 5–10 minutes. IM administration of diazepam is an option, but is felt to be less efficacious than rectal dosing. *(McMillan, 703, 2296; Brunton, 4–7)*

3. **(C)** Prolonged administration (from an infusion error) resulted in the abnormally low peak of this scenario. Several steps can be taken to minimize problems with intravenous drug administration to infants and children. These include the following: standardization and documentation of the total administration time; documentation of the volume and content of the solution used to "flush" an intravenous dose; standardization of specific infusion techniques (infusion duration, volumes) for drugs with a narrow therapeutic index; standardization of dilution and infusion volumes for drugs given by intermittent IV injection; avoidance of attaching lines for drug infusion to a central hub with other solutions infused concurrently at widely disparate rates; preferential use of large-gauge cannula; maintenance of the recommended solution at a specified height above the infusion site for use with a gravity-based controller; and the use of low-volume tubing and the most distal sites for access of the drug into an existing intravenous line. *(Behrman, 333–336; Brunton, 4–7)*

4. **(A)** The case describes a child with tinea corporis and tinea capitus. These infections are caused by dermatophytes of the genera *Trichophyton* and *Microsporum*. These are infections of the dermis that can invade hair follicles when found in hair-containing areas such as the scalp. The typical

presentation is a circular rash with raised borders and a scaling interior. This diagnosis can be confirmed by a potassium hydroxide testing of a scraping of the lesion. Tinea capitus needs to be treated with a systemic antifungal—most commonly griseofulvin is used (A). In tinea capitus (scalp infection), the fungus invades the hair follicle and topical creams will not effectively treat the organism (B, D, E). Tinea corporis (body infection) can be treated with topical antifungal creams. Amoxicillin (C) is an antibiotic effective against bacterial infections and will not treat fungal infection. *(McMillan, 870–872)*

5. **(C)** Patients with severe asthma exacerbations often need admission to the hospital for administration of medications and supportive care. In very rare circumstances a patient with very severe asthma and poor air exchange will become obtunded and will need endotracheal intubation. The medications used to facilitate intubation in this scenario have two additional goals over routine intubation: first, it should not worsen the bronchospasm; and second, it should allow the physician/patient to ventilate once the endotracheal tube is placed as soon as possible. Ketamine and lidocaine can be used to prevent or reduce bronchoconstriction. Ketamine has been shown to have direct bronchodilatory effects, and lidocaine blunts the airway responsiveness, such as the coughing reflex. Rocuronium is one of the nondepolarizing muscle relaxants that does not cause bronchospasm and is indicated in rapid sequence intubation. The other medication combinations listed are not ideal because they do not incorporate medications that help to reduce bronchospasm and to achieve rapid return to spontaneous ventilation (A, B, D). Intubating without medication (E) in this case would be inappropriate. *(McMillan, 2682; Brunton, 346–375)*

6. **(C)** More than 800 cough and cold remedies are available over the counter in the United States. The majority of these medications contain some form of antihistamine, decongestant, antitussive, expectorants, and analgesics. A review article of the use of over-the-counter medications from 1950–1991 showed no good evidence for the effectiveness of over-the-counter medications for preschool-age children. A 2000

report from the American Association of Poison Control Centers showed that 5% of poisonous exposures to children under 6 years of age were related to cough and cold preparation exposure. Parents should always be counseled to consult a physician for dosing and safety of any over-the-counter medication (C). All over-the-counter medications whether or not they are labeled pediatric or children's possess some risk, therefore they are not safe (A, B). Most over-the-counter medications do contain acetaminophen (D). It is not safe to give over-the-counter medications containing acetaminophen, along with additional acetaminophen; there is risk for an overdose (E). *(McMillan, 764; Kelly, 25(4):115–123)*

7. **(A)** A Pediatric Fleet Enema is a hypertonic solution with high levels of phosphate. If these enemas are retained or are given in quick succession, there is a chance of inducing hyperphosphatemia, especially in conjunction with renal failure, although this can happen even without renal insufficiency. Hyperphosphatemia often manifests with the signs of an induced hypocalcemia—which are lethargy, tetany, and occasionally seizures. An albuterol overdose would most likely present as tachycardia, sweating, and tachypnea (B). Sepsis would likely present with fever, hypotension, and tachycardia (C). An asthma exacerbation would present with tachypnea and wheezing (D). Anaphylaxis would present with hypotension, wheezing, hives, and difficulty breathing (E). *(McMillan, 672–673;Maraffa, 20(7):453–456.)*

8. **(D)** Many allergy medications use decongestants which are often a form of an adrenergic agonist. Pseudoephedrine acts to release norepinephrine and causes a sympathetic surge. One of the useful effects of this as a decongestant is that it causes constriction of blood vessels and decreases edema by allowing less blood flow to the lining of the nose and sinuses. The systemic side effects manifest as tachycardia, restlessness, and hypertension (D). Intranasal pseudoephedrine will act locally, but does not have the degree of systemic action of oral pseudoephedrine. Diphenhydramine or Benadryl is an antihistamine. The most common side effect is drowsiness (B). Intranasal steroid sprays

have limited systemic side effects (C). Cromolyn is a mast cell stabilizer that blocks the release of histamine. Adverse effects are typically GI upset and throat irritation (E). *(McMillan, 2428–2432)*

9. **(B)** Atropine is one of the medications that can be delivered via endotracheal tube. It is an anticholinergic used to block vagal stimulation to the heart and raise the heart rate in bradycardic neonates. Other medications that can be administered via endotracheal tube are lidocaine, epinephrine, atropine and naloxone—the acronym LEAN can be used to remember these medications. Recently, vasopressin has been added as another agent that may be given via the endotracheal tube during cardiac arrest. This route can be an effective way to administer medication before IV access is obtained in any setting. Calcium chloride, amiodarone, dopamine, and phenobarbital should not be administered via endotracheal tube (A, C, D, E). *(McMillan, 208–210)*

10. **(D)** Topical benzocaine has been associated with methemoglobinemia. Methemoglobin is an oxidized form of hemoglobin that is not capable of carrying oxygen. This can manifest as cyanosis without showing a drop in the pulse oximeter. This state can be reversed by administering methylene blue. Acetaminophen overdose can manifest as hepatic dysfunction, not with cyanosis (A). Ibuprofen overdose can manifest with platelet dysfunction and renal impairment, not cyanosis (B). Pseudoephedrine has the side effect of tachycardia and hypertension (C). Aspirin side effects are metabolic acidosis and ringing in the ears (tinnitus). *(McMillan, 2696; Dahshan, 117:806–809)*

11. **(D)** The case describes a patient with mild persistent asthma. Asthma severity is classified by frequency of symptoms during the day and symptoms at night.

TABLE 9-1.

Classification	Days with Symptoms	Nights with Symptoms
Mild intermittent	″ 2/week	″ 2/month
Mild persistent	3-6/week	3-4/month
Moderate persistent	Daily	≥ 5/month
Severe persistent	Continuous	Frequent

The treatment of mild persistent asthma is the initiation of a controller medication plus the use of albuterol as needed—the most effective controller is a low dose inhaled corticosteroid twice daily (D). Albuterol alone will not control the persistent nature of this patient's symptoms (A). Over the counter cough medication does not address the root of the problems and symptoms will persist (B). Albuterol twice daily may help with symptoms, but albuterol should be given on an as needed basis and a controller medication given twice daily (C). Systemic steroids daily are used for acute exacerbations of asthma for a short course and for severe persistent asthma as a long term therapy (E). *(McMillan, 2407)*

12. **(C)** The above case describes mucocutaneous lymph node syndrome or Kawasaki disease. This is a disease of unknown etiology which has a set of diagnostic criteria that need to be met to make the diagnosis. The presence of high spiking fever for 5 days plus at least four or five of the following: (1) bilateral bulbar conjunctival injection; (2) mucous membrane changes; (3) extremity changes—erythema, edema, desquamation; (4) polymorphous rash—primarily truncal; (5) single large cervical lymph node. The treatment of choice after recognition is a combination of IVIG and high-dose aspirin. This treatment has been shown to decrease the complication rate of coronary artery aneurysm if administered during the first 10 days of fever (C). Acetaminophen and ibuprofen will lower the fever, but will not lessen the complication rate (A, D). IV antibiotics have no role in the treatment of Kawasaki disease (B). Steroids are generally not considered part of the initial treatment for Kawasaki disease (E). *(McMillan, 1015–1020)*

13. **(C)** The use of local anesthetic with epinephrine is contraindicated in areas that have an end-organ arterial supply. These areas include the ear, tip of the nose, distal extremities, and the digits. The epinephrine will cause vasoconstriction and will allow the local anesthetic to work more effectively and longer, however vasoconstriction in an end-organ vascular bed can cause ischemia. The shoulder, cheek, neck,

and forehead would be appropriate places to use local anesthetic mixed with epinephrine (A, B, D, E). *(McMillan, 2672)*

14. **(A)** Magnesium sulfate is used as a smooth muscle relaxant and can be used to help control bronchospasm in severe asthma and cause vasodilatation (A). Calcium chloride, sodium phosphate, potassium chloride, and sodium bicarbonate do not have any bronchodilating properties (B, C, D, E). *(McMillan, 699)*

15. **(D)** Children with epilepsy often will outgrow their seizure disorder and be medication free in later life. Some patients have a progressive neurologic disorder that will require escalating medication doses and the addition of medications. In a child with increasing seizure frequency who is on a medication, it is important to check the serum drug level to be sure that it is in a therapeutic range. If the medication is subtherapeutic, it may indicate noncompliance with the medication or that the dose needs to be increased due to increasing volume of distribution or changes in metabolism (D). Adding a second agent at this time would not be the next best step in the management before knowing if the phenytoin level is normal (A, B, C). Performing an EEG is unlikely to be helpful because you already know that the patient has a seizure disorder and the child's clinical presentation is consistent with seizures (E). *(McMillan, 2288)*

16. **(A)** The diagnosis of ADHD is made by observing the symptoms of impulsivity and hyperactivity in more than one setting. This child clearly exhibits these behaviors in school and in the home. Occasionally it is worth a trial of a stimulant medication to see if this helps to control these behaviors and allows the child to perform better in the school setting. Stimulants are reported to be effective in 70% of individuals with ADHD. Methylphenidate is one stimulant medication that is commonly prescribed. Common side effects include decreased appetite and decreased sleep (A). Imipramine is a tricyclic antidepressant (TCA) and paroxetine is a selective serotonin reuptake inhibitor (SSRI), both used to treat major depressive disorder (B, D). Haloperidol is an antipsychotic

used to treat acute psychosis (C). Phenytoin is an antiepileptic used to treat seizure disorders (E). *(McMillan, 674–680)*

17. **(C)** A patent ductus arteriosus is a common abnormality seen in premature infants secondary to hypoxia, acidosis, and increased pulmonary pressure from significant lung disease. The ductus arteriosus should close within the first 2–3 days of life, when this does not occur properly the patient can exhibit signs of pulmonary edema and heart failure. One medical option for assisting the ductus to close is the initiation of indomethacin. Indomethacin inhibits prostaglandin synthesis and allows the ductus to close. Repeat courses may be needed. If this is ineffective, surgical correction may be needed. A dopamine infusion would be needed if the patient were hypotensive, and is not appropriate in this case (A). Administration of 100% oxygen may cause a lowering of the pulmonary vascular resistance and cause more pulmonary blood flow, worsening pulmonary edema (B). A prostaglandin infusion is used to keep a ductus arteriosus open in the case of cyanotic heart disease (D). Corticosteroids have no role in the closure of a patent ductus arteriosus (E). *(McMillan, 226)*

18. **(D)** This is most likely a dystonic reaction caused by the antiemetic, metoclopramide. This is an uncommon side effect of metoclopramide administration. Dystonia often manifests with head turning (acute torticollis) and severe back arching (opisthotonos). Acute dystonia should be treated with IV diphenhydramine or benztropine. This is unlikely to be hypocalcemia or tetany, given the time relationship to the medication administration (A, B). This is unlikely to be a seizure because he is awake and alert during the episode and has no mention of a seizure history (D). This is unlikely to be meningitis; the child is awake and alert and does not show meningeal signs (E). *(McMillan, 2372–2373)*

19. **(D)** Neuromuscular blocking agents are classified as either nondepolarizing or depolarizing agents. Nondepolarizing agents act as competitive antagonists for acetylcholine at the acetylcholine receptor of the neuromuscular

junction. By blocking the receptor without stimulating it, they stop neuromuscular transmission from occurring. Pancuronium, vecuronium, atracurium, and rocuronium are examples of nondepolarizing neuromuscular blockers (A, B, C, E). The depolarizing agents such as succinylcholine interact with the receptor and cause the muscle end-plate to depolarize. Unlike acetylcholine, succinylcholine is resistant to degradation by acetylcholinesterase and as such continues to occupy the receptor preventing the muscle from repolarizing. The depolarizing neuromuscular blockers, succinylcholine, are contraindicated in patients with muscular dystrophy. (*McMillan, 2682; Brunton, 196–199*)

20. **(B)** Long-term therapy with thiazide diuretics has been shown to be beneficial in the management of CLD-related pulmonary edema (also called, bronchopulmonary dysplasia or BPD). A thiazide diuretic acts by blocking the reabsorption of sodium and chloride in the thin portion of the ascending limb of the loop of Henle. In addition, they block the reabsorption of calcium leading to hypercalciuria, which can lead to the production of nephrocalcinosis and eventual renal failure. Increased urinary excretion of potassium can result in hypokalemia. The thiazides block the excretion of uric acid and can lead to hyperuricemia with symptomatic gout in susceptible patients. (*McMillan, 323–324*)

21. **(C)** While daily administration of phenobarbital may reduce the recurrence rate for febrile seizures, the continuous administration of phenobarbital is not necessary or recommended. The therapy does not prevent the development of epilepsy. In addition, undesirable side effects (rashes, hyperactivity, irritability, lethargy) are found in at least 20% of patients taking continuous phenobarbital. Phenytoin has not been shown to be effective. Although valproic acid and phenobarbital are effective, the potential toxicities outweigh the benefit and their routine use. Intermittent therapy with phenobarbital is ineffective. (*McMillan, 2298*)

22. **(C)** Nitrite poisoning can result from medication overdose or ingestion (amyl nitrate, nitroglycerin, nitrate food additives, or contaminated well water). Nitrites increase the oxidation of hemoglobin, resulting in methemoglobinemia. Methemoglobin contains oxidized iron (ferric or Fe^{3+}) as opposed to reduced iron (ferrous or Fe^{2+}) found in normal hemoglobin. Methemoglobin can be converted to hemoglobin by a reducing agent such as methylene blue, which is administered intravenously as a 1% solution. (*Behrman, 1610*)

23. **(A)** Although many organisms can cause endocarditis following a dental procedure, *Streptococcus viridans* remains the most common. Penicillin is highly effective, with a longer half-life, and is the drug of choice. For those allergic to penicillins or amoxicillin against this organism, but amoxicillin, the use of cephalexin or another first-generation oral cephalosporin, clindamycin, or a macrolide such as azithromycin, or clarithromycin is recommended. (*McMillan, 1652–1655*)

24. **(C)** Penicillins and cephalosporins are ineffective against *Mycoplasma*. Erythromycin, azithromycin, and tetracycline are all effective. However, tetracycline causes discoloring deposited in growing bone and teeth and is generally not recommended for those under 8 years of age. Although deposits have not been shown to have significant pathophysiologic effects, it does cause staining of the teeth that is cosmetically unacceptable. Chloramphenicol is effective; however, the infrequent but lethal side effect of aplastic anemia restricts use of this drug to certain serious infections. (*McMillan, 540, 1399*)

25. **(A)** The sodium nitroprusside molecule contains cyanide which is released following the metabolism of the parent compound. Cyanide normally is converted by the rhodanese enzyme of the liver to thiocyanate, which is then excreted by the kidneys. The risk of cyanide toxicity increases with the dose and the duration of administration of sodium nitroprusside. Cyanide binds to cytochrome oxidase and inhibits oxidative phosphorylation leading to a metabolic acidosis. Cyanide also increases the effects of catecholamines on the smooth muscle of the arterioles leading to an increase in blood pressure and a need to increase the dose of nitroprusside (tachyphylaxis). Treatment of

cyanide toxicity includes discontinuation of sodium nitroprusside and administration of thiosulfate. Thiosulfate provides a sulfur donor for the rhodanese enzyme to convert cyanide to thiocyanate. In extreme cases, amyl nitrite or sodium nitrite is administered to induce methemoglobinemia since cyanide will bind to the methemoglobin instead of the cytochrome oxidase. (Brunton, 88–90)

26. **(B)** Ethosuximide is one of the drugs of choice in the treatment of absence (petit mal) seizures. Amotrigine (Lamictal) or valproic acid (Depakene, Depakote) are other commonly prescribed anticonvulsants for absence seizure. (McMillan, 2289)

27. **(B)** Many rodent poisons contain warfarin, an anticoagulant that inhibits the production of prothrombin by the liver, leading to hemorrhage. Symptoms typically are delayed for 12–24 hours following ingestion. The degree and duration of toxicity is variable depending on the size of the child, amount of ingestion, and formulation of the rodenticide. The hepatic toxicity can be effectively counteracted by large doses of vitamin K. (McMillan, 1747–1748; Brunton, 1529–1531)

28. **(C)** Ingestion of toxic doses of acetaminophen (> 140 mg/kg) results in the depletion of hepatic glutathione stores and the production of the toxic intermediate metabolite, N-acetylbenxoquinoneimine. The toxic intermediate metabolite covalently binds to hepatocytes and leads to cellular death. N-acetylcysteine acts as a surrogate glutathione or sulfate donor and thereby prevents the binding of the toxic intermediary to the hepatocyte. Therapy is indicated based on the history and should be administered regardless of the level. N-acetylcysteine is most effective if administered within 12–24 hours postingestion. (McMillan, 759–764)

29. **(A)** The most likely diagnosis is congenital adrenal hyperplasia or CAH. CAH results from an enzymatic defect in the adrenal cortical production of corticosteroids. Ninety percent of cases and the one presenting as outlined above result from deficiency of the 21-hydroxylase enzyme. Without this enzyme, there is deficiency of corticosteroids resulting in an Addisonian-like state and deficiency of aldosterone resulting in hyperkalemia. The overproduction of adrenal androgens can result in virilization of female infants. Careful physical examination is necessary to be certain that the testes are palpable and that the infant in question is not a virilized female. (McMillan, 2138–2140)

30. **(E)** Stimulant drugs such as methylphenidate (Ritalin), amphetamines, and atomoxetine (Strattera) have been shown to have a beneficial effect in many children with attention-deficit hyperactivity disorder. The seemingly paradoxical calming action of stimulant drugs in these children may be related to increased awareness of, and therefore response to, external stimuli, permitting sustained attention. The drugs have no role in the management of seizure disorders, temper tantrums, or breath-holding spells. Appetite suppression often is a side effect of these drugs. (McMillan, 678–680)

31. **(B)** The increasing percentage of *Streptococcus pneumoniae* resistant to penicillin has followed widespread overuse of antibiotics. Isolates which are nonsusceptible to penicillin (including both intermediate and resistant strains) are defined by minimum inhibitory concentration (MIC) testing and the definition of nonsusceptible varies depending on whether or not the isolate is from a meningeal or nonmeningeal source. Meningitis or septicemia potentially caused by *S pneumoniae* should be initially treated with a third-generation cephalosporin plus either vancomycin. Therapy should be appropriately tailored based on susceptibility testing of the organism isolated. Cefuroxime is a second-generation cephalosporin and is not recommended in the treatment of meningitis. (McMillan, 929–930)

32. **(C)** Although a diagnosis of sepsis should not be eliminated immediately, hypoplastic left heart syndrome or other obstructive left-sided cardiac lesions are most likely, given this neonate's clinical presentation. The most common clinical presentation of hypoplastic left heart syndrome is respiratory distress on the second or third day of life. Prostaglandin E_1 maintains patency of the ductus arteriosus and thereby preserves blood flow to the systemic

circulation. Although this is deoxygenated blood due to total mixing, there is adequate oxygen delivery to maintain life. Milrinone is a phosphodiesterase inhibitor whose cardiovascular effects include increased inotropy and peripheral vasodilatation. These effects are similar to dobutamine which acts through $beta_{1,2}$-adrenergic receptors. (*McMillan, 1558–1561*)

33. **(A)** Octreotide is a somatostatin analogue that increases the resistance in the splanchnic vasculature and reduces portal venous pressure, thereby decreasing the bleeding from esophageal varices. It has replaced vasopressin in this clinical situation as octreotide has less of an effect on systemic blood pressure. (*McMillan, 2064–2066*)

34. **(E)** Cystic fibrosis is the most common cause of pancreatic insufficiency in childhood. Most patients with this disease have less steatorrhea and improved weight gain when receiving pancreatic replacement therapy. (*McMillan, 1436*)

35. **(E)** Neonatal meningitis and sepsis most commonly are caused by group B streptococcus, gram-negative enteric bacilli, or *Listeria monocytogenes*. Initial combination therapy with ampicillin plus gentamicin; or ampicillin plus cefotaxime is recommended though the latter regimen is preferred if meningitis is present. Neither the cephalosporins nor gentamicin provides coverage against *L monocytogenes*. Cefuroxime is not recommended for treatment of meningitis because of reports of delayed CSF sterilization. (*McMillan, 493–495*)

36. **(A)** In addition to treating oncologic conditions, cyclophosphamide is used in immunosuppressive regimens for autoimmune disorders and organ transplantation. High doses of cyclophosphamide results in bladder epithelial dysplasia, hemorrhagic cystitis, and sterility. (*Brunton, 1395–1396*)

37. **(B)** Erythromycin has historically been the drug of choice to prevent spread of pertussis though currently, azithromycin is generally preferred as therapy. On rare instances *Bordetella pertussis* has been found to be macrolide resistant; in such a case, trimethoprim-sulfamethoxazole is an alternative but its efficacy is less well documented. Treatment of the index case generally will eradicate the organism from the tracheobronchial tree and reduce spread. Although erythromycin alters the clinical course of pertussis when given early in the paroxysmal stage, it does not seem to alter the clinical course if started later in the illness. A 14-day course of erythromycin is recommended for prevention and treatment of pertussis; a 5 day course is recommended for azithromycin. (*McMillan, 1094–1097*)

38. **(A)** This case describes an 8-year-old with primary nocturnal enuresis. The male to female ratio is 3:2 for this disorder. About 15% of 5-year-olds and 5% of 10-year-olds have enuresis. There are many therapy options; however behavioral conditioning has been shown to have the best success rate of 70%–80% (A). DDAVP (B) is used to decrease urine output for 1–7 hours, is very expensive therapy, and has been shown to have a 40%–60% success rate with a high rate of relapse after discontinuation (B). Imipramine is a tricyclic antidepressant which is FDA approved to treat enuresis, it has been shown to be 30%–50% effective (C). Motivational therapy, such as a reward system for not wetting the bed has been shown to be only 25% effective (D). Furosemide is a diuretic and would not be useful in the treatment of enuresis (E). (*McMillan, 670–672*)

39. **(B)** Minimal change disease is characterized by nephrotic syndrome without systemic disease. Two-thirds of the cases present between the ages of 2 to 6. The recommended treatment regiment is to start a course of high-dose corticosteroids and to follow urine protein to see if there is a response. Severe cases may need hospitalization for diuretic therapy; however most cases caught early can be treated as an outpatient. IVIG (A) is not indicated as a first-line therapy for minimal change disease, it is a first-line treatment for Kawasaki disease. A kidney biopsy (C) is not indicated with this presentation of nephrotic syndrome. Minimal change disease is by far the most likely diagnosis and a kidney biopsy will be of little help and a high morbidity. If the patient does not respond to the course of steroids, a biopsy may be appropriate.

Cyclophosphamide (D) is a second-line therapy for minimal change disease. Antibiotic therapy (E) is not indicated for minimal change disease; however an early presentation may be confused with a peri-orbital cellulitis. *(McMillan, 1867–1868)*

40. **(C)** Idiopathic thrombocytopenia purpura (ITP) is an autoimmune-mediated disease that leads to the destruction of platelets via the reticuloen-dothelial system. Serious complications are rare; however with a platelet count of less than 20,000 there is a risk for intracranial hemorrhage. Anti-d immunoglobulin (or Rhogam) is the treatment of choice for patients with ITP who are Rh positive. The mechanism of action is not fully understood, however the theory is that the anti-d coats red blood cells and these antibody-coated red blood cells compete with the platelets for destruction by the reticuloendothelial system. A complication of this therapy is a mild anemia from the red cell destruction. This therapy only works in patients who are Rh-positive blood type. IVIG (A) is a second-line therapy for patients with Rh-positive blood type and first line for patients who are Rh negative. Amoxicillin (B) and antibiotics have no role in the treatment of ITP. A platelet transfusion (D) is not indicated in the acute setting of ITP, the transfused platelets will be destroyed via the same mechanism outlined above and will offer little benefit. Observation (E) is not a good option in this patient. With a platelet count of less than 20,000 and small mucosal bleeding, there is a risk of intracranial hemorrhage. *(McMillan, 1731–1733)*

41. **(D)** The child in the case has the diagnosis of acute chest syndrome. The diagnosis of acute chest syndrome is made in children with sickle cell disease when a new infiltrate is found on chest x-ray. Acute chest syndrome can have serious short- and long-term complications and lead to respiratory failure. Antibiotics should be started in a timely manor and both a third-generation cephalosporin and a macrolide are recommended (D). Amoxicillin, ceftriaxone, and azithromycin alone would not be sufficient therapy (A, B, C). Withholding antibiotic therapy would not be appropriate in this case, even if this is a viral process, acute chest syndrome should be treated with antibiotics. *(McMillan, 1697)*

42. **(D)** Notification to the local poison center can provide guidance and follow-up of all forms of toxic exposures, including acetaminophen toxicity. Acetaminophen toxicity can occur in a child if the dose is in the range of 150 mg/kg per 24 hour period. It should be treated with either oral or IV *N*-acetylcysteine as soon as the elevated acetaminophen level is detected, regardless of hepatic enzyme levels. This treatment can help prevent further liver dysfunction and avoid liver transplantation (D). Steroids and furosemide have no role in the treatment of acetaminophen toxicity (A, B). Naloxone is used to reverse opioid toxicity (C). Providing no treatment to this child may allow the liver dysfunction to worsen and the child may progress toward fulminate liver failure and liver transplant (E). *(McMillan, 751–752)*

43. **(D)** Pelvic inflammatory disease is caused by *Chlamydia* and gonococcal infection of the upper reproductive tract. It can have long-term complications if not treated properly, such as infertility, ectopic pregnancy, and abdominal adhesions. Since PID can be polymicrobial infections, it is important to treat all potential causes. Ceftriaxone and doxycycline (D) is an acceptable outpatient treatment regimen for PID. Clindamycin in conjunction with gentamicin is an acceptable inpatient treatment regimen; however clindamycin alone is not sufficient (A). Neither ceftriaxone nor doxycycline alone is an adequate treatment regimen. Metronidazole is used to treat trichomonal infections and can be used in conjunction with an accepted treatment regimen, but should not be used as a single agent (E). *(McMillan, 587–590)*

44. **(C)** Dysfunctional uterine bleeding (DUB) is common during adolescence and can be concerning to the patients, but is often self-resolving over time. If the patient is having frequent bleeding and wants to become regular, the best therapy is an oral contraceptive pill with estrogen and progestin (C). A platelet disorder may manifest as heavy menses, but often has other signs of bleeding and low platelets, this patient does not have any other signs (B). Testosterone cream is not indicated for dysfunctional uterine bleeding (A). NSAIDs are the first-line therapy

for dysmenorrhea, or painful menses, not for DUB (D). Careful observation may be a potential choice for a patient with DUB as most cases will self-resolve. This patient is looking for an intervention that will help make her menses more regular and oral contraceptives are the clear choice. *(McMillan, 564–565)*

45. **(E)** Careful examination, close observation, and reliable follow-up represent an important approach to many pediatric complaints. This case describes erythema toxicum neonatorum which is a benign rash of the neonate that is self-resolving and requires no treatment (E). The rash typically starts out as papules of 2–3 mm in diameter and progresses to vesicles and then resolves over 2 weeks. The vesicles are noted to contain a large number of eosinophils when looked at under a microscope. Acyclovir (A) is the treatment for cutaneous herpes simplex infection, this patient's history and microscopic findings are not consistent with this diagnosis. Topical steroids are often used for eczema and atopic dermatitis (B). Antidandruff shampoo is the first-line treatment for seborrhea (cradle cap). Phototherapy is the first-line treatment for hyperbilirubinemia (D). *(McMillan, 461)*

46. **(C)** Intraosseous needle insertion is often the quickest means to vascular access, however, this patient's status provides for a reasonable attempt at peripheral venous access. Intracardiac (D) and arterial access (B) are not appropriate for this patient. Surgical cut down (E) should only be pursued when intraosseous and central venous access methods have failed or cannot be pursued (such as multiple trauma). *(McMillan, 2675–2677)*

47. **(B)** This case scenario describes a child with sciatic nerve injury following intramuscular injection into the gluteal region. Although postinjection injury can occur in both adults and children, children appear to be at higher risk. The degree of nerve injury appears to be related to direct nerve trauma by the needle, host response to the trauma (inflammation), and toxicity of the agent injected. For instance, Penicillin G is considered to be more toxic to the nerve. An allergic reaction to penicillin would not cause these symptoms (A). The

anterolateral thigh (C) and deltoid (D) muscle appear to have the lowest risk for complications such as bleeding, muscle contracture, and nerve injury. Though cerebral vascular accident (E) is within the differential for new onset of neurologic findings, it does not best describe this clinical scenario. *(McMillan, 2685–2687)*

48. **(B)** Cardiomyopathy most commonly is an adverse effect related to the administration of anthracyclines such as doxorubicin. Children are at higher risk for cardiac toxicity and those younger than 5 years are at higher risk than older children. Both acute and chronic cardiac toxicity can occur. The acute phase is characterized by arrhythmias and conduction abnormalities. Chronic cardiomyopathies can occur early (within a year of anthracycline therapy) and late (greater than a year after completing anthracycline therapy). The early form of cardiomyopathy is related to the cumulative dose of anthracyclines. A high-dose rate and preexisting cardiac disease can also increase the risk. *(Brunton, 1428; Behrman, 2112)*

49. **(E)** Neurotoxicity in this form of peripheral neuropathy is a dose-limiting toxicity that can occur with the use of vincristine. It is related to the cumulative dose and occurs more commonly on a weekly schedule. It often presents as a peripheral mixed neuropathy involving both the sensory and motor nerves. Loss of deep tendon reflexes, paresthesias, and wrist and foot drop are the most common manifestations. *(Behrman, 1967, 21126, Brunton, 1418–1419)*

50. **(C)** Although steroids are first-line therapy for acute graft-versus-host disease (GVHD), they are not without their risks, particularly in this patient population that may require long-term therapy to suppress GVHD symptoms. Infection, hypertension, hyperglycemia, weakness, and HPA-axis suppression are common side effects of corticosteroids. Growth retardation, psychosis, osteoporosis, central obesity, moon facies, acne, hirsutism, pseudotumor cerebri, and glaucoma can also occur. Cataracts can occur with long-term therapy. *(Behrman, 930–931; McMillan, 1765)*

51. (E) The patient has a head injury and is at risk for increased intracranial pressure. Ketamine increases ICP and is relatively contraindicated in patients with intracranial hypertension, and should be avoided in this patient. All of the other agents decrease the cerebral metabolic rate for oxygen and thereby decrease cerebral blood flow and intracranial pressure, which could be beneficial if there is a head bleed increasing the ICP. *(Behrman, 466; McMillan, 2682)*

52. (D) Nitric oxide (NO) is a naturally occurring vasodilator. PPHN occurs in term and post-term infants. Predisposing factors include birth asphyxia, meconium aspiration pneumonia, early-onset sepsis, HMD, hypoglycemia, polycythemia, maternal use of nonsteroidal anti-inflammatory drugs with in utero constriction of the ductus arteriosus, and pulmonary hypoplasia as a result of diaphragmatic hernia, amniotic fluid leak, oligohydramnios, or pleural effusions. PPHN is often idiopathic. Some patients with PPHN have low plasma arginine and nitric oxide metabolite concentrations and polymorphisms of the carbamoyl phosphate synthase gene, findings suggestive of a possible subtle defect in nitric oxide production. Exogenous surfactant therapy has been beneficial in some patients. iNO (inhaled nitric oxide), a potent and selective pulmonary vasodilator (equivalent to endothelium-derived relaxation factor), when given at an initial dose of 1–20 ppm, has improved oxygenation in patients with PPHN and reduce the need for ECMO. Although brief exposure to higher doses (40–80 ppm) appears to be safe, long-term treatment with 80 ppm increases the adverse effects. Responses to iNO include no improvement; initial improvement but not sustained, with ECMO being required; initial and sustained improvement, usually weaned by the fifth day of therapy; and an initial response but prolonged dependency, possibly as a result of pulmonary hypoplasia or alveolar capillary dysplasia. Methemoglobinemia is a rare but possible complication of iNO. The maximal safe duration of iNO therapy is unknown. *(McMillan, 316–318)*

53. (E) The treatment of acidosis is critical in the management of salicylate intoxication. Acidosis enhances the passage of salicylate (nonionized form) from the extracellular space into the cells, including the blood–brain barrier, where it disrupts mitochondrial function. Salicylates are weak acids that in an alkaline medium dissociate to the ionized form and can be "trapped" there. Sodium bicarbonate's alkalinization effect occurs solely in the extracellular space and increases the level of ionized drug in the extracellular plasma. The intracellular-to-extracellular gradient of diffusible, nonionized drug is increased, thus enhancing the trapping of salicylate in the extracellular plasma. Alkalinization of the blood with sodium bicarbonate can prevent salicylates from entering the brain and CSF, alkalinization of the urine results in enhanced urinary salicylate excretion. CNS status may improve as the plasma pH increases, because of a shift of salicylate equilibrium from brain to blood despite a lack of urine alkalinization. Cardiac arrhythmias and seizures are not common in salicylate poisoning. Sodium bicarbonate alone will not worsen his hydration status, but fluids should be replaced as needed and fluid status and urine output should be carefully monitored. *(McMillan, 757)*

54. (B) Morphine is a commonly used opioid for the treatment of sickle cell disease both chronically and for acute pain crises. It is available as an intravenous medication, and can be given on a PCA pump for those old enough to use them. It is also available in several long-acting and short-acting preparations for chronic pain and breakthrough pain as needed. Fentanyl is the shortest acting of the agents listed and is available intravenous, as a lozenge, or as a transdermal long-acting patch, but oral formulations are not available. Oxycodone comes as long- and short-acting oral preparations, but is not available IV. Meperidine is available IV or as a short-acting oral preparation, but should be avoided due to the adverse effects of its active metabolite, normeperidine. Methadone is available as IV and oral, but has the longest half-life and is not used as a short-acting medication. *(Berhman, 2027–2028, 479–480)*

55. (E) This child is most likely under volume resuscitated and requires an intravascular fluid bolus. In the setting of high insensible losses (such as a burn injury), low urine output suggests low intravascular fluid volume. For most children with burns, the Parkland formula is an appropriate starting guideline for fluid resuscitation (4 mL lactated Ringer/kg/% BSA burned). One-half of the fluid is given over the first 8 hours calculated from the time of onset of injury. The remaining half is given at an even rate over the next 16 hours. The rate of infusion is adjusted according to the patient's response to therapy. Pulse and blood pressure should return to normal, and an adequate urine output (1 mL/kg/h) should be accomplished by varying the intravenous infusion rate. Inadequate urine output reflects depleted intravascular volume. Although it will temporarily increase urine output, the use of diuretics will only further decrease the intravascular volume. (*Behrman, 452–454; McMillan, 711–712*)

56. **(C)** Management strategies of infants born with HLHS classically have been divided into three basic approaches: staged palliative reconstruction, cardiac transplantation, and supportive care only. Immediate medical management is centered on maintaining ductal patency and optimizing the balance between systemic and pulmonary vascular resistance. Intravenous prostaglandin E$_1$ is effective in maintaining patency of the ductus arteriosus and enables the neonate to have optimized cardiac hemodynamics and a normalized acid-base balance before surgical intervention. Intravenous indomethacin and ibuprofen will close the ductus arteriosus. Preoperative management should avoid excessive pulmonary blood flow; oxygen administration, hyperventilation, and high-dose inotropic agents should be avoided if possible so as not to alter the tentative balance between the pulmonary and systemic vascular beds. (*McMillan, 1560; Behrman, 1926–1928*)

57. **(E)** Lyme disease is the most common vector-borne disease in the United States. Most cases occur in southern New England, the eastern parts of the Middle Atlantic states, and the upper Midwest, with a smaller endemic focus of Lyme disease along the Pacific coast. Lyme disease is a zoonosis caused by the transmission of the spirochete *Borrelia burgdorferi* to humans through the bite of an infected tick of the *Ixodes* species. The first clinical manifestation of Lyme disease is the typical annular rash,

named erythema migrans. The initial lesion occurs at the site of the bite. The rash may be uniformly erythematous, or it may appear as a target lesion with central clearing; rarely, there may be central vesicular or necrotic areas. Erythema migrans may be associated with systemic features including fever, myalgia, headache, or malaise. Without treatment, the rash gradually expands (hence the name *migrans*) to an average diameter of 15 cm and remains present for at least 1–2 weeks. No clinical trials of treatment for Lyme disease have been conducted in children. Recommendations for the treatment of children are extrapolated from studies of adults. Doxycycline (100 mg twice daily × 14-21 days) for older children or amoxicillin (50 mg/kg/day divided three times daily × 14–21 days) are first-line therapy. Patients who are treated with doxycycline should be alerted to the risk of developing dermatitis in sun-exposed areas while taking the medication. Cefuroxime is also approved for the treatment of Lyme disease and is an alternative for persons who cannot take doxycycline and who are allergic to penicillin. Preliminary results with azithromycin have been disappointing. There is little need to use newer agents because the results of treatment with either amoxicillin or doxycycline have been good. (*McMillan, 1046–1049; Behrman, 1274–1278*)

58. **(E)** The most common organisms causing meningitis in children are *Streptococcus pneumoniae* and *Neisseria meningitidis*. After the introduction of *Haemophilus influenzae* type b conjugate vaccine in 1988, there was a greater than 99% decline in invasive disease caused by *H influenzae* type b, including meningitis. Penicillin remains the drug of choice for the treatment of meningococcal meningitis. It is highly effective, inexpensive, and generally free of significant side effects, except for allergic reactions. Ceftriaxone, cefotaxime, or ampicillin are acceptable alternatives. Several of the third-generation cephalosporins are useful for the treatment of bacterial meningitis (including *H influenzae* and S. pneumoniae meningitis) prior to identification of the infecting organism. However, once *N meningitides* has been identified, penicillin becomes the antibiotic of choice. Penicillin G should be administered IV at a

dose of 250,000–400,000 units/kg/day divided every 4–6 hours. *(Behrman, 2514–2519, 1164–1168)*

59. **(B)** Deferoxamine is the chelating agent of choice for iron poisoning. Deferoxamine binds with iron to form a water-soluble compound, ferrioxamine, which can be renally excreted or dialyzed. Deferoxamine may also limit the entrance of iron into the cell and help chelate intracellular iron. Because of its short half-life, it is administered as a continuous infusion at a dose of 15 mg/kg/h for up to 24 hours. Rapid administration of deferoxamine can lead to hypotension, which should be treated by reducing the infusion rate. Deferoxamine is indicated for severe intoxication (ingestion of more than 25 mg/kg of elemental iron or severe illness) or a serum iron concentration greater than 350 mg/dL. The use of activated charcoal, ipecac, and gastric lavage for iron poisoning are no longer recommended for acute iron ingestion. Dimercaprol (BAL) actually enhances the toxicity of iron and is contraindicated in cases of iron ingestion. EDTA is used for lead poisoning, not iron poisoning. *(McMillan, 751–752)*

60. **(D)** The most likely diagnosis is acute pancreatitis, given this clinical scenario. Though the differential diagnosis includes gastritis and peptic ulcer, the epigastric pain with radiation into the back is more characteristic of pancreatitis. The most likely etiologies of pancreatitis in the pediatric age group include trauma, viral infections, gallbladder disease, drugs, and toxins. The latter groups include corticosteroids, alcohol, valproic acid, tetracycline, and furosemide. Diagnostic evaluation should include a serum amylase and lipase. *(Behrman, 1652–1654)*

61. **(E)** Treatment of gonococcal urethritis depends on achieving a high antimicrobial level in the serum for a short time; prolonged treatment is not required. Benzathine penicillin should never be used as it will not achieve sufficiently high blood levels. Procaine penicillin 4.8 million units IM with 1 g of probenecid is effective against penicillin-sensitive strains. However, penicillin resistance is so common that a single dose of ceftriaxone, 125 mg IM, is generally the treatment of choice and provides high bactericidal levels in the blood. Extensive clinical experience indicates that ceftriaxone is safe and effective for the treatment of uncomplicated gonorrhea at all anatomic sites, curing 98.9% of uncomplicated urogenital and anorectal infections in published clinical trials. Patients infected with *Neisseria gonorrhoeae* frequently are coinfected with *Chlamydia trachomatis*; this finding has led to the recommendation that patients treated for gonococcal infection also be treated routinely with a regimen that is effective against uncomplicated genital *C trachomatis* infection. To maximize compliance with recommended therapies, medications for gonococcal infections should be dispensed on site. Azithromycin 1 g as a single oral dose or doxycycline 100 mg PO bid for 7 days are effective for the treatment of chlamydial infections, not gonococcal infections. Either regimen should be added to the ceftriaxone to treat the possible coinfection with chlamydia. *(McMillan, 584–590)*

62. **(A)** Liver injury is the major toxic effect of acetaminophen poisoning and generally is seen only with large overdoses or poisonings. In adults, greater than 150mg/kg is considered toxic, whereas in children, greater than 200 mg/kg is considered toxic. Generally, children less than 2 years old tend to have the least toxicity. The hepatic damage is not caused by the acetaminophen itself, but rather by the toxic metabolic product. The metabolic pathway producing the hepatotoxic metabolite is less well developed in infants and young children, and therefore, the risks of liver injury are actually somewhat less in young children. Treatment involves administration of N-acetylcysteine, either oral or IV, which minimizes metabolism of the acetaminophen to the toxic metabolite. Treatment is most effective if started within 24 hours of ingestion. Alkalinization of the urine and dialysis are ineffective treatment modalities. *(McMillan, 759–764)*

63. **(B)** Ampicillin plus an aminoglycoside is the initial treatment of choice for a newborn infant with presumptive group B streptococcus infection. However, once group B streptococcus has been identified and demonstrated to be susceptible, then switching to penicillin G is the drug of choice to treat group B streptococcal infections, including meningitis. Treatment should be continued for 14–21 days. *(McMillan, 505)*

64. (A) The most important toxic effect of the tricyclic antidepressants is sodium channel blockade. The cardiac sodium channel is responsible for cardiac cell depolarization (action potential phase 0); its inhibition leads to slowed depolarization of individual cardiac cells. This, in turn, leads to slowing of the wave of depolarization across the myocardium. The ECG manifestation of slowed depolarization is prolongation of the QRS complex, the hallmark of TCA overdose. QRS prolongation serves as a marker for TCA ingestion and the risk of adverse cardiac or central nervous system events; such as ventricular tachycardia or seizures. This is true not just because QRS prolongation identifies patients who have ingested a substantial overdose, but also because slowed cardiac conduction is the proximate cause of much of the cardiovascular toxicity of these drugs. Additional toxic effects of TCAs include alpha-adrenergic blockade (causing systemic vasodilation/hypotension), and cholinergic muscarinic receptor blockade may cause an "anticholinergic syndrome," including sinus tachycardia, delirium, coma, mydriasis, impaired gut motility, urinary retention, impaired sweating, and dry mucosa. *(McMillan, 753–754)*

65. (B) The most effective intervention for the cardiovascular toxicity of TCA overdose is sodium bicarbonate ($NaHCO_3$ = 1 molar, or 1 meq/mL). $NaHCO_3$ is useful in stabilizing cardiac membranes and consequently reduces arrhythmias. $NaHCO_3$ is effective in reducing TCA-induced QRS prolongation, reversing hypotension, and treating ventricular dysrhythmias. $NaHCO_3$ is generally administered as intravenous boluses of 1 meq/kg up to adult dose of 50 meq as needed to correct acidosis if pH less than 7.1, QRS greater than 0.16 seconds, arrhythmias are present or hypotension is not responding to fluids. In general, antiarrhythmics should be avoided in TCA ingestion, and supportive care provided including admission to a monitored setting, intravenous fluids, and inotropic support. *(McMillan, 754)*

66. (D) A gram-negative rod, non-lactose fermenter, oxidase positive is most concerning for *P aeruginosa*. Children with leukemia or other debilitating malignancies, particularly those who are receiving immunosuppressive therapy and who are neutropenic, are extremely susceptible to septicemia by *P aeruginosa* usually from endogenous seeding from the patient's respiratory or gastrointestinal tract. Empiric therapy should include an antipseudomonal agent tailored to the antibiotic resistance patterns of *P aeruginosa* for the hospital. Many strains are susceptible to the antipseudomonal penicillins (ticarcillin or piperacillin), fourth-generation cephalosporins (cefepime), carbapenems (imipenem or meropenem), aztreonam, ciprofloxacin, and aminoglycosides. Ceftazidime is a third-generation cephalosporin that has good activity against *P aeruginosa*, other third-generation cephalosporins, including ceftriaxone, have limited activity against *P aeruginosa*. Fluoroquinolones other than ciprofloxacin have variable activity against *P aeruginosa*. Aminoglycosides should not be used as monotherapy. Due to the rapid emergence of resistance, double therapy (usually a semisynthetic penicillin and aminoglycoside) is often recommended, but the evidence to support this is not robust. *(Behrman, 1208–1210)*

67. (E) Tumor lysis syndrome results when the intracellular contents released from dying leukemic blasts exceeds the ability of the body to adequately metabolize and excrete them. This is most frequently associated with leukemia presenting with a very high WBC counts. Hyperuricemia, a result of the metabolism of excess amounts of released nucleic acids, can result in renal failure that then can further worsen the patient's ability to excrete other metabolites. Hyperphosphatemia and secondary hypocalcemia may lead to further renal failure and the danger of seizures. Hyperkalemia may lead to alterations in the electrocardiogram with increased amplitudes of T waves, arrhythmia, and cardiac arrest. Patients presenting with tumor lysis syndrome or those at high risk with induction of chemotherapy require immediate intervention with intravenous hydration to maintain urine flow and alkalinization with intravenous sodium bicarbonate and allopurinol or other agents to increase the solubility and renal excretion of insoluble urate. Allopurinol inhibits the enzyme that accelerates the conversion of xanthine and hypoxanthine to uric acid and is used to prevent hyperuricemia in children at risk for the tumor lysis syndrome when receiving chemotherapy. Frequent monitoring of serum electrolytes, in addition to potassium, calcium, phosphorus, creatinine, and urine output, is critical. (McMillan, 1756–1757)

68. **(D)** *Clostridium difficile*–associated diarrhea, also known as pseudomembranous colitis or antibiotic-associated diarrhea, usually occurs in patients receiving antimicrobial therapy. Virtually all known antibiotics have been implicated; penicillins, broad-spectrum cephalosporins, and clindamycin are the most frequent offenders. The classic picture of pseudomembranous colitis is diarrhea with blood and mucus accompanied by fever, cramps, abdominal pain, nausea, and vomiting. Disease occurs during and as long as weeks after antibiotic therapy. The first and essential step in treatment is the discontinuation of the current antibiotics, if possible. In most instances, this course combined with appropriate fluid and electrolyte replacement is sufficient. Metronidazole is preferred as primary therapy, (20–40 mg/kg/24 h divided q 6–8 hours PO for 7–10 days) because oral therapy with this agent is similar in efficacy to vancomycin given orally for mild and moderate cases of disease, has lower cost (about $20 versus $200), and avoids the emergence of enterococcal resistance to vancomycin. If parenteral therapy is the only option, metronidazole is preferred because achievable colonic concentrations are superior, and because clinical failure has been reported with the use of parenteral vancomycin. Oral vancomycin (25–40 mg/kg/24h divided q 6 hours PO) is preferred for severe or complicated disease and for direct instillation in treatment of intestinal obstruction or adynamic ileus. (Behrman, 1230–1231; McMillan, 1038–1040)

69. **(E)** Malignant hyperthermia (MH) has occurred in association with several forms of myopathy, especially central core disease. MH is characterized by symptoms of rapidly rising body temperature, tachycardia, tachypnea, cyanosis, and respiratory and metabolic acidosis. Many patients with malignant hyperthermia have no obvious clinical symptoms of muscle disease. Usually, affected patients experience rigidity and myoglobinuria. Unexplained fevers, muscle

cramps, and increased serum creatine kinase values may represent clinical clues to the presence of malignant hyperthermia. The clinical syndrome can be aborted by the intravenous administration of dantrolene. Dantrolene can prevent or reduce the increase in myoplasmic calcium ion concentration that activates the acute catabolic processes associated with malignant hyperthermia. (McMillan, 2326)

70. **(B)** Ciprofloxacin and the other fluoroquinolones exert their antibacterial activity based on their peak/MIC ratio, termed concentration-dependent activity. Higher concentrations above the MIC exert greater killing activity. Fluoroquinolones do not have the nephrotoxic and ototoxic effects that aminoglycosides do; therefore therapeutic drug monitoring by levels is not necessary to ensure high peaks for efficacy and low troughs for toxicity. Recommended doses of fluoroquinolones ensure adequate peak levels. Other antibiotics exert their efficacy based on the time the antibiotic concentration exceeds the MIC (termed time dependent), and these drugs are typically dosed more frequently to ensure efficacy. Examples of time-dependent drugs include beta-lactams, macrolides, and clindamycin. (Behrman, 334–336; Brunton, 1182, 1225–1226)

71. **(D)** The concept of a steady-state concentration after repeated doses of a drug is important for the appropriate timing of serum sampling in monitoring drug therapy. Blood levels measured before a steady state is reached do not represent or predict drug concentrations at steady state. Dosage adjustments based on such premature data can result in serious dosage errors. Steady-state blood levels are achieved after approximately five drug half-lives have elapsed since the first dose, if no loading dose is given. A loading dose of drug may be necessary or desirable to rapidly achieve adequate therapeutic drug concentrations. (McMillan, 49)

72. **(E)** Phenytoin has been associated with IUGR as well as other congenital anomalies. IUGR is associated with medical conditions that interfere with the circulation and efficiency of

the placenta, with the development or growth of the fetus, or with the general health and nutrition of the mother. IUGR is often classified as reduced growth that is symmetric (head circumference, length, and weight equally affected) or asymmetric (with relative sparing of head growth). Symmetric IUGR often has an earlier onset and is associated with diseases that seriously affect fetal cell number, such as conditions with chromosomal, genetic, malformation, teratogenic, infectious, or severe maternal hypertensive etiologies. Asymmetric IUGR is often of late onset and is associated with poor maternal nutrition or with late onset or exacerbation of maternal vascular disease (preeclampsia, chronic hypertension). Other drugs such as narcotics, alcohol, cigarettes, cocaine, and antimetabolites are commonly a cause of IUGR. *(Behrman, 692)*

73. **(E)** Theophylline is rarely used in pediatric asthma because of its potential toxicity. Theophylline, when used chronically, can reduce asthma symptoms and need for supplemental beta-agonist use. Because theophylline may have some glucocorticoid-sparing effects in individuals with oral glucocorticoid-dependent asthma, it is still sometimes used in this group of asthmatic children. Theophylline has a narrow therapeutic window; therefore, serum theophylline levels need to be routinely monitored, especially if the patient has a viral illness associated with a fever or is placed on a medication known to delay theophylline clearance, such as macrolide antibiotics, cimetidine, oral antifungals, oral contraceptives, and ciprofloxacin. Toxic effects include both mild symptoms (nausea, vomiting, abdominal pain, headache, irritability) and severe and life-threatening reactions (intractable convulsions, tachyarrhythmia). Both therapeutic and toxic effects are dose dependent, and it is difficult to maintain therapeutic effects without some toxicity. *(Behrman, 961–965; McMillan, 2406–2409)*

74. **(D)** 75. **(B)** 76. **(F)** 77. **(E)** 78. **(C)**

TABLE 9-2.

Drug	Indications	Pharmacology	Dose range

Dopamine	(1) Hypotension
	(2) Low cardiac output
		Dopaminergic effects
		  (vasodilatation at 1–5 µg/kg/min)
		β-adrenergic effects
		  (inotropy at 5–10 µg/kg/min)
		α-adrenergic effects
		  (vasoconstriction at >15 µg/kg/min)
			2–20 µg/kg/min

Epinephrine	(1) Cardiogenic and septic shock (2) Low cardiac output with low systemic vascular resistance (3) Bradycardia	$\beta_1 > \beta_2 > \alpha$ adrenergic effects but all are present.	0.1–1 µg/kg/min
Dobutamine	(1) Myocardial dysfunction (2) Low cardiac output in setting of elevated pulmonary resistance	β_1-adrenergic effects	2–20 µg/kg/min
Isoproterenol	(1) Slow heart rate (2) Myocardial dysfunction with normal systemic vascular resistance	β_1-adrenergic effects with some β_2 effects at higher doses.	0.05–0.5 µg/kg/min
Norepinephrine	(1) Hypotension (2) Spinal shock (3) Inadequate cardiac output (4) α-adrenergic blockade (5) Low cardiac output with low systemic vascular resistance	α_1-adrenergic effects (vasoconstriction) β_1-adrenergic effects (increased inotropy)	0.1–2 µg/kg/min
Milrinone	(1) Cardiogenic shock (2) Low cardiac output with elevated pulmonary and systemic vascular resistance	Phosphodiesterase type III inhibitor	Load: 50 µg/kg Infusion: 0.75–1 µg/kg/min

These drugs are usually administered in an intensive care setting, where the dose can be carefully titrated to hemodynamic response. Continuous determinations of arterial blood pressure and heart rate are performed; measuring cardiac output at the bedside with a pulmonary thermodilution (Swan-Ganz) catheter may also be helpful in assessing drug efficacy.

Dopamine is a predominantly beta-adrenergic receptor agonist, but it has alpha-adrenergic effects at higher doses. Dopamine has less chronotropic and arrhythmogenic effect than the pure beta-agonist isoproterenol. In addition, it results in selective vasodilatation at lower dosages (< 5 μg/kg/min) via its interaction with dopamine receptors. At an intermediate dose of 5–10 μg/kg/min, dopamine results in increased contractility via its beta-adrenergic effects with little peripheral vasoconstrictive effect. However, if the dose is increased beyond 15 μg/kg/min, its peripheral alpha-adrenergic effects may result in vasoconstriction.

Dobutamine, a derivative of dopamine, is useful in treating low cardiac output conditions. Infusions cause direct inotropic effects with a moderate reduction in peripheral vascular resistance. Dobutamine can be used as an adjunct to dopamine therapy to avoid the vasoconstrictive effects of high-dose dopamine. Dobutamine is also less likely to cause cardiac rhythm disturbances than isoproterenol. The usual dose is 2–20 μg/kg/min.

Isoproterenol is a pure beta-adrenergic agonist that has a marked chronotropic effect; it is most effective in patients with slow heart rates and should be used with caution in those who already have significant tachycardia. Children receiving isoproterenol must be carefully monitored for arrhythmias.

Epinephrine is a mixed alpha- and beta-adrenergic receptor agonist that is usually reserved for patients with cardiogenic shock and low arterial blood pressure. Although epinephrine can raise blood pressure effectively, it also increases systemic vascular resistance and therefore increases the afterload against which the heart has to work.

Milrinone is useful in treating patients with low cardiac output who are refractory to standard therapy. It works by inhibition of phosphodiesterase, which prevents the degradation of intracellular cyclic adenosine monophosphate. Milrinone has both positive inotropic effects on the heart and significant peripheral vasodilatory effects and has generally been used as an adjunct to dopamine or dobutamine therapy in the intensive care unit. It is given by intravenous infusion at 0.5–1 μg/kg/min, sometimes with an initial loading dose of 50 μg/kg. A major side effect is hypotension secondary to peripheral vasodilatation, especially when a loading dose is used. The hypotension can generally be managed by the administration of intravenous fluids to restore adequate intravascular volume. *(McMillan, 2582–2587)*

79. (E) 80. (B) 81. (F) 82. (D) 83. (C) 84. (D) Although several recent studies have failed to demonstrate the effectiveness of intravenous theophylline in hospitalized children receiving frequent inhaled beta-agonist and systemic glucocorticoid therapy, theophylline may still have a role in the treatment of children with severe, life-threatening asthma exacerbations. If a child responds poorly to intensive therapy with nebulized albuterol, ipratropium, and parenteral glucocorticoids, then adding intravenous theophylline may be a consideration. It is important to remember that the therapeutic window for theophylline is narrow and patients treated with this therapy must have serum levels routinely checked.

The indications for the administration of nebulized epinephrine include moderate-to-severe stridor at rest, respiratory distress, hypoxia, and when stridor does not respond to cool mist. The duration of activity of racemic epinephrine is less than 2 hours. The mechanism of action is believed to be constriction of the precapillary arterioles through the β-adrenergic receptors causing fluid reuptake from the interstitial space and a decrease in the laryngeal mucosal edema. The symptoms of croup may reappear, but racemic epinephrine does not "cause" rebound worsening of the obstruction. *(McMillan, 2406–2407, 1505–1506; Brunton, 961–968)*

85. (C) 86. (A) 87. (E) 88. (D) Opioids act by mimicking actions of endogenous opioid peptides in binding to receptors located in the brain, brainstem, spinal cord, and peripheral nervous system. Opioids have dose-dependent respiratory depressant effects and directly blunt ventilatory responses to hypoxia and hypercarbia. The respiratory depressant effects of opioids can be increased with coadministration of other sedating drugs, such as benzodiazepines or barbiturates. Other common side effects can include constipation, nausea, vomiting, urinary retention, and pruritus. Optimal use of opioids requires proactive and anticipatory management of these side effects. Constipation is the most common side-effect of opioid usage in all age groups. *(Behrman, 466; Brunton, 569–575)*

89. **(C)** 90. **(B)** 91. **(A)** Serum concentration of drugs can reflect the route of administration. Continuous infusions (C) to obtain steady serum concentrations and effect can minimize the adverse effects seen with bolus administration (A) and intermittent administration (B) of drugs. *(McMillan, 45–46; Brunton, 4–7)*

92. **(B)** 93. **(A)** Alcohol (ethyl alcohol or ethanol) is rapidly absorbed in the stomach and is transported to the liver and metabolized by two pathways. The primary pathway involves removal of two hydrogen atoms to form acetaldehyde, a reaction catalyzed by alcohol dehydrogenase through reduction of a cofactor nicotinamide-adenine dinucleotide. Some drugs, such as phenytoin, salicylate, and alcohol, saturate their elimination pathways. When these pathways become "saturated," the resultant drug concentration in the blood changes disproportionately to the dose administered. These drugs follow the principles of zero-order, or Michaelis-Menten, kinetics. The classic principles of elimination half-life ($t_{1/2}$) and clearance (Cl) do not apply to drugs that exhibit zero-order kinetics.

In contrast, the behaviors of most clinical drugs follow the principles of linear or first-order pharmacokinetics. This means that the serum concentration or amount of drug in the body is directly proportional to the dose administered. For example, if dosing of a drug which follows linear pharmacokinetics is doubled, the resulting drug concentration in the

blood (at steady state) also doubles. Such predictable behaviors of a drug become the basis for serum drug level monitoring and dose adjustment. *(McMillan, 47; Brunton, 1886-87)*

94. **(C)** 95. **(D)** 96 **(A)** Pharmacokinetic interactions between drugs can occur through a variety of mechanisms. Such interactions may affect the absorption, distribution, metabolism, and/or excretion of any given drug. Dose-response curves are a useful way to observe the impact of one drug on the pharmacodynamic profile or effect of a drug or group of drugs. Potency relates to the relative concentration of a drug to achieve an effect. In the graph, A is greater than B is greater than C. Efficacy is the maximal effect of the drug. In the graph, efficacy between drugs is A = B = C; and all are more efficacious than D. *(Brunton, 24–29)*

97. **(A)** 98. **(B)** 99. **(A)** 100. **(B)** The clinical response to recommended dose of a drug can vary considerably, even when the dose is administered relative to a patient's body weight, surface area, and age. This variation is a result of inter-individual differences in drug pharmacokinetics and pharmacodynamics and a number of biologic variables, including genetic differences in drug metabolism or drug receptors, and concurrent pathophysiology (such as renal or hepatic insufficiency). Individual variability with respect to drug efficacy and possible toxicity frequently necessitates the adjustment of dosage regimens for specific patients, especially when prescribing drugs with a narrow therapeutic window. Problems with clearance and elimination of the drug can result in a steady rise in serum drug concentration. Often, such medications must be adjusted for this problem in clearance, such as in renal insufficiency. "Cumulative" properties refer to the administration of a "routine" dose at an interval that precludes adequate clearance of the drug. This can be addressed by adjusting the dose amount and/or dosing interval. The CYP-450 enzyme system represents more than 13 primary enzymes and a number of isozymes of specific gene families. Activity of this system is affected by genetic polymorphisms, normal

development, and presence of other drugs. An understanding of the substrates for specific isozymes and the effects certain drugs may have on isozyme activity (eg, induction, inhibition) allows the clinician to predict the possibility of clinically important metabolic-based drug-drug interactions. *(McMillan, 47)*

Case Diagnosis
and Management

Joseph Y. Allen, MD

This chapter contains clinical scenarios followed by a set of questions. These "real life" scenarios and questions are designed to assess the examinee's clinical judgment and practical thinking ability as well as her or his fund of knowledge. Case-based questions are common on national examinations, so it is important to become comfortable with them. To maximize your learning experience, answer all of the questions about the case before looking at the answers. And, refrain from looking ahead at the next question about the case in hopes of obtaining additional information for the question at hand. Not only would this negate the learning-testing experience, it might actually lead to an incorrect answer! For example, diagnostic or therapeutic steps that might be correct later in the case might by considered incorrect earlier when certain information was not available.

Questions

DIRECTIONS: This part of the test consists of a series of cases. Each case is followed by a group of related questions. For each of the multiple choice questions in this section select the one lettered answer that is the best response in each case.

Questions 1 through 3

An 18-month-old male toddler presents with pallor. He drinks 64 oz of cow milk per day. The examination is significant only for an obese and playful male with pallor. Stool is negative for blood.

1. Which laboratory test would most likely reveal the diagnosis?

   (A) chest x-ray
   (B) examination of stool for ova and parasites
   (C) complete blood count
   (D) serum haptoglobin
   (E) bone marrow aspirate

2. Testing reveals a mean corpuscular volume of 60 fL (nL 72–86 fL) and an elevated red cell distribution width. The most likely diagnosis is

   (A) vitamin B_{12} deficiency
   (B) B-cell leukemia
   (C) hemosiderosis
   (D) iron deficiency anemia
   (E) sickle cell disease

3. Appropriate therapy is started for this patient. When should reticulocytosis peak?

   (A) 12–24 hours
   (B) 1–3 days
   (C) 5–10 days
   (D) 2–4 weeks
   (E) 1–2 months

Questions 4 through 6

A 10-month-old female presents in winter with 2 days of rhinorrhea, tachypnea, and wheezing. She has respirations of 60 breaths per minute, HR of 160 beats per minute, and an oxygen saturation of 90% on room air. Examination reveals an alert infant in mild respiratory distress with mild intercostals retractions and coarse bilateral expiratory wheezing.

4. Appropriate therapy for this infant should begin with which of the following?

   (A) intravenous access and a 20 cc/kg bolus of normal saline
   (B) oxygen by nasal canula
   (C) bag-valve mask followed by rapid-sequence intubation
   (D) posterior-anterior and lateral chest radiographs
   (E) intravenous corticosteroids

5. Chest radiography reveals bilateral air trapping, chest hyperexpansion, and peribronchial thickening. Which of the following is the most likely diagnosis?

   (A) congestive heart failure
   (B) acute respiratory distress syndrome (ARDS)
   (C) pneumococcal pneumonia
   (D) *Mycoplasma pneumoniae* pneumonia
   (E) viral bronchiolitis

6. Which of the following is the best additional therapeutic option for this patient?

   (A) inhaled beta agonist therapy
   (B) ribavirin
   (C) extracorporeal membrane oxygenation
   (D) palivizumab (Synagis)
   (E) Heliox

Questions 7 through 9

A 6-year-old previously well male presents with 1 week of worsening elbow swelling and fever. He denies trauma. Examination reveals a male in mild distress with a temperature to 102°F. His left elbow is warm, erythematous, edematous, and tender around the joint. He is holding it in mid-flexion and strongly resists passive movement.

7. Which is the most likely offending organism for his condition?

   (A) *Neiserria gonorrheae*
   (B) Group B streptococcus
   (C) *Pseudomonas aeruginosa*
   (D) *Mycobacterium tuberculosis*
   (E) *Staphylococcus aureus*

8. Which of the following should be performed first?

   (A) administration of oral antibiotics
   (B) arthrocentesis of left elbow
   (C) administration of nonsteroidal anti-inflammatory agents
   (D) fasciotomy of the affected limb
   (E) laboratory evaluation for immunologic deficiencies

9. Which of the following is a poor prognostic factor for this condition?

   (A) age greater than 6 months
   (B) gram-positive infection
   (C) absence of physeal involvement
   (D) positive Gram stain of joint fluid
   (E) hip or shoulder involvement

Questions 10 and 11

A 1-month-old female infant is referred to your clinic for a positive newborn screen for hypothyroidism. On history, the mother reports she is "a good baby who sleeps all the time but is a slow eater." She was jaundiced for the first 2 weeks and stools twice a week. Examination reveals an alert infant with a large tongue, cool skin, a large umbilical hernia, edematous extremities, and hypotonia.

10. The most likely cause of this infant's condition is which of the following?

    (A) maternal ingestion of propylthiouracil
    (B) thyroid dysgenesis
    (C) iodide transport defects
    (D) thyrotropin deficiency
    (E) thyrotropin receptor–blocking antibodies

11. Which of the following management options should be initiated next?

    (A) levothyroxine therapy at a dose of 10–15 mcg/kg/day
    (B) thyroid scintiscan at the next available date
    (C) neurodevelopmental consultation
    (D) radiographs of the legs
    (E) confirmation of the state screen findings with a TSH level

Questions 12 through 14

A 4-year-old previously healthy boy presents with 1 day of scrotal swelling. His mother noted his scrotum to be markedly swollen and thinks his eyes are puffy. Examination reveals an afebrile child with a BP of 90/50 mm Hg. He is alert with significant bilateral periorbital edema. His abdomen has ascites with no organomegaly. His scrotum and lower extremities have tense pitting edema.

12. The initial laboratory test most likely to point to the etiology of his illness is as which of the following?

    (A) chest radiograph
    (B) liver biopsy
    (C) urine analysis
    (D) hepatitis panel
    (E) stool guaiac and pH

13. Subsequent testing reveals a serum albumin of 1 g/dL, a cholesterol level of 560 mg/dL (nL 109–189 mg/dL), and normal complement and liver enzyme levels. The most likely diagnosis for this patient is which of the following?

    (A) membranous glomerulonephritis
    (B) focal segmental glomerulosclerosis
    (C) poststreptococcal glomerulonephritis
    (D) membranoproliferative glomerulonephritis
    (E) minimal-change disease

14. Which of the following statements regarding this patient's most likely condition is true?

    (A) It almost never responds to steroid therapy.
    (B) Spontaneous bacterial peritonitis is not a concern.
    (C) These patients have an increased tendency to hemorrhage.
    (D) A low-salt diet is essential during flares of the illness.
    (E) Nonresponse to therapy for at least 1 year should prompt a nephrology referral for biopsy.

Questions 15 through 17

A 7-year-old well female presents to your emergency department with episodic headache and hypertension. During the episodes she is sleepy, complains of headaches, vomits, and becomes sweaty. Her current vital signs are: T 101°F, HR 150 beats per minute, BP 220/130 mm Hg. She is diaphoretic, sleepy but arousable, and clutches her head. Pupils are reactive and papilledema is present. There is no organomegaly and femoral pulses are normal.

15. After determining that her airway is intact and breathing sufficient, the first course of action should be which of the following?

    (A) immediate CT scan of the head to evaluate for a mass lesion
    (B) lumbar puncture to rule out meningitis
    (C) administration of an antihypertensive medication

    (D) administration of a benzodiazepine to relieve the patient's anxiety
    (E) placement of a large bore central catheter for dialysis

16. Her vital signs are stabilized on the appropriate therapy. Now happy and interactive, she is transferred to the ICU. Which option is most likely to lead to a diagnosis?

    (A) magnetic resonance imaging of the brain
    (B) urine for catecholamines
    (C) ECG and echocardiography
    (D) inquiry into a family history of essential hypertension
    (E) surgical consult for laparotomy

17. The urinary vanillyl mandelic acid level returns at 400 mg/g creatinine (nL < 8 mg/g creatinine). Which of the following is the best treatment for this condition?

    (A) surgical removal of all tissue
    (B) radiologic injection of cyclophosphamide directly
    (C) watchful waiting as most regress spontaneously
    (D) oral mineralcorticoid therapy
    (E) oral propylthiouracil therapy

Questions 18 through 20

You are seeing a 7-day-old male infant for a well-child check. The baby is breastfeeding well. He has had no fever or emesis. He passed his first stool at 3 days of age, and has not passed another stool. Examination reveals an afebrile, well appearing, and vigorous baby. The abdomen is firm and slightly distended with bowel sounds present. The perianal area is slightly erythematous and rectal examination reveals increased tone with no stool present in the rectal vault.

18. Of the following, which is the best initial diagnostic test?

    (A) stool assay for *Clostridium difficile* toxin
    (B) abdominal ultrasound
    (C) serum TSH
    (D) barium enema
    (E) diagnostic trial of mineral oil

19. The initial diagnostic approach is unsuccessful. Which test to should you perform next to diagnose this patient?

   (A) serum TSH
   (B) stool for esosinophils
   (C) anal manometry
   (D) upper gastrointestinal series with small bowel follow through
   (E) rectal biopsy

20. Testing reveals an absence of the Meissner and Auerbach plexus. With proper treatment, what is the most likely prognosis for this patient?

   (A) he will likely be continent
   (B) he will need a colostomy for his entire childhood
   (C) he will need a total colectomy and likely have serious incontinence problems
   (D) he will need a small bowel transplant and require lifelong parenteral nutrition
   (E) he will be at great risk for frequent life-threatening intra-abdominal infections

Questions 21 and 22

A previously well 2-year-old girl is brought to you for evaluation of a "broken elbow." The father reports swinging her round and round by her left arm and leg. She now is crying and not moving her left arm as it is held in a flexed and slightly pronated position at her side. No effusions or point tenderness are discernible.

21. Which of the following is the most appropriate initial management?

   (A) intravenous line placement for sedation and reduction
   (B) hyperpronation or supination-flexion of the arm
   (C) complete blood count and erythrocyte sedimentation rate
   (D) social work evaluation for abuse
   (E) radiographic evaluation of the left elbow

22. When counseling the father regarding his child's condition, you should tell him which of the following?

   (A) recurrence is unlikely
   (B) splinting at bedtime is desirable
   (C) gymnastics should be avoided
   (D) suspicion of abuse requires that you report this injury
   (E) children outgrow predisposition for this condition

Questions 23 through 25

A 16-year-old female living in a shelter presents with 3 days of worsening lower abdominal pain. She reports multiple unprotected sexual encounters. She is febrile to 39°C and is ill appearing. She has bilateral lower quadrant tenderness without rebound. Her pelvic examination reveals purulent vaginal discharge with adnexal and cervical motion tenderness. Pregnancy test is negative.

23. What is the most appropriate management strategy at this time?

   (A) inpatient admission with intravenous antibiotics for pelvic inflammatory disease
   (B) social service referral for in loco parentis designation prior to initiation of therapy
   (C) initiation of antibiotic therapy in the emergency department and discharge with close outpatient follow-up
   (D) urine analysis and empiric intramuscular antibiotic therapy for cystitis
   (E) nonsteroidal therapy and oral contraceptive pills for pregnancy prophylaxis

24. The patient remains febrile and has worsening abdominal pain despite 72 hours of antibiotic therapy. At this time what is the best next step?

   (A) continue therapy at the scheduled doses
   (B) add diphenhydramine for a potential drug reaction
   (C) consult gynecology for imaging and drainage of a possible tubo-ovarian abscess
   (D) repeat blood cultures and obtain a C-reactive protein to help monitor response to therapy
   (E) consult infectious disease for evaluation of the possibility of methicillin-resistant *S aureus* infection

25. The patient improves and is ready for discharge. Which of the following is true about this patient's condition?

  (A) recurrence is rare

  (B) recurrence is associated with an increased risk of infertility

  (C) douching and oral contraceptives may decrease the risk of recurrence

  (D) male partners with *N gonorrheae* are always symptomatic

  (E) ectopic pregnancies are not a concern after PID

Questions 26 and 27

An 11-year-old boy presents after cutting his ankle on a rusty piece of metal at the junkyard. His father reports he is positive his son's immunizations are current because the patient received booster doses just prior to kindergarten at 5 years of age. Examination reveals a healthy boy in no distress with a 4 cm bleeding laceration on the posterior aspect of the lower leg.

26. What should be the first step in management of this wound?

  (A) radiography to evaluate for metallic particles

  (B) irrigation of the wound with normal saline

  (C) intravenous antibiotics directed against gram-positive organisms

  (D) surgery assistance for this complicated injury

  (E) direct pressure on the wound for hemostasis

27. The wound is treated. For tetanus prophylaxis, which of the following should this patient receive?

  (A) no prophylaxis

  (B) Td only

  (C) Td and tetanus immune globulin (TIG)

  (D) DTaP

  (E) TIG only

Questions 28 and 29

A 6-month-old boy is brought in by his mother for crying. Your examination reveals a thin boy with tender swelling around the midshaft of his left femur. He cries when the leg is manipulated, but is comfortable when left alone. An x-ray reveals a transverse midshaft femur fracture. The father tells you the patient's 16-month-old brother lifted him off the bed and dropped him on the floor earlier that evening.

28. What should be the next step in the management of this patient?

  (A) review with parents the history of the injury

  (B) MRI of left lower extremity

  (C) skeletal survey

  (D) internal fixation of the fracture

  (E) fibroblast assay

29. During the evaluation the father asks that they be discharged immediately as he has to be at work early. What is the most appropriate course of action?

  (A) let them go home and follow-up with their pediatrician the next day

  (B) splint the child with follow-up by an orthopedist

  (C) call security to forcibly incarcerate the father

  (D) directly confront the parents of their complicity in allowing this to happen

  (E) inform the family that the safety of the child may be at risk as the history given does not match with his pattern of injuries

Questions 30 and 31

A 3-month-old female presents with 2 days of crying and decreased oral intake. She is afebrile, HR is 280 beats per minute, and BP is 85/40 mm Hg. Her saturations are 99% on room air. She is alert and easily consolable, her lungs are clear, and she is tachycardic with no murmurs audible. There is no organomegaly and the peripheral pulses are normal in strength.

30. Which test should you order first to confirm the diagnosis?

  (A) complete blood count and differential

  (B) echocardiogram

  (C) blood glucose

(D) thyroxine and TSH levels

(E) electrocardiogram

31. Her heart rate and blood pressure remain unchanged after testing. The initial treatment for the most likely cause of her condition is which of the following?

(A) adenosine

(B) defibrillation

(C) verapamil

(D) digoxin

(E) ibuprofen

Questions 32 and 33

A 15-year-old previously well female presents with 1 week of hair loss. She denies fever, weight loss, or medications. On examination, she is pleasant but nervous about her hair loss. Her scalp reveals patches of complete hair loss with small broken hair that easily pull out at the edges. The scalp is smooth and no inflammation is seen. Microscopic examination of the shafts reveals the stubs to resemble exclamation points.

32. What illness does this patient most likely have?

(A) tinea capitis

(B) alopecia areata

(C) trichotillomania

(D) hair traction alopecia

(E) chemical exposure

33. You tell the patient the likely course of this illness is which of the following?

(A) spontaneous resolution

(B) resolution after chemotherapy

(C) difficult to predict

(D) progression to total hair loss and then resolution

(E) improvement with dietary change

Questions 34 through 36

A 6-month-old female develops a persistent cough with progressively worsening paroxysms and cyanosis. There is occasional posttussive emesis. The child is afebrile. Between coughing spells, the physical examination is normal.

34. At this time, what would be most important question to ask the family regarding patient history?

(A) birth weight

(B) immunizations

(C) consanguinity

(D) early infant deaths in relatives

(E) family history of reactive airways disease

35. The white blood cell count on the patient is 32,000/mm^3, with 80% lymphocytes and 2% mononuclear cells. What is the most appropriate next step at this time?

(A) order a bone marrow examination

(B) prescribe intravenous gammaglobulin

(C) prescribe oral azithromycin

(D) perform a lumbar puncture

(E) repeat the blood count in 24 hours

36. The most appropriate method to identify the responsible organism is via which of the following?

(A) throat swab

(B) nasopharyngeal swab

(C) blood culture

(D) sputum culture

(E) bronchoscopy

Questions 37 through 39

A 17-year-old female presents to your clinic with complaints of recurrent headaches for 6 months. They are described as circumferential; onset is not associated with time of day. There has been no emesis and the headaches have not interfered with activities. Her weight is 140 kg and her BP is 140/90 mm Hg. Her examination reveals bilateral papilledema, and an otherwise normal neurologic examination.

37. What is the best next step in management of this patient?

(A) oral administration of nifedipine

(B) determination of renin levels

(C) intravenous nitroprusside drip

(D) computerized tomography of the head

(E) intravenous mannitol and furosemide

38. The imaging study is normal, reveals no mass and normal-sized ventricles. At this point you should do which of the following?

(A) perform lumbar puncture

(B) treat with dexamethasone

(C) treat with acetazolamide

(D) refer her for opthalmalogic evaluation

(E) refer her for psychiatric evaluation

39. You proceed and she has relief from her symptoms. Despite appropriate care she begins to develop visual loss and optic nerve atrophy is suspected. Your best course of action is to do which of the following?

(A) increasing the dose of dexamethasone

(B) increasing the frequency of lumbar punctures

(C) increasing the dose of acetozolamide

(D) refer her to a surgeon for gastric banding to speed up weight loss

(E) refer to an ophthalmologist for evaluation for optic nerve fenestration

Questions 40 through 42

A 10-month-old female presents to the emergency department with a 2-day history of runny nose and fever to 102°F. On examination, her temperature is 103°F, HR 140 beats per minute, and a RR 30 times per minute. She is alert and playful with copious rhinorrhea. After the examination is complete, she becomes stiff and displays tonic-clonic movements of all four extremities.

40. Which of the following should be your first task?

(A) obtain whole blood glucose

(B) administer intravenous lorazepam (Ativan)

(C) perform lumbar puncture

(D) establish airway patency

(E) administer intramuscular fosphenytoin (Cerebyx)

41. After 5 minutes, the seizure ceases and the respiratory rate is 30 breaths per minute. The patient is sleepy but arousable. Fundoscopic examination is normal as is the remainder of the physical examination. Rectal acetaminophen is given. Which of the following tests should be performed at this time?

(A) electroencephalogram

(B) skull radiographs

(C) arterial blood gas

(D) computerized tomography scan of the head

(E) lumbar puncture

42. The patient quickly becomes alert, happy, and playful. She is afebrile and has a normal examination. All ordered tests are normal. Which of the following management plans is most appropriate at this time?

(A) discharge home after instructions regarding home management of fever and seizures

(B) discharge home on phenytoin

(C) discharge home on phenobarbital

(D) discharge home with alternating doses of ibuprofen and acetaminophen every 3 hours for the next 3 days

(E) admission for observation and MRI

Questions 43 through 45

A 6-year-old female presents with short stature. Her family reports she has been well and has had no other medical problems. Her diet and review of systems is unremarkable.

43. Which of the following would be most important to know at this time?

(A) maternal age at menarche

(B) parental growth rate and height

(C) paternal age at conception

(D) maternal age at conception

(E) sibling growth rate and height

44. The physical examination reveals a pleasant girl at less than the 5th percentile for height and 10th percentile for weight. In addition to her short stature, she has a broad chest, cubitum valgum, and 2/6 systolic ejection murmur at the right upper sternal border. Which test is most likely to confirm the etiology of her short stature at this time?

(A) serum LH/FSH levels

(B) abdominal ultrasound

(C) growth hormone levels

(D) karyotype

(E) bone age analysis of the nondominant hand

45. Of the following management options, which is indicated for this patient?

(A) transthoracic echocardiogram

(B) halo bracing for cervical laxity

(C) counseling regarding the likelihood of severe mental deficiency

(D) hysterectomy to prevent the development of endometrial carcinoma

(E) initiation of thyroid hormone replacement therapy

Questions 46 through 48

A 13-month-old boy presents with 5 days of fever to 103°F. His temperature is 102.8°F, HR 160 beats per minute, and RR 36 times per minute. On examination, he is found to be irritable with markedly injected conjunctiva, a strawberry tongue, and red, cracked lips. A 2-cm lymph node is present in the left anterior cervical chain. There is no meningismus. His lungs are clear and he is tachycardic. A diffuse erythematous blanching rash is present on his chest and extremities. No desquamation of the fingertips is noted.

46. Among the following, which diagnostic test is most important in establishing the disease most likely to be causing this constellation of symptoms?

(A) complete blood count

(B) erythrocyte sedimentation rate

(C) viral culture

(D) clinical judgment

(E) presence of antinuclear antibody

47. After the diagnosis is confirmed, therapy is initiated with improvement in symptoms within 24 hours. Which of the following complications is most likely to occur in this illness?

(A) thrombocytopenia

(B) sterility

(C) hydrops of the gallbladder

(D) ulcerative colitis

(E) transverse myelitis

48. Prior to discharge, the parents state that their child needs his immunizations updated. You should counsel the parents that their son should follow which course of treatment?

(A) stay on schedule for his vaccinations

(B) have measles and varicella immunizations deferred for 11 months after IVIG

(C) not be given diphtheria-tetanus-acellular pertussis vaccine because it may potentiate a relapse of his illness

(D) not receive influenza vaccine because he will be on chronic aspirin therapy

(E) have his primary series of vaccines repeated

Questions 49 and 50

A 2-year-old is brought to your emergency department for refusal to walk after he tripped and fell while running. Examination reveals a well-appearing afebrile child in no distress. His left leg has full range of motion and some point tenderness in the distal tibia.

49. The most appropriate first step in your evaluation is to obtain which of the following?

(A) a C-reactive protein

(B) a blood culture

(C) radiographs of the tibia

(D) a social work consultation

(E) a serum alkaline phosphatase

50. Your initial evaluation confirms your suspicion. At this point you should perform which task next?

(A) make a referral to child protective services for abuse

(B) place a long-term intravenous catheter for intravenous antibiotics

(C) arrange an immediate orthopedic referral

(D) perform a needle aspirate of the affected area

(E) immobilize the affected limb in a splint with outpatient follow-up

Questions 51 through 53

You are called to the nursery to evaluate a 3-day-old, full-term male infant with lethargy. The nurse reports the infant was feeding well on standard formula until 4 hours previously. He has had no emesis. There is no maternal history of fever or rash. The infant currently is afebrile with a HR 110 beats per minute, RR of 50 times per minute, and a BP of 80/45 mm Hg. He is lethargic but the examination is otherwise unremarkable. There are no dysmorphic features. Whole blood glucose is normal. Serum calcium and electrolyte results are pending.

51. What should be your next step in the evaluation of the patient?

    (A) obtain emergent abdominal ultrasound
    (B) obtain complete blood count, urine analysis and lumbar puncture as well as cultures of blood, urine, and CSF
    (C) urine drug screen
    (D) obtain emergent upper gastrointestinal series with small bowel follow-through
    (E) obtain emergent magnetic resonance imaging of the head to evaluate for an intracranial hemorrhage

52. The neonatal evaluation for sepsis is complete and the neonate is placed on antibiotics. The next day there is no evidence of infection and the infant has not improved. Additional studies are obtained, including a serum ammonia which is 1150 mmol/L (nL 64–107) and a blood pH of 7.36. Medical therapy is initiated. The urinary orotic acid level returns and is markedly elevated as well. Which of the following is the most likely diagnosis?

    (A) ornithine transcarbamylase deficiency
    (B) carbamoyl synthetase deficiency
    (C) methylmalonic academia
    (D) carnitine palmitoyl transferase deficiency
    (E) glycogen synthetase deficiency

53. Six hours after institution of treatment with appropriate intravenous doses of arginine, the serum ammonia is 1200 mmol/L. The best course of action at this time is which of the following?

    (A) increase the rate of IV arginine to clear ammonia faster

    (B) begin a double volume exchange transfusion
    (C) transfer the patient to a center where hemodialysis can be performed
    (D) discuss DNR status with the family
    (E) allow another 6 hours of therapy as ammonia in tissue needs to be metabolized first and therapy can be toxic as well

Questions 54 through 56

A 3-year-old girl is seen in the emergency department for bruising. Her family denies fever or weight loss but states she had a "cold" 3 weeks ago. She is afebrile and the remaining vital signs are normal. She is happy and playful and has generalized ecchymoses and petechiae.

54. What should be the first test you obtain?

    (A) bone marrow aspirate
    (B) *Neiserria meningitidis* latex assay of the cerebrospinal fluid
    (C) *Rickettsia rickettsiae* serology
    (D) skeletal survey looking for healing fractures
    (E) complete blood count and differential

55. The laboratory results return and the platelets are 10,000/mm³. A bone marrow aspirate demonstrates increased megakaryocytes but is otherwise normal. Which of the following is an indication for WinRho (anti-RhoD antibodies)?

    (A) platelet count less than 100,000/mm³
    (B) fever greater than 39°C
    (C) splenomegaly
    (D) epistaxis
    (E) bone marrow with megakaryocyte hypoplasia

56. Which of the following would be an indication for splenectomy in this patient?

    (A) platelet count below 10,000/mm³
    (B) gingival bleeding
    (C) persistence of thrombocytopenia for more than 1 month

(D) persistence of thrombocytopenia for more than 1–2 years

(E) presence of splenomegaly and anemia

Questions 57 and 58

A 4-year-old boy presents to the emergency department with a chief complaint of pallor. He was well until 1 week previously when he developed bloody diarrhea that resolved with oral antibiotics. He is afebrile with a BP of 150/100 mm Hg and a HR of 130 beats per minute. He is alert and fundoscopic examination is normal. His examination is significant for pallor.

57. Which test is most likely to reveal the diagnosis?

(A) complete blood count and smear

(B) stool culture

(C) computerized tomography of the head

(D) renal ultrasound

(E) urine myoglobin levels

58. The laboratory results reveal a hemoglobin of 8 g/dL, a BUN and creatinine of 40 and 1.8, respectively. The urine output is normal. What should you tell the family regarding the treatment of this disease?

(A) aggressive medical management and dialysis result in the majority of the patients doing well

(B) high-dose steroids are essential in the treatment of this illness

(C) most patients eventually require renal transplantation

(D) antibiotics need to be continued for 21 days

(E) recurrence of this illness is frequent

Questions 59 and 60

An 18-month-old female presents to the emergency department with fever up to 102°F, a barky cough, and stridor. The examination shows an RR of 60 breaths per minute with an oxygen saturation of 95% while breathing room air, marked stridor, moderate substernal retractions, and equal aeration without wheezes or rhonchi.

59. As the patient is being evaluated, initial therapy for this patient should begin with which of the following?

(A) acetaminophen per rectum

(B) nebulized dexamethasone

(C) nebulized racemic epinephrine

(D) humidified air only in a position of comfort

(E) stat portable AP and lateral neck films

60. Despite therapy the patient becomes more toxic appearing and is drooling. The parents subsequently report the child has received no immunizations. Her respiratory rate is now 70 breaths per minute and she appears sleepy. At this point the best intervention is which of the following?

(A) blind intubation with a laryngeal mask airway

(B) humidified oxygen and observation with the patient in a position of comfort

(C) rapid sequence intubation in the emergency department

(D) anesthesia assistance for intubation in the operating room with surgical availability

(E) prompt administration of intravenous cefotaxime

Questions 61 and 62

A 4-year-old male presents to the office with wheezing and increased work of breathing for the fifth time in the past year. On examination, his RR is 30 breaths per minute and oxygen saturation is 98% while breathing room air. He is talking in complete sentences and there is expiratory wheezing with a prolonged expiratory phase.

61. What is the first treatment he should receive?

(A) nebulized beta agonist therapy

(B) intravenous beta agonist therapy

(C) subcutaneous epinephrine

(D) oxygen via 15 L nonrebreather

(E) intramuscular steroids

62. The patient improves after receiving the treatment selected. Further history reveals that the patient has been using inhaled albuterol three times per week to control wheezing. He awakens each night with coughing, but seems better in the morning. In addition to albuterol and a short course of oral steroids what is the best additional medicine he should receive at this time?

(A) epinephrine auto injector (Epi-Pen) to be used as needed

(B) salmeterol to be used in divided doses daily

(C) fluticasone to be used in divided doses daily

(D) theophylline to be used in divided doses daily

(E) cetirizine to be used in divided doses daily

Questions 63 through 65

A previously well 9-year-old Hispanic male presents with 2 days of yellow eyes and abdominal pain. He visited Mexico 1 month previously. On examination he is febrile to 101°F, has scleral icterus, and moderate right upper quadrant tenderness. The liver is moderately enlarged.

63. What would be the most helpful additional history?

(A) sickle cell disease in the family

(B) excessive carrot intake

(C) history of malar rash

(D) acetaminophen usage

(E) vaccination status prior to travel

64. What test would most likely confirm his diagnosis?

(A) hepatitis A serology

(B) hepatitis B serology

(C) 24-hour copper excretion

(D) abdominal ultrasound

(E) acetaminophen level

65. Diagnostic testing confirms the diagnosis and the family has questions about the disease. You should tell them which of the following?

(A) an effective vaccine is not routinely available

(B) the recurrence risk is approximately 25%

(C) if he were to contract hepatitis D simultaneously, he would likely need a liver transplant

(D) fulminant hepatitis is uncommon in children with hepatitis A infection

(E) intimate sexual contact is the most common route of transmission

Questions 66 through 68

You are called to see a 2-hour-old male with cyanosis and tachypnea. Oxygen saturation is 80% while breathing room air and the RR is 60 breaths per minute with BP of 80/50 mm Hg. The baby is cyanotic and there are no murmurs. The rest of the examination is unremarkable. The baby is placed in on an FiO_2 of 1.0 by head hood and arterial blood gases reveal the PaO_2 to be 30 mm Hg.

66. What is the most likely etiology of the hypoxemia?

(A) methemoglobinemia

(B) cyanotic congenital heart disease

(C) sepsis

(D) pneumonia

(E) arteriovenous fistula

67. A chest x-ray shows normal lung fields, slightly generous cardiothymic silhouette, and a narrow upper mediastinum. An electrocardiogram is normal. What would the most likely diagnosis based on this information?

(A) transposition of the great arteries

(B) tetralogy of Fallot

(C) ventricular septal defect

(D) endocardial fibroelastosis

(E) total anomalous pulmonary venous return

68. The airway is stabilized and prostaglandin E_1 therapy is initiated. Echocardiography confirms the diagnosis. At this point what is the best intervention?

(A) emergent cardiac catheterization and atrial septostomy

(B) nothing until the patient's hypoxemia improves

(C) empiric antibiotics for sepsis

(D) emergent cardiovascular surgery consultation for immediate arterial switch

(E) dobutamine and milrinone to enhance cardiac function

Questions 69 through 71

A 6-year-old previously well African American child presents with new-onset jaundice, dark urine, and pallor. There is a history of a recent mild upper respiratory tract infection. Vital signs are normal. Physical examination is remarkable for icterus and pallor. Laboratory examination reveals hemoglobin of 7 g/dL with a normal platelet and white blood cell count. The total bilirubin is 4 mg/dL.

69. Which of the following historical findings is most likely to indicate the diagnosis?

(A) His father has sickle cell trait.

(B) Baby aspirin given to him last year was associated with dark urine.

(C) His grandmother was diagnosed with leukemia last year.

(D) He was diagnosed as being iron deficient 4 years ago.

(E) His healthy cousin returned from a trip to Mexico 1 month ago.

70. The bilirubin is predominantly unconjugated and the reticulocyte count is 12%. Further history reveals that for the past 2 days he has been given an antibiotic that his grandfather was taking for a urinary tract infection. What is the most likely diagnosis?

(A) sickle cell disease

(B) preleukemia

(C) infectious hepatitis

(D) spherocytosis

(E) glucose-6-phosphate-dehydrogenase deficiency

71. What is the most appropriate management at this time?

(A) immediate transfusion to bring the hemoglobin to 14 g/dL

(B) immediate transfusion to bring the hemoglobin to 10 g/dL

(C) withhold transfusion and follow vital signs and hemoglobin level

(D) initiate prednisone at 2 mg/kg/day

(E) transfusion to bring the hemoglobin to 10 g/dL and prednisone at a dose of 2 mg/kg/day

Questions 72 and 73

A 16-year-old female presents with leg weakness after recovering from an upper respiratory illness. On examination her vital signs are normal. She is unable to stand alone. Motor strength is 5/5 in the arms and 2/5 in the legs. Deep tendon reflexes are absent in the legs.

72. What finding is classically associated with this illness?

(A) hydrocephalus

(B) elevated serum C-reactive protein

(C) myoglobulinuria

(D) elevated cerebrospinal fluid protein

(E) presence of *Clostridium* species on stool culture

73. Testing demonstrates marked slowing of nerve conduction velocity. What would the most appropriate intervention be at this time?

(A) administration of intravenous immune globulin

(B) discharge and reassurance about the overall benign nature of this disease

(C) administration of intravenous fresh frozen plasma

(D) supplemental oxygen via nasal cannula

(E) administration of intravenous interferon-beta

Questions 74 and 75

A 5-year-old male presents with a 5-lb weight loss over the previous 2 weeks and nighttime enuresis. On examination, he is alert and talkative with a BP of 90/60 mm Hg and a HR of 130 beats per minute. Mucous membranes are sticky and respirations are rapid and deep. The bedside whole blood glucose is 750 mg/dL. Intravenous access is obtained.

74. What should the first step in management be?

(A) regular insulin 0.1 U/kg IV push
(B) bicarbonate 1 meq/kg IV over 1 hour
(C) endotracheal intubation
(D) 20 cc/kg isotonic crystalloid solution over 1 hour
(E) a diet soda

75. After your intervention, the whole blood glucose is 485 mg/dL. Intravenous fluids and insulin are given, and the patient is admitted for further care. Which of the following metabolic abnormalities is most likely to occur during insulin therapy?

(A) hypokalemia
(B) hyperkalemia
(C) hyperphosphatemia
(D) hypercalcemia
(E) hypermagnesemia

Questions 76 through 78

A 13-month-old female in day care presents to the outpatient clinic with 3 days of rhinorrhea, cough, and fever to 101°F. Her examination is significant for clear nasal congestion and red tympanic membranes that are mobile with insufflation. The mother asks for antibiotics.

76. What is the most appropriate therapy at this time?

(A) amoxicillin 80–90 mg/kg/day for 10 days
(B) amoxicillin 40–50 mg/kg/day for 5 days
(C) ceftriaxone 50 mg/kg IM in one dose
(D) otorhinolaryngology consult for tympanocentesis
(E) acetaminophen and fluids

77. The mother brings her child in 6 days later for persistent fever (up to 103°F) and pulling at the left ear. On examination, the left tympanic membrane is bulging and immobile. The bony landmarks are not visible. The mother states the day care won't let her back in without antibiotics. The most appropriate therapy at this time is which of the following?

(A) amoxicillin 80–90 mg/kg/day for 10 days
(B) erythromycin 40–50 mg/kg/day for 10 days
(C) ceftriaxone 50 mg/kg IM in one dose
(D) otorhinolaryngology consult for drainage
(E) acetaminophen and fluids

78. The patient returns again in 2 days with continued fevers to 104°F. The child is still fussy. There is redness, swelling, and tenderness posterior to the left ear and the pinna is displaced forward. The most appropriate therapy at this time is which of the following?

(A) amoxicillin 80–90 mg/kg/day for 10 days
(B) amoxicillin 40–50 mg/kg/day for 5 days
(C) ceftriaxone 50 mg/kg IM in one dose
(D) otorhinolaryngology consult for drainage
(E) acetaminophen and fluids

Questions 79 through 81

A mother brings her 17-year-old daughter to your clinic for evaluation of 6 weeks of fatigue, 10-lb weight loss, and listlessness. The vital signs include a HR of 70 beats per minute and BP of 90/50 mm Hg. Examination reveals a thin girl with a flat affect, but no other abnormalities.

79. The best next step in this patient's management would be which of the following?

(A) obtain a serum beta-human chorionic gonadotrophin (b-HCG)
(B) a referral to an oncologist for a bone marrow aspirate
(C) obtain stat urine drug screen
(D) reassure the mother that this is normal behavior
(E) interview the patient alone

80. Further discussion with the patient reveals signs of depression. However, she is interactive and denies any drug use or suicidal ideation. She has friends and makes As and Bs in school. The results of screening laboratory work are normal. Appropriate initial management should be which of the following?

(A) immediate psychiatry consultation due to the medicolegal risk posed by the patient

(B) immediate inpatient admission with 24-hour suicide watch

(C) urine collection for illicit substances against the patient's will

(D) initiation of a selective serotonin reuptake inhibitor (SSRI) and scheduling of outpatient counseling with a therapist

(E) reassurance to the patient that it is a sign of puberty and the feelings will pass

81. You are called 3 weeks later as the patient is brought to an outside emergency department because of increasing hyperactivity, loquaciousness, and 3 days of insomnia. The patient's parents state that she purchased a large amount of goods. Urine toxicology is negative. This patient most likely has which of the following?

(A) a drug reaction

(B) bipolar disorder

(C) schizophrenia

(D) reaction to sexual abuse

(E) normal adolescent behavior

Questions 82 through 84

A 7-year-old girl presents with a 3-week history of fatigue, 5-lb weight loss, and listlessness. Examination is significant for a thin girl who appears tired. Petechiae and ecchymoses are present over her trunk and extremities. The complete blood count reveals a white blood cell count of $85,000/mm^3$, hemoglobin of $7\ g/dL$, and platelets of $15,000/mm^3$. The differential reveals 80% blasts and 20% lymphocytes. She is febrile to 103°F and has a BP of $90/50$ mm Hg.

82. Appropriate empiric antibiotic therapy would begin with which of the following?

(A) intramuscular ceftriaxone

(B) intravenous clindamycin and cefuroxime

(C) intravenous ceftazidime

(D) intravenous amphotericin and voriconazole

(E) oral ciprofloxacin

83. Bone marrow examination confirms the diagnosis of acute lymphocytic leukemia. Which of the following would indicate a poor prognosis?

(A) patient's age (7 years)

(B) patient's initial white blood count $(85,000/mm^3)$

(C) hyperdiploidy

(D) absence of the Philadelphia chromosome (9:22)

(E) absence of blasts in the cerebrospinal fluid

84. Induction chemotherapy is begun. Which of the following patterns of metabolic abnormalities might be expected to occur?

(A) hypokalemia, hypouricemia, hypophosphatemia

(B) hypokalemia, hypouricemia, hyperphosphatemia

(C) hyperkalemia, hyperuricemia, hyperphosphatemia

(D) hyperkalemia, hypouricemia, hypophosphatemia

(E) hypokalemia, hyperuricemia, hypophosphatemia

Questions 85 through 87

A first-time mother brings her 6-week-old full-term male infant in because of excessive crying. She states he is feeding well and has had no fever but seems to cry "all the time" for the last 3 weeks. Examination reveals an alert and vigorous infant who has gained weight very well since the 2-week check-up and is currently cooing with no abnormalities noted on examination.

85. What should the initial approach to management be?

(A) a full sepsis evaluation

(B) a skeletal survey

(C) a radioisotope milk scan

(D) a urine analysis and urine culture

(E) counseling, reassurance, and close follow-up

86. What would be the most appropriate management option at this time?

   (A) suggesting that a single individual, preferably the mother, act as the sole caregiver
   (B) swaddling of the infant
   (C) warm water feedings three times a day to decrease gastric upset
   (D) vigorous shaking of the baby back and forth to simulate uterine movements
   (E) oral paregoric to calm the infant's immature nervous system

87. If this infant had presented with acute onset of irritability and crying and an episode of bilious emesis, differential diagnosis should focus on which of the following diagnoses?

   (A) hair tourniquet around a digit
   (B) milk protein intolerance
   (C) occult fracture
   (D) gastroesophageal reflux
   (E) malrotation with volvulus

Questions 88 and 89

A 10-month-old female is brought to the emergency department for evaluation of streaks of blood on the surface of the stools. The parents deny any history of travel, diarrhea, or fever.

88. What additional history would be most likely to point to a specific diagnosis in this patient?

   (A) family history of hemophilia
   (B) dietary iron intake
   (C) history of constipation
   (D) presence of rotavirus in day care contacts
   (E) family history of Crohn disease

89. Examination reveals a small fissure without erythema in the posterior area of the anus. What is the most appropriate treatment at this time?

   (A) prescribing milk of magnesia
   (B) encouraging the use of a rectal dilator to stretch the internal anal sphincter
   (C) prescribing a stool softener and titrating the dose to desired stool consistency

   (D) prescribing an oral antibiotic to prevent secondary infection of the fissure
   (E) referral to a naturopathic practitioner for colonic irrigation

Questions 90 and 91

An 8-year-old girl presents with a 3-month history of intermittent joint swelling and stiffness and is subsequently diagnosed with juvenile idiopathic arthritis (JIA).

90. Which of the following types of JIA is most commonly associated with development of severe arthritis?

   (A) systemic onset JIA
   (B) pauciarticular JIA without ocular involvement
   (C) pauciarticular JIA with associated ocular involvement
   (D) polyarticular rheumatoid factor positive JIA
   (E) polyarticular rheumatoid factor negative JIA

91. Vision loss associated with JIA is most commonly due to which of the following?

   (A) optic neuritis
   (B) retinal artery thrombosis
   (C) retinal detachment
   (D) beta carotene malabsorption
   (E) chronic iridocyclitis/uveitis

Questions 92 through 94

A 4-month-old male infant presents with 3 days of profuse watery nonbloody diarrhea and nonbilious emesis. He was being fed milk, orange juice, and rice water. Vital signs are T 99°F, HR 170 beats per minute, and BP 66/40 mm Hg. His eyes and fontanelle are sunken and he has poor skin turgor with a capillary refill time of 3–4 seconds; pulses are normal.

92. This description is most consistent with which of the following?

   (A) hypovolemic shock, compensated
   (B) hypovolemic shock, uncompensated
   (C) cardiogenic shock, compensated

(D)   septic shock, uncompensated

(E)   normal cardiovascular state

93.   His weight just prior to intravenous fluid therapy is 6.3 kg. His fluid deficit is approximately what measurement?

(A)   50 cc

(B)   250 cc

(C)   650 cc

(D)   850 cc

(E)   1100 cc

94.   Assuming normal kidney function, the initial hydrating fluid bolus in this patient should be which of the following?

(A)   sodium 140 meq/L

(B)   sodium 100 meq/L

(C)   sodium 80 meq/L

(D)   sodium 40 meq/L

(E)   glucose 10 mg%

Questions 95 through 97

An 8-day-old full-term neonate presents with 1 day of vesicular lesions of the skin and mouth. She is afebrile and alert. There are multiple 3–5 mm vesicles on an erythematous base present on her trunk and mouth. The pregnancy was uncomplicated and the parents have no history of genital lesions.

95.   Which of the following is the best course of action at this time?

(A)   discharge home and follow up in 72 hours

(B)   culture the lesions and begin treatment with oral clindamycin (Cleocin)

(C)   check a complete blood count and urine analysis and, if normal, discharge patient after intramuscular ceftriaxone (Rocephin)

(D)   perform bacterial cultures of blood, urine, cerebrospinal fluid, bacterial and viral cultures of the lesions, and initiate broad-spectrum antibacterial therapy

(E)   perform bacterial cultures of blood, urine, cerebrospinal fluid, bacterial and viral cultures of the lesions, and initiate broad-spectrum antibacterial therapy and acyclovir

96.   Viral shedding due to maternal HSV reactivation is associated with transmission to the fetus in approximately what proportion of cases?

(A)   2%–5%

(B)   10%–15%

(C)   35%–40%

(D)   70%–75%

(E)   90%

97.   Risk factors for vertical transmission of HSV type 2 include which of the following?

(A)   maternal coinfection with HSV type 1

(B)   physician rupture of membranes just prior to delivery

(C)   scalp electrode usage

(D)   coinfection with the human immunodeficiency virus

(E)   delayed administration of acyclovir to the mother in labor

Questions 98 and 99

A 15-day-old, full-term, large-for-gestational age infant is brought to your clinic for evaluation of a chest mass. Examination reveals an afebrile vigorous baby with a firm, nontender mass palpable over the middle third of the right clavicle.

98.   What is the most appropriate course of action for this patient?

(A)   reassurance to the family about the condition

(B)   weight-bearing and comparison views of the clavicles

(C)   skeletal survey to rule out abuse

(D)   fibroblast assay for osteopetrosis

(E)   report to child protective services for failure to seek care in a timely fashion

99.   Risk factors for this condition include which of the following?

(A)   congenital syphilis

(B)   breech presentation

(C)   maternal drug use

(D)   female gender

(E)   thanatophoric dysplasia

Questions 100 through 102

You are called to evaluate the cause of hypotonia in a 1-day-old full-term female infant born to a 28-year-old mother. The baby is alert and moves all extremities well but is hypotonic. She has upward slanting palpebral fissures, speckled irides, a large tongue, short fifth digits, and bilateral transverse palmar creases. Karyotype is 46,XX.

100. What is the most likely reason for this result?

(A) the number of chromosomes was miscounted

(B) she has a partial translocation involving chromosome 21

(C) there is no chromosomal abnormality

(D) interference of the test by maternal-fetal blood transfusion

(E) she has Turner syndrome

101. What is the frequency of Down syndrome?

(A) 1/12 live births

(B) 1/600 live births

(C) 1/4000 live births

(D) 1/8000 live births

(E) 1/20,000 live births

102. Patients with Down syndrome are at increased risk for which of the following?

(A) hyperthyroidism

(B) arthritis of the cervical spine

(C) streak gonads

(D) cardiac malformations

(E) rhabdomyosarcoma

103. You are seeing a previously well 22-month-old male with fever to 102°F, rhinorrhea, and cough for 3 days. His parents report that he remains playful with no alteration in his activity. Your examination reveals rhinorrhea and is otherwise unremarkable. The complete blood count reveals a white blood count (WBC) of 6000/mm³, normal hemoglobin and platelet count; WBC differential is 8% neutrophils, 40% lymphocytes, 50% monocytes, 2% basophils. The best course of action at this time is which of the following?

(A) hospitalization and treatment with intravenous ceftazidime and tobramycin

(B) intramuscular dosages of ceftriaxone for a 7-day period

(C) bone marrow aspirate to rule out leukemia

(D) initiation of treatment with granulocyte colony-stimulating factor

(E) close outpatient follow-up and repetition of the complete blood count in 1–2 days

Questions 104 through 106

A 3-year-old boy with sickle cell disease (hemoglobin SS) presents with a 1-hour history of right-sided weakness. Examination reveals right hemiparesis. A CT scan of the brain is normal.

104. Acute treatment for this patient's condition is which of the following?

(A) observation

(B) anticoagulation with heparin

(C) exchange transfusion

(D) intravenous tissue plasminogen activator

(E) hydroxyurea

105. The patient recovers completely, but prior to discharge develops a fever to 102°F. He appears otherwise well. Infection with which of the following organisms would be of most concern in this patient?

(A) *Mycobacterium tuberculosis*

(B) *Clostridium botulinum*

(C) group A beta-hemolytic streptococcus

(D) *Streptococcus pneumoniae*

(E) influenza A

106. The patient's father inquires about the possibility that his son's children will have sickle cell disease. You should you inform him which of the following about the risk?

(A) is negligible

(B) is approximately 25%

(C) is approximately 50%

(D) approaches 100%

(E) cannot be determined at this time

Questions 107 through 109

During a well-child examination, the mother of a previously healthy 5-year boy inquires whether you think her child is unusually clumsy. The mother thinks her son is going to be strong as he has "big calves," but her family tells her he seems to trip a lot. Your examination reveals a pleasant male with a slightly waddling gait and mildly enlarged calves.

107. Which of the following physical examination findings would suggest the diagnosis of Duchenne muscular dystrophy?

(A) Rovsing sign
(B) opisthotonus
(C) Gower sign
(D) Chovstek sign
(E) Grey-Turner sign

108. Complications of Duchenne muscular dystrophy most commonly include which of the following?

(A) renal failure from myoglobinuria
(B) ophthalmoplegia
(C) seizures
(D) immunosuppression
(E) aspiration pneumonia

109. The mother is devastated to learn the diagnosis and that she carries the affected gene. A true statement about Duchenne muscular dystrophy inheritance is which of the following?

(A) 50% of her daughters will be affected with the disease
(B) about 25% of the cases are from new mutations
(C) women are never affected with the disease
(D) the risk of recurrence is minimal
(E) an affected male will pass the illness on to all his sons

Questions 110 and 111

An 8-year-old girl is seen in the emergency department with a complaint of 1-week worsening shortness of breath. She denies fever or cough. Vital signs include HR 140 beats per minute and BP 78/40 mm Hg. She is alert with mild tachypnea and is most comfortable leaning forward. Cardiac examination reveals tachycardia and muffled heart tones.

110. What finding is the most suggestive of pericardial tamponade?

(A) pulsus paradoxus of greater than 10–20 mm Hg
(B) electrocardiogram with low voltages in all leads
(C) chest radiograph demonstrating an enlarged cardiothymic silhouette
(D) egophany over the left anterior chest
(E) bounding carotid pulses

111. Echocardiography confirms a large pericardial effusion compromising left ventricle function. After ensuring that the airway is stable, what should the next intervention be?

(A) intravenous solumedrol 30 mg/kg rapid infusion
(B) continuous intravenous milrinone infusion
(C) thoracotomy and placement of a pericardial window
(D) pericardiocentesis under ultrasound guidance
(E) intravenous albumin and furosemide

Questions 112 through 114

A previously healthy 7-day-old, full-term infant presents to your clinic with jaundice which began on the first day of age. He is afebrile with normal vital signs and growth indices. He is breastfeeding well and has five gray stools and six wet diapers per day. Examination reveals a vigorous infant with marked scleral icterus and jaundice to the level of the umbilicus. The liver is palpable 3 cm below the right costal margin. Your nurse was only able to obtain a limited sample of blood.

112. What are the most important tests to direct further evaluation at this time?

(A) complete blood count and culture
(B) total and direct bilirubin
(C) blood type and Coomb test
(D) aspartate aminotransferase and alanine aminotransferase
(E) alpha$_1$-antrypsin levels

113. The child is sent to the emergency department, and testing reveals the total bilirubin to be 16 mg/dL with a conjugated fraction of 14 mg/dL. Which of the following tests would be most likely to reveal the cause of this infant's conjugated hyperbilirubinemia?

(A) urine analysis and culture
(B) urine succinylacetone
(C) sweat chloride test
(D) abdominal ultrasound
(E) thoracolumbar films

114. The above test is ordered and is abnormal. A subsequent liver biopsy to confirm the diagnosis reveals a paucity of biliary channels and plugging with the channel diameter of greater than 150 mm. What is the best treatment for this condition?

(A) phenobarbital to promote bile flow
(B) immediate liver transplant using a parental split liver graft
(C) hepatocyte infusion directly into the residual portal vein
(D) Kasai hepatoportoenterostomy after 6 months of life to make it technically easier
(E) Kasai hepatoportoenterostomy as soon as possible after diagnosis

Questions 115 and 116

A 4-year-old boy is brought in for evaluation because of perianal irritation and itching and parental concern that this might be a manifestation of sexual abuse. Examination reveals a playful boy; inspection of the perianal region demonstrates several superficial excoriations and several thread-like worms.

115. What is the best next step in management?

(A) antiparasitic treatment and reassurance about the benign nature of the condition
(B) stool for ova and parasite examination
(C) social work evaluation and child protective services referral
(D) instructions to the family regarding improved hygiene
(E) antiparasitic treatment of household pets, the most likely reservoir for this parasite

116. Which of the following should you treat this condition with?

(A) mebendazole
(B) metronidazole
(C) diethylcarbamazine
(D) praziquantel
(E) thiabendazole

Questions 117 through 119

A 2-year-old 13-kg female is brought to the emergency department by her parents after they found her with an empty bottle of cherry-flavored acetaminophen drops about 2 hours prior. You note that the bottle contained 1 oz at a concentration of 80 mg/0.8 cc. The parents report they just purchased it earlier in the day for her 2-month-old brother. No treatment was given prior to arrival at the emergency department. The patient's vital signs are normal, and her physical examination is unremarkable.

117. What should the next step in this patient's management be?

(A) intubate to secure the airway
(B) do nothing until 4 hours have elapsed since the purported time of ingestion
(C) give activated charcoal with sorbitol at a dose of 1 g/kg orally or via nasogastric tube
(D) induce emesis with syrup of ipecac
(E) proceed with gastric lavage using a 12-French orogastric tube

118. You proceed with management. The 4-hour acetaminophen level is 200 mg/kg. What is the best next step?

(A) continue observation in the emergency department for 6 hours and discharge if the patient remains asymptomatic
(B) start the antidote, N-acetylcysteine
(C) continue activated charcoal every 4 hours in addition to the antidote, N-acetylcysteine
(D) begin preparations for liver transplant
(E) place a hemodialysis catheter for initiation of hemodialysis

119. The toxicity of acetaminophen comes from which of the following?

    (A) its renal metabolite
    (B) acetaminophen directly
    (C) its glucoronidate metabolite
    (D) its sulfated metabolite
    (E) its cytochrome P-450 metabolite

Questions 120 and 121

A previously healthy 3-year-old male is brought in by his parents with a chief complaint of increased sleepiness, which began during a visit to his grandmother's house earlier that day. The patient's vital signs are HR of 50 beats per minute, temperature of 97°F, RR of 8 times per minute, and a BP of 98/65 mm Hg. Examination reveals an obtunded male toddler who is unresponsive to sternal rub and lacks a gag reflex. He also has miosis.

120. The first step in managing this patient is

    (A) bedside whole blood glucose
    (B) urinary catherization to obtain urine drug screen
    (C) intravenous flumazenil
    (D) securing an airway and insuring adequate breathing
    (E) intravenous epinephrine for bradycardia

121. The grandmother reports that she has multiple medications in her house and is concerned that the patient's problems may be due to an ingestion. Which one of her medicines would most likely cause the symptoms reported?

    (A) clonidine
    (B) nifedipine
    (C) meperidine
    (D) labetalol
    (E) diazepam

Answers and Explanations

1. **(C)** Given the history of excessive intake of milk, a food known to be low in iron, and the presentation of pallor, initial testing should focus on the hemoglobin and iron status. The reticulocyte count and the mean corpuscular volume (MCV) generally are low in iron deficiency. Chest radiography and stool smears for ova and parasites are not indicated. Serum haptoglobin is low in state of hemolysis, but that is not the most likely cause of anemia in this case. A bone marrow biopsy is not indicated at this time. *(Behrman, 2014–2016)*

2. **(D)** In iron deficiency anemia, the red blood cells are smaller than normal and are variable in size; therefore a decreased MCV and elevated red cell distribution width (RDW) are classic with this history. Vitamin B12 deficiency from a poor diet or intrinsic factor deficiency presents with an elevated MCV. No blasts indicating leukemia or stippling suggesting hemosiderosis were noted on the smear. Additionally, there is no evidence of sickled cells. *(Behrman, 1469–1471)*

3. **(C)** When iron deficiency anemia is suspected, elemental iron at a dose of 6 mg/kg/day divided into two or three doses should be initiated. Appetite will return to normal in 12–24 hours. Bone marrow response will begin in 36–48 hours. Reticulocytosis will peak around 5–7 days. Repletion of stores will occur in 1–3 months depending on the severity of the anemia. Contrary to common belief, iron does not constipate patients. Increasing vitamin C intake via diet or supplementation can increase iron absorption. Parents should be counseled regarding the importance of a diverse diet. Milk intake should be limited to 16–24 oz/day. *(Behrman, 1469–1471)*

4. **(B)** The initial step in the management of patients presenting in respiratory distress is assessment of the "ABCs" (airway, breathing, and circulation). The presence of hypoxemia is an indication for administration of supplemental oxygen. There is no indication of a compromised airway (eg, stridor) in this patient. While there is mild distress, there is no indication at this time of respiratory failure necessitating emergent intubation. Chest radiographs and administration of corticosteroids may be necessary, but are not the first priority in this patient's management. *(Behrman, 1388–1390, 1773–1777)*

5. **(E)** The age, physical findings, and season all point to bronchiolitis, most likely due to respiratory syncytial virus (RSV), as the most likely cause of this patient's problem. RSV is the etiologic agent in about 70% of patients with bronchiolitis and results in approximately 70,000 inpatient admissions yearly in the United States. Congestive heart failure likely would be associated with other physical findings such as hepatomegaly, or have demonstrable cardiomegaly on the chest radiograph. Respiratory distress syndrome typically has a ground-glass appearance on chest radiography and presents with more severe clinical symptoms. Pneumococcal pneumonia classically presents with a more focal infiltrate with consolidation, is unilateral, and is not associated with wheezing. Mycoplasmal infections are not common at this age. *(Behrman, 991–993, 1285–1287)*

6. **(A)** A trial of beta agonist therapy, such as albuterol or racemic epinephrine should be offered to all patients with bronchiolitis with symptoms of distress; however, not all patients will respond. Ribavirin aerosal treatment is available but not recommended routinely. Guidelines as delineated by the American Academy of Pediatrics suggest that the high cost, technical issues associated with aerosal administration, potential toxic effects among exposed health care workers, and lack of convincing efficacy data limit its usefulness and at this time. It may be best utilized in the immunocompromised host (eg, bone marrow transplant recipient with RSV infection). A humanized mouse monoclonal antibody product (palivizumab) is licensed for prevention of infection with RSV, but has no well-defined role in treatment of confirmed infections. Heliox (70/30 mixture of helium/oxygen) has been used for upper airway obstructions and extracorporeal membrane oxygenation may be utilized in severe bronchiolitics but is not indicated here. *(Behrman, 991–993, 1285–1287)*

7. **(E)** Gram-positive organisms, in particular *S aureus*, are a significant source of soft tissue infections in the immunocompetent child. Spread to deep tissues can occur directly or hematogenously. Arthritis due to infection with *Neisseria* typically presents as a monoarticular septic joint in sexually active individuals. Group B streptococcal arthritis is most commonly seen in neonates. *P aeruginosa* or other gram negatives should be considered in drug users or immunodeficient individuals. Arthritis due to *M tuberculosis* is uncommon and would have a more indolent course. *(Behrman, 2845–2847)*

8. **(B)** The examination is very concerning for a septic arthritis of the left elbow. Erosion and permanent damage of the joint can occur quickly. Obtaining fluid for cultures by arthrocentesis prior to antibiotic therapy is preferred, particularly in light of the increasing frequency of antibiotic-resistant organisms. Oral antibiotics are inappropriate for initial treatment of septic arthritis. Nonsteroidal anti-inflammatory agents provide symptomatic relief only and are not a primary treatment modality in septic arthritis. *(Behrman, 777–780)*

9. **(E)** Young infants, patients with hip and shoulder involvement, and those whose antibiotic therapy is delayed are at increased risk of a poor outcome following bacterial arthritis. Additionally, septic arthritis due to gram-negative and fungal organisms is more difficult to eradicate. The Gram stain is only positive in approximately 50% of cases, and the presence or absence of organisms on Gram stain is of no prognostic value in septic arthritis. *(Behrman, 777–780)*

10. **(B)** Thyroid dysgenesis accounts for 85% of the cases of congenital hypothyroidism. Maternal ingestion of propylthiouracil causes a transitory hypothyroidism, but history should reveal maternal use of this drug. The other causes of congenital hypothyroidism are uncommonly seen. *(Behrman, 2319–2325)*

11. **(A)** When a patient presents with a state screen that is positive and has obvious clinical symptoms of hypothyroidism, initiating thyroxine prior to confirmation is essential. Therapy initiated prior to 2–4 weeks of life can ensure near-normal intelligence. Dosing for infants starts at 10–15 mcg/kg/day. Older children require about 4 mcg/kg/day and adults require only 2 mcg/kg/day. A scintiscan to look for ectopic thyroid tissue is helpful. Close neurodevelopmental follow-up is necessary. Radiography of the distal femur of patients with congenital hypothyroidism frequently reveals absent distal epiphysis. This finding is occasionally used as a quick indirect screen for hypothyroidism. *(Behrman, 1698–1703)*

12. **(C)** Edema results from two pathophysiologic conditions: increased venous hydrostatic pressure or decreased oncotic pressure. Increased hydrostatic pressure, resulting in extravasation of fluid into the interstitial space, results from conditions such as venous thrombosis and congestive heart failure. Reduced oncotic pressure most commonly results from hypoalbuminemia due to decreased production of albumin (eg, liver failure) or increased loss of albumin (eg, via the gastrointestinal tract or kidneys); reduction in oncotic pressure in turn results in fluid extravasation into the interstitial tissues. Of the choices given, a urine analysis for protein is the quickest, cheapest, least invasive, and most helpful initial test to direct further evaluation. *(Behrman, 2190–2194)*

13. **(E)** In conjunction with proteinuria, elevated serum cholesterol, hypoalbuminemia, and edema constitute the nephrotic syndrome. Membranous glomerulonephritis, focal segmental glomerulosclerosis, membranoproliferative disease, and acute poststreptococcal glomerulonephritis all may be associated with the nephrotic syndrome. However, minimal-change disease is much more common in children, accounting for 85% of protein-losing nephropathies. *(Behrman, 1592–1595)*

14. **(D)** Fortunately, 90% of patients with minimal-change disease respond rapidly to steroids. Loss of properdin factor B that opsonizes bacteria can occur, leading to an increased risk of spontaneous bacterial peritonitis. Antithrombin III is also lost in the urine, so children are at increased risk of thrombosis, not hemorrhage. During flares low-sodium diets, combined with diuretics and albumin infusions may be necessary to decrease edema. A referral and renal biopsy should be performed after 1 month (not 1 year) of nonresponse to steroid therapy to determine the etiology of the illness. *(Behrman, 1592–1595)*

15. **(C)** Hypertension presenting with symptoms (headache, altered mental status, papilledema) requires immediate antihypertensive therapy. Causes of severe hypertension (> 95th percentile) include renal artery stenosis, malignant hyperthyroidism, aldosteronism, pheochromocytoma, and a coarctation of the aorta. An intracranial mass with Cushing triad causing hypertension should present with bradycardia but this can be a late presenting sign. An LP should be deferred in a patient with papilledema until imaging demonstrates the absence of an intracranial mass. *(Behrman, 1990, 2372–2373)*

16. **(B)** Determination of urine level of vanillyl mandelic acid (VMA, a metabolite of epinephrine), thyroid function analysis, and CT imaging of the abdomen for a mass as well as renal artery caliber delineation are all essential in looking for the etiology of her hypertension. Laparotomy may be needed for eventual therapy but is not a part of the initial evaluation. *(Behrman, 1184, 1741–1742)*

17. **(A)** An elevated VMA level with this patient's symptoms point to a pheochromocytoma as the cause of her hypertension. Pheochromocytomas arise from the chromaffin cells of the sympathetic nervous system; they can arise in the adrenal medulla or anywhere along the sympathetic chain. They can be inherited sporadically or as a component of types IIA and IIB multiple endocrine neoplasia syndromes from a mutation in the RET proto-oncogene. The definitive treatment is surgical with exquisite detail to peri- and postoperative hypertension. *(Behrman, 1184, 1741–1742)*

18. **(D)** Ninety-nine percent of healthy neonates pass their first stool (meconium) within 48 hours after birth. Delayed passage of the meconium raises concern for Hirschsprung disease. Barium enema may demonstrate a "transition zone" at the junction of the dilated normal bowel proximally and the narrowed aganglionic segment distally. As frequent rectal stimulation and digital examination may alter the radiographic appearance, the barium enema should be delayed until 2–3 days after these procedures, if feasible. Botulism and hypothyroidism may present with constipation, but this neonate's vigorous appearance and history of feeding make these unlikely. Mineral oil should not be given to infants because of the risk of aspiration and subsequent lipoid pneumonia (see Figure 10-1). *(Behrman, 1565–1567)*

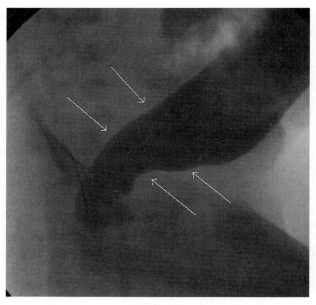

Figure 10-1
(Courtesy of Doug Rivard, DO)

19. **(E)** The diagnostic ability of the barium enema depends on demonstration of a transition zone of narrow distal bowel expanding into more normal caliber proximal bowel. However, false-negative studies occur, especially if performed after previous rectal stimulation (eg, digital examination). Biopsy above the dentate line remains the gold standard for diagnosis; in Hirschsprung disease, it reveals a lack of the neuronal plexus (Meissner and Auerbach), hypertrophied nerve bundles, and increased acetylcholinesterase levels. Stool examination for eosinophils may be useful in cases of milk protein allergy, but is not indicated in this breastfed baby. Anal manometry to measure pressure changes of the rectum is technically challenging in young infants but can be performed in older patients. Upper GI series with small bowel follow through is useful in the diagnosis of intestinal malrotation, but is not indicated in the patient described. *(Behrman, 1139–1141)*

20. **(A)** The prognosis for surgically treated HD generally is satisfactory with a majority of patients achieving fecal continence. In 75% of patients, the aganglionic segment is limited to the distal rectosigmoid area. Colostomy placement is rare and is only temporary until the proximal segment recovers from its dilated state. A total colectomy is necessary in fewer than 10% of patients. A small bowel transplant is needed only if a large proportion of the small bowel is aganglionic (total intestinal Hirschsprung disease). Enterocolitis can occur in untreated Hirschsprung disease, but is uncommon following surgical correction. *(Behrman, 1139–1141)*

21. **(B)** The history of longitudinal traction in a child less than 4 years old, the lack of tenderness or effusion on examination, and the characteristic posture (arm flexed at elbow and slightly pronated) point to nursemaid elbow (radial head subluxation) as the most likely diagnosis. This occurs when the radial head is subject to longitudinal traction causing the developing annular ligament to remain partially entrapped in the radiohumeral joint. In patients with a typical history and physical examination, maneuvers to reduce the subluxation are both diagnostic and therapeutic. Hyperpronation or supination/flexion of the forearm are two maneuvers that can reduce the subluxation. Although causing brief pain, reduction does not require sedation. On successful reduction a "clunk" can be felt over the lateral portion of the elbow, and the patient will generally begin using the arm normally within a short period. Radiographs are not indicated as they will be normal. While nonaccidental trauma may result in a nursemaid elbow, the history given is compatible with the injury and, in the absence of other suspicious findings, is not an indication for social service evaluation. *(Behrman, 2827)*

22. **(E)** Recurrence of nursemaid's elbow has been reported in as many as 30% of children. Therefore, counseling the parents on the mechanism of this injury is important. No splints are necessary and physical activity as tolerated should be permitted. A radial head subluxation by itself typically is not indicative of abuse. The annular ligament and radial head strengthen with age and radial head subluxation is rare after 4 years of age. *(Behrman, 2092)*

23. **(A)** This adolescent has several risk factors that make her a candidate for admission. The fever and toxic appearance suggest that she has an illness beyond a cystitis or simple cervicitis caused by *N gonorrhea* or *C trachomatis*. Residence in a shelter also suggests increased difficulty with outpatient follow-up. Treatment for an emergent condition as well as for sexually transmitted diseases does not require legal proceedings. Appropriate pain control will be necessary, but admission and intravenous antibiotic therapy are the first critical step in this patient with pelvic inflammatory disease (PID). Prior to discharge from the hospital and hopefully after this patient has developed a trusting professional relationship with her physician, counseling regarding contraception and further protection as well as lifestyle choices are indicated. *(AAP:Red Book,493–498)*

24. (C) Complications of PID including chronic pelvic pain, perihepatitis, ectopic pregnancies, infertility, and tubo-ovarian abscess should be worsening signs and symptoms despite appropriate antimicrobial therapy. These are suggestive of tubo-ovarian abscess. Consultation with a gynecologist and diagnostic imaging (usually ultrasound) is appropriate at this time. A C-reactive protein to monitor therapy is not needed when the clinical picture clearly suggests lack of response to therapy. Methicillin-resistant *S aureus* is an uncommon cause of PID. (*AAP:Red Book,493–498*)

25. (B) PID causes scarring of the reproductive tract and can lead to many complications later in life. There is a 10% risk of tubal infertility after a single episode of PID, with a 50% risk after three or more episodes. Patients who have had PID are at increased risk for repeat infections, and douching or oral contraceptives do not prevent them. Male carriers are not always symptomatic. PID is a risk factor for future ectopic pregnancies. (*AAP:Red Book, 493–498*)

26. (E) The first step in management of any laceration is hemostasis. Once this is achieved, irrigation, evaluation of the wound for foreign bodies, and antimicrobial therapy can begin. If the wound injury is found to involve tendons, ligaments, vessels, or may be associated with severe cosmetic imperfection, surgical assistance for repair is appropriate. (*AAP:Red Book,649*)

27. (B) Two questions to ask when confronted with tetanus prophylaxis are (1) has the patient received three or more doses of tetanus toxoid and (2) is the wound clean. Tetanus immune globulin is necessary in those who have a dirty wound and fewer than three doses of tetanus-containing vaccine or those with a history of HIV infection. In those with greater than or equal to three tetanus-containing vaccines, TIG is not necessary but the age-appropriate tetanus vaccine should be given if immunization is incomplete (see Table 10-1). (*AAP:Red Book, 650–651*)

TABLE 10-1   Guide to Tetanus Prophylaxis in Routine Wound Management (Centers for Disease Control and Prevention. Manual for the Surveillance of Vaccine-Preventable Diseases 4th Edition, 2008. Published 2008. Updated April 8, 2009. http://www.cdc.gov/vaccines/pubs/surv-manual/chpt16-tetanus.htm)

History of adsorbed tetanus toxoid (doses)	Clean minor wounds		All other wounds[a]	
	Tdap or Td[b]	TIG[c]	Tdap or Td[b]	TIG[c]
<3 or unknown	Yes	No	Yes	Yes
≥3 doses[d]	No[e]	No	No[f]	No

[a]Such as (but not limited to) wounds contaminated with dirt, feces, soil, and saliva; puncture wounds; avulsions; and wounds resulting from missiles, crushing, burns, and frostbite.

[b]For children younger than 7 years of age, DTaP is recommended; if pertussis vaccine is contraindicated, DT is given. For persons 7–9 years of age or 65 years or older, Td is recommended. For persons 10–64 years, Tdap is preferred to Td if the patient has never received Tdap and has no contraindication to pertussis vaccine. For persons 7 years of age or older, if Tdap is not available or not indicated because of age, Td is preferred to TT.

[c]TIG is human tetanus immune globulin. Equine tetanus antitoxin should be used when TIG is not available.

[d]If only three doses of fluid toxoid have been received, a fourth dose of toxoid, preferably an adsorbed toxoid, should be given. Although licensed, fluid tetanus toxoid is rarely used.

[e]Yes, if it has been 10 years or longer since the last dose.

[f]Yes, if it has been 5 years or longer since the last dose. More frequent boosters are not needed and can accentuate side effects.

28. (C) The injury this child suffered is not consistent with the story that is presented. Other "red flags" suggesting nonaccidental trauma include stories that are developmentally impossible or change over time, reticence on the part of one caregiver to speak, and delay in seeking medical care. This child clearly is at risk and needs an evaluation with a skeletal survey. Findings suggestive of abuse are multiple healing injuries, rib fractures, bucket handle fractures, or healing long bone fractures. A hip spica is the treatment for a femur fracture in infants; internal fixation is not indicated. Although osteogenesis imperfecta may present with long bone fractures, it is rare and evaluation for more common conditions such as abuse takes precedence. Eighty percent of inflicted skeletal trauma occurs in children under 18 months of age. Among fractures resulting from abuse, skull fractures are most common followed by fractures of the extremities. (*Rudolph, 463–469, 561*)

29. **(E)** When confronted with possible nonaccidental trauma, the safety of the affected child as well as other members of the household is of primary importance. Evaluation for factors that may contribute to the potential for abuse should be undertaken. The assistance of a social worker is often valuable in this regard. All states mandate that physicians report any case of suspected abuse. Mandated reporters are immune from prosecution, even if abuse is not proven, as long as the report is made in good faith. Direct confrontation and accusation are not productive and may hinder further efforts in the investigative process. Incarcerating the father is not appropriate as he has made no threats, nor is there sufficient evidence to implicate him as the perpetrator of the injury. However, this child should not be discharged until there is sufficient investigation of the social situation to permit safe placement. *(Rudolph CD 463–469, 561)*

30. **(E)** A patient with this degree of tachycardia needs immediate assessment of her cardiorespiratory status. As her airway, breathing, and circulation are intact with no evidence of impending failure, a brief evaluation can be performed to evaluate her tachycardia. Obtaining an electrocardiogram during the episode likely will be valuable for analysis of the rhythm and determining the best treatment modality. The other tests are helpful in evaluating sinus tachycardia, which usually peaks around 220–230. A tachycardia over 230 is more suggestive of a supraventricular tachycardia (SVT), which is the most common dysrhythmia requiring medical intervention in children. *(Rudolph CD 1854–1856)*

31. **(A)** Once the diagnosis of supraventricular tachycardia is made, adenosine 0.1 mg/kg (maximum 6 mg) rapid intravenous push is the treatment of choice. If the initial attempt is unsuccessful, the dose can be doubled and repeated (to a maximum of 12 mg). Side effects include transient headache, flushing, and chest pain. Serious side effects of adenosine include atrial fibrillation, apnea, bronchospasm, brief asystole, accelerated ventricular rhythms, and wide complex tachycardia. Cardioversion (not defibrillation) is indicated if the patient is

unstable. Digoxin is also used for recalcitrant SVT. Calcium channel blockers are contraindicated for children under 1 year of age as they may precipitate cardiovascular collapse. Ibuprofen would be useful for sinus tachycardia due to fever, but this patient had no fever and the heart rate is above that seen with sinus tachycardia. *(Rudolph CD, 1854–1856)*

32. **(B)** All of the listed answers may cause hair loss. Tinea capitis generally has more patchy hair loss and may have "black dots," representing broken hair. Trichotillomania will have bizarre patterns of hair loss in linear bands that has stubs of varying length. Hair traction alopecia occurs in areas of stress where the hair is pulled into braids or ponytails. It may become permanent if scarring occurs. Chemical exposure should be elicited from history. Alopecia areata is the most likely cause in this patient, given the complete hair loss and the characteristic exclamation point appearance of the hair. *(Rudolph CD, 1210–1212)*

33. **(C)** Alopecia areata occurs when hair that is in a growing phase (anagen) abruptly stops growing, causing the hair shafts to taper and lose adhesion to the follicle. Round patches of hair anywhere on the body can be affected, but are most noticeable when on the scalp. Clues to diagnosis include lack of inflammation, easily removed hair at the borders, and the exclamation point appearance of the hair under the microscope. Unfortunately the course is difficult to predict, a fact that should be stressed to the patient. Treatments with steroids, minoxidil, and immunomodulators such as cyclosporine have shown some success, but their use should be undertaken in consultation with a dermatologist. *(Rudolph CD, 1210–1212)*

34. **(B)** This history is highly suggestive of pertussis. The clinical course is divided into three stages: (1) the catarrhal stage, 2–10 days in duration, characterized by rhinorrhea, lacrimation, and sometimes low-grade fever; (2) the paroxysmal stage, lasting 1–6 weeks, during which there are intermittent episodes of coughing that may terminate with a forced inspiration against a partially closed glottis resulting in a "whoop"

or may terminate with vomiting; (3) the convalescent stage, lasting up to 6 months, during which the coughing episodes gradually resolve. Infants with pertussis often do not whoop because of their inability to generate sufficient inspiratory forces. Between episodes of cough, the examination is often normal. Of the choices given, the immunization status is of most importance. *(McMillan, 1094–1097)*

35. **(C)** A high white blood count with a marked lymphocytosis is characteristic of pertussis. Therefore, prescribing a macrolide, specifically azithromycin, is the most appropriate choice. A repeat CBC is not needed to follow the treatment. In fact, antibiotics do not hasten the resolution of the illness, but will decrease spread to other household members. Even so, all household contacts should also be treated prophylactically. *(McMillan, 1094–1097)*

36. **(B)** *Bordetella pertussis* is most likely to be recovered from the nasopharynx and more likely to be positive early in the illness. Throat swabs are less likely to be positive and sputum is almost never obtainable from infants. Bronchoscopy is not necessary to make the diagnosis and bacteremia does not occur. Special media are needed for cultivation of the organism. *(McMillan, 1094–1097)*

37. **(D)** This history and the finding of papilledema is strongly suggestive of pseudotumor cerebri, also known as benign intracranial hypertension, a condition marked by overproduction of cerebrospinal fluid leading to increased intracranial pressure. However, imaging to rule out a mass or a sinus thrombosis should be performed. A history of ingestion of vitamin A, tetracycline, or steroids, or a history of pregnancy would further support the diagnosis of pseudotumor cerebri. Her blood pressure is mildly elevated, but does not warrant treatment at this time with oral or intravenous antihypertensive agents. Mannitol and furosemide would be used in the emergent management of suspected herniation, but the patient currently has no signs to suggest that problem. *(Rudolph CD, 2398; Behrman, 2525–2526)*

38. **(A)** The next step would be lumbar puncture with determination of opening and closing pressures. Removal of sufficient fluid to reduce the CSF pressure is therapeutic. At times a nonsteroidal drug or even a narcotic may be necessary to temporarily relieve the headaches associated with pseudotumor cerebri. Serial lumbar punctures may be needed for continued symptomatic relief. Medications to reduce CSF production include acetazolamide and steroids. *(Rudolph CD,2398; Behrman, 1862)*

39. **(E)** Indications for surgical interventions include vision loss despite adequate therapy or inability to tolerate treatment. Surgical options include optic nerve fenestrations or placement of a lumboperitoneal shunt; repeat or additional (MRI) imaging should also be performed in case a small tumor was missed initially. *(Rudolph CD, 2398; Behrman, 1862)*

40. **(D)** The first priority in managing this patient is ensuring that the airway is patent and ventilation/oxygenation is adequate. Suction of vomitus may be needed as well. *(McMillan, 702–704, 2297–2299; Pediatrics, 97:769–772, 1996)*

41. **(E)** Given the patient's age, fever, and paucity of abnormal physical findings, the most likely diagnosis is febrile seizure. The most pressing need is to rule out meningitis. The American Academy of Pediatrics strongly recommends consideration of a lumbar puncture in all patients less than 12 months of age who present with a simple febrile seizure. In the absence of signs of increased intracranial pressure, a head CT is not indicated prior to lumbar puncture. Skull x-rays, arterial blood gas, and electroencephalograms have very low yield in this clinical situation and are not routinely warranted. *(McMillan, 702–704, 2297–2299; Pediatrics, 97:769–772, 1996)*

42. **(A)** It is reassuring that this patient's physical examination has returned to normal, compatible with the diagnosis of a simple febrile seizure. The parents should be counseled that about one-third of children experiencing a febrile seizure will have at least one recurrence. The risk is higher in children experiencing the first seizure before the age of 1 year. Chronic

anticonvulsant prophylaxis is not indicated for simple febrile seizures. While attempts to control fever are certainly warranted in patients with a history of febrile seizures, the use of antipyretics alone has not proven effective in the prevention of recurrence. In particular, there is no evidence that the use of alternating doses of acetaminophen and ibuprofen is necessary or effective in seizure prevention. Hospital admission and neuroimaging are not necessary in patients whose examination returns to normal prior to discharge from the emergency department. *(McMillan, 702–704, 2297–2299; Pediatrics, 97:769–772, 1996)*

43. **(B)** Before a lengthy and expensive diagnostic evaluation is undertaken, the growth patterns of the biological parents should be evaluated, as they are predictive of the child's growth pattern. Sibling height may be helpful, but is not predictive. Parental age does not affect offspring height per se, but may be indirectly associated in cases of age-related disorders such as Down syndrome. Social factors may influence growth rate as psychosocial dwarfism is seen in institutionalized and maltreated children. *(Behrman, 2386–2389)*

44. **(D)** The physical findings described suggest the diagnosis of Turner syndrome. Girls with Turner syndrome often present with short stature without typical stigmata including webbed neck, low hairline, and a broad chest with widely spaced nipples. Other findings include dysgenic ovaries, and estrogen levels are low resulting in a lack of negative feedback on the pituitary gland. Consequently, luteinizing- and follicle-stimulating hormone levels are high. An abdominal ultrasound will reveal the streak ovaries. Growth hormone levels are low and the bone age is delayed. Although all of the tests listed will likely reveal abnormalities, it is the karyotype that will ultimately confirm the diagnosis. *(Behrman, 1753–1754)*

45. **(A)** Echocardiography is indicated in patients with Turner syndrome because of the association with various cardiac anomalies, including bicuspid aortic valve, aortic stenosis, and anomalous pulmonary venous return. While characteristic of Down syndrome, cervical laxity is not

a feature of Turner syndrome. Growth hormone may increase adult height, and estrogen replacement therapy can improve bone density, growth, and sexual maturation. However, thyroid hormone replacement is not routinely indicated. The risk of endometrial carcinoma is not increased in these patients. Although Turner syndrome is associated with increased risk for some learning problems, mental retardation is not a feature of the disorder. Psychosocial support is important as well; the Turner Syndrome Society has chapters in the United States that can provide a support network for patients and their families. *(Behrman, 1753–1754)*

46. **(D)** The constellation of these symptoms is strongly suggestive of Kawasaki disease (Figure 10-2). The disease is most commonly seen in children under 5 years of age. Diagnostic criteria include fever of at least 5 days' duration together with at least four of the following features: (1) conjunctival injection; (2) oral changes, including erythema of the oral mucosa and pharynx, strawberry tongue, and red, cracked lips; (3) an erythematous, generalized rash; (4) changes in the peripheral extremities consisting of swelling of the hands or feet, erythematous palms or soles, or desquamation of the fingertips; and (5) a unilateral lymph node at least 1.5 cm in diameter. In addition, other potential causes of the illness (eg, measles, scarlet fever, and Stevens-Johnson syndrome) must be excluded. *(AAP:Red Book, 412–415)*

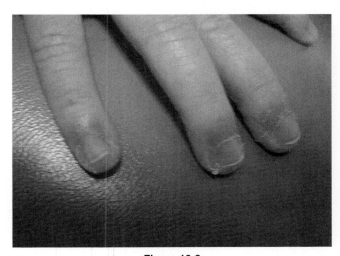

Figure 10-2

47. **(C)** Kawasaki manifestations and complications include arthralgias, irritability, vomiting, sterile pyuria, mild hepatic dysfunction, aseptic meningitis, pericardial effusion, myocarditis, and coronary artery ectasia and aneurysms. In addition to these problems, hydrops of the gallbladder is a well-described complication. Although thrombocytopenia has rarely been described in association with this disease, thrombocytosis is the more characteristic finding. Sterility, ulcerative colitis, and transverse myelitis are not associated with this disease. *(AAP:Red Book,412–415)*

48. **(B)** Receipt of IVIG may interfere with the immune response to some live viral vaccinations. Therefore, measles and varicella immunization should be deferred for 11 months following IVIG administration. Other routine vaccines should be given as scheduled. Influenza vaccine should be encouraged, as there is a potential for Reye syndrome when aspirin is given. No repetition of previously administered vaccines is necessary. *(AAP:Red Book,415)*

49. **(C)** The history of trauma with the presence of localized tenderness on examination and the lack of systemic symptoms such as fever make infection unlikely. Therefore, C-reactive protein and blood culture are not indicated. At this point there is no indication of underlying metabolic bone disease and alkaline phosphatase is not warranted. Although a high index of suspicion for nonaccidental trauma is appropriate, the history given is consistent with the physical findings described, and social service consultation is not warranted at this time. Given the possibility of fracture, performance of radiographs would be the most appropriate choice. *(Behrman, 2839)*

50. **(E)** The history and physical findings described are suggestive of a "toddler's fracture," also termed childhood accidental spiral tibial (CAST) fracture. These fractures occur most commonly in the distal tibia, often following relatively minor trauma. They are not suggestive of abuse. The diagnosis is confirmed by radiographs; occasionally, the fracture may be radiographically occult or demonstrable only on oblique films. Immobilization of the limb in a posterior short leg splint will provide support and reduce the pain that occurs with movement of the limb. Casting can occur later when swelling has subsided. Healing typically occurs in 4–6 weeks. *(Behrman, 2097)*

51. **(B)** The differential diagnosis of the lethargic neonate is extensive and includes infection, effect of maternal medications, electrolyte disturbances, metabolic abnormalities, congenital abnormalities, and trauma. The delay in onset of symptoms until day 3 of life make maternal medications an unlikely cause of lethargy in this neonate. There is no history of abdominal distention or bilious emesis to suggest an intraabdominal emergency such as midgut volvulus and diagnostic imaging is therefore not indicated. If there were reason to suspect head trauma or intracranial bleeding, CT would be the imaging modality of choice. Of the options presented, performance of an evaluation for infection is the most appropriate first step. *(Rudolph CD,106–107)*

52. **(A)** Inborn errors of metabolism are likely in this patient. While rare individually, these disorders in aggregation approximate the incidence of sepsis. Therefore, consideration of one of these disorders, particularly when the evaluation for infection does not yield any definite evidence of infection, should not be delayed. In a male with an elevated ammonia level, especially without acidosis, a urea cycle defect is the most likely possibility. Elevation of urine orotic acid, a by-product produced in increased amounts due to a lack of ornithine transcarbamylase, is consistent with ornithine transcarbamylase deficiency. Inheritance is X-linked dominant, and there are over 20 variants. Females with the defective gene typically have milder forms of the illness. *(Behrman, 558–559)*

53. **(C)** Therapy for suspected urea cycle defects involves parenteral nutrition with glucose, lipids, and essential amino acids to promote anabolism. Arginine hydrochloride intravenously is essential to supply the urea cycle

with ornithine, which now becomes an essential amino acid. Additional emergent medications to lower the ammonia include sodium benzoate, that combines with glycine to form hippuric acid, and sodium phenylacetate, that combines with glutamine to form phenylacetylglutamine, both of which are more easily excreted by the kidney than ammonia. Citrulline is necessary as 1 mol of citrulline will remove 1 mol of ammonia. Frequent monitoring of ammonia levels is necessary. If no appreciable change in ammonia is noted within a few hours, the only therapeutic option left is dialysis, which may be technically difficult or impossible if access cannot be obtained. Increasing arginine infusion rates or prolonging an ineffective therapy will provide no benefit to this child. Exchange transfusion has little effect on lowering total body ammonia. While many children do suffer permanent debilitating effects of the initial hyperammonemia, consideration of DNR status at this time is inappropriate. *(Behrman, 367–370)*

54. **(E)** In a well-appearing child with a recent viral illness and without fever, toxicity, or systemic signs of illness who presents with unexplained petechiae and ecchymoses, idiopathic thrombocytopenic purpura (ITP) is the most likely diagnosis. A complete blood count is indicated to establish the presence of thrombocytopenia and assess the other cell lines. When other cell lines are affected, a bone marrow may be needed to rule out leukemia and other hematologic disorders. Trauma presenting only with generalized petechiae would be rare. rickettsial or neisserial infections can cause petechiae but most affected patients have other symptoms. *(Rudolph CD,1556–1557)*

55. **(D)** The presence of isolated thrombocytopenia and increased megakaryocytes on bone marrow examination establishes the diagnosis of idiopathic thrombocytopenic purpura. If examination of the bone marrow reveals a lack of megakaryocytes, the diagnosis is not ITP and other causes of thrombocytopenia should be pursued. Several treatment options for ITP exist, including simple observation. Corticosteroids,

intravenous immunoglobulin, and anti-Rho antibodies have all been used with success. Indications for treatment include evidence of bleeding, thrombocytopenia less than 50,000, or prolonged thrombocytopenia. The presence of fever is not relevant to the treatment decision. The mechanism of action of anti-Rho antibodies is uncertain. However, it is thought that reticuloendothelial Fc receptor blockade is involved. This type of therapy will only be effective in patients that are Rh-positive. *(Rudolph CD, 1556–1557)*

56. **(D)** ITP resolves completely within 6 months in 80%–90% of cases. Splenectomy is seldom necessary, and usually is reserved for chronic cases lasting greater than 6–9 months. Splenectomy may also be required for control of severe recalcitrant bleeding. Low platelet counts, bleeding, splenomegaly, and anemia are not in themselves indications for splenectomy. *(Rudolph CD, 1556–1557)*

57. **(A)** In a patient presenting with hypertension and pallor following a history of hemorrhagic enteritis, the presence of hemolytic-uremic syndrome (HUS) should be considered. The most frequent cause is infection with *E coli* O157:H7. The primary event in this condition is endothelial injury from verotoxin release, resulting in a microangiopathic hemolytic anemia. Renal vascular involvement results in hypertension. The CBC and smear will show anemia, thrombocytopenia, and schistocytes. The other tests may be abnormal but will not establish the diagnosis. *(Behrman, 2181–2182)*

58. **(A)** Additional evidence for HUS is manifested by the elevated BUN and creatinine. Care for HUS is primarily careful medical management in conjunction with early and frequent dialysis to control fluid overload, manage electrolyte abnormalities, and remove plasminogen activator inhibitor-1 so that endogenous fibrinolytic mechanisms can dissolve vascular thrombi. Plasmapheresis and fresh frozen plasma have been used with some success as well. Steroids and antibiotics have no ameliorative effect, and the illness rarely recurs. Ninety percent of patients survive the

acute phase and the majority of patients regain normal renal function. *(Behrman, 367–370)*

59. **(C)** This patient has typical signs and symptoms of croup which is caused primarily by parainfluenza viruses. Infection results in tracheal airway inflammation and edema. In mild cases, positive intrathoracic airway pressure generated by coughing generates a high-pitched, seal-like barky cough. As narrowing continues, the negative thoracic pressure generated by the diaphragm will cause the airway to collapse, requiring more accessory muscle effort to generate airflow. Nebulized epinephrine provides immediate effect in relief of edema, primarily through its alpha agonist effect. Steroids are effective in relieving the edema of croup, but typically take several hours for effects to be seen. The hypoxia and degree of respiratory distress this child is manifesting requires more than just humidified air. While the other options presented may all be useful in the management of croup, racemic epinephrine will provide the fastest relief. *(Behrman, 1762–1765)*

60. **(D)** If a patient is not responsive to initial therapies, other etiologies of upper airway obstruction must be considered. Of those (a foreign body, retropharyngeal abscess, epiglottitis, peritonsillar abscess, or Ludwig angina), epiglottitis is the diagnosis suggested by the clinical presentation in this patient. Compared to patients with viral croup, patients with bacterial epiglottitis typically are more toxic appearing. They present with lethargy, drooling, and a rapid onset of respiratory failure. When the diagnosis of bacterial epiglottitis is highly suspected, intervention (intubation) should not be delayed to await radiographic confirmation (*thumb print sign*), antibiotic administration, or observation. Because of the risk of the development of complete airway obstruction, establishment of an artificial airway is the first priority. Controlled endotracheal intubation, performed in the operating suite if possible, should be undertaken with immediate surgical backup. Rapid-sequence intubation in the emergency department may become necessary, but is not preferred

to the more controlled environment of the operation suite. *(Behrman, 836, 1275–1278)*

61. **(A)** The patient described is not in severe distress as indicated by the ability to talk in complete sentences and the lack of hypoxia. The recurrent episodes of wheezing suggest asthma as the most likely etiology. An initial trial of an inhaled beta agonist is the most appropriate choice. These agents' primary mode of action is relaxation of airway smooth muscle. The other therapies listed are sometimes used, but not as the initial management for acute exacerbations of mild-to-moderate asthma. *(Rudolph CD, 1950–1963; Behrman, 958–969)*

62. **(C)** An expert panel report provides guidelines for management of asthma based on the severity of the disease. For infants and young children who have had four or more episodes of wheezing in the past year that lasted more than 1 day and impaired sleep plus additional risk factors for developing persistent asthma, including parental history of asthma, physician diagnosis of atopic dermatitis, or evidence of sensitization to aeroallergens, two of the following including evidence of sensitization to foods, greater than or equal to 4% peripheral blood eosinophilia, or wheezing apart from colds, long-term control therapy is recommended. The patient described has persistent asthma. Recommended management includes the daily use of an anti-inflammatory agent. Therefore, inhaled fluticasone is the most appropriate choice given. Autoinjectable epinephrine should be used for anaphylaxis and is not indicated in the routine management of asthma. Salmeterol, a long-acting beta$_2$-adrenergic agonist, is indicated for patients with more severe asthma. Because of its narrow therapeutic index and need for frequent monitoring, theophylline's use has declined and currently is considered only a second line-agent for patients with asthma refractory to standard therapy. Antihistamines do not decrease bronchoconstriction and are not routinely part of chronic asthma management (see Table 10-2). *(Rudolph CD, 1950–1963; Behrman, 674–679; http://www.nhlbi.nih.gov/guidelines/asthma/asthgdln.htm)*

TABLE 10-2. National Heart Lung and Blood Institute. National Asthma Education and Prevention Program Expert Panel Report 3. Guidelines for the Diagnosis and Management of Asthma (epr-3). http://www.nhlbi.nih.gov/guidelines/asthma/asthsumm.pdf. Published July 2007. Updated 2002.

Classifying Asthma Severity and Initiating Therapy in Children

Components of Severity	Intermittent — Ages 0-4	Intermittent — Ages 5-11	Persistent: Mild — Ages 0-4	Persistent: Mild — Ages 5-11	Persistent: Moderate — Ages 0-4	Persistent: Moderate — Ages 5-11	Persistent: Severe — Ages 0-4	Persistent: Severe — Ages 5-11
Impairment								
Symptoms	≤2 days/week	≤2 days/week	>2 days/week but not daily	>2 days/week but not daily	Daily	Daily	Throughout the day	Throughout the day
Nighttime awakenings	0	≤2x/month	1-2x/month	3-4x/month	3-4x/month	>1x/week but not nightly	>1x/week	Often 7x/week
Short-acting beta$_2$-agonist use for symptom control	≤2 days/week	≤2 days/week	>2 days/week but not daily	>2 days/week but not daily	Daily	Daily	Several times per day	Several times per day
Interference with normal activity	None	None	Minor limitation	Minor limitation	Some limitation	Some limitation	Extremely limited	Extremely limited
Lung Function — FEV$_1$ (predicted) or peak flow (personal best)	N/A	Normal FEV$_1$ between exacerbations; >80%	N/A	>80%	N/A	60-80%	N/A	<60%
Lung Function — FEV$_1$/FVC		>85%		>80%		74-80%		<75%
Risk — Exacerbations requiring oral systemic corticosteroids (consider severity and interval since last exacerbation)	0-1/year (see notes)	0-1/year (see notes)	≥2 exacerbations in 6 months requiring oral systemic corticosteroids, or ≥4 wheezing episodes/1 year lasting >1 day and risk factors for persistent asthma	≥2x/year (see notes); Relative annual risk may be related to FEV$_1$				
Recommended Step for Initiating Therapy (See "Stepwise Approach for Managing Asthma" for treatment steps.)	Step 1 (for both age groups)	Step 1 (for both age groups)	Step 2 (for both age groups)	Step 2 (for both age groups)	Step 3 and consider short course of oral systemic corticosteroids	Step 3: medium-dose ICS option and consider short course of oral systemic corticosteroids	Step 3 and consider short course of oral systemic corticosteroids	Step 3: medium-dose ICS option or step 4 and consider short course of oral systemic corticosteroids

The stepwise approach is meant to assist, not replace, the clinical decisionmaking required to meet individual patient needs.

In 2-6 weeks, depending on severity, evaluate level of asthma control that is achieved.
- Children 0-4 years old: If no clear benefit is observed in 4-6 weeks, stop treatment and consider alternative diagnoses or adjusting therapy.
- Children 5-11 years old: Adjust therapy accordingly.

Key: FEV$_1$, forced expiratory volume in 1 second; FVC, forced vital capacity; ICS, inhaled corticosteroids; ICU, intensive care unit; N/A, not applicable

Notes:
- Level of severity is determined by both impairment and risk. Assess impairment domain by caregiver's recall of previous 2-4 weeks. Assign severity to the most severe category in which any feature occurs.
- Frequency and severity of exacerbations may fluctuate over time for patients in any severity category. At present, there are inadequate data to correspond frequencies of exacerbations with different levels of asthma severity. In general, more frequent and severe exacerbations (eg, requiring urgent, unscheduled care, hospitalization, or ICU admission) indicate greater underlying disease severity. For treatment purposes, patients with ≥2 exacerbations described above may be considered the same as patients who have persistent asthma, even in the absence of impairment levels consistent with persistent asthma.

63. (E) The history of recent travel to a country with high rates of contagious illness makes an infectious etiology more likely in this previously healthy child. His icterus and hepatomegaly point to an infectious hepatitis. Whether he had received the hepatitis A vaccine would be most useful to know. Sickle cell may be associated with jaundice, but is most common in individuals of African descent. Consumption of large amounts of carotene-containing vegetables such as carrots may result in carotenemia. This may cause cutaneous discoloration resembling jaundice, but would not cause scleral icterus or systemic symptoms. Malar rash might suggest the possibility of systemic lupus erythematosis which might be associated with hepatitis, but the constellation of findings presented is more suggestive of an infectious illness. Acetaminophen can result in hepatic dysfunction but generally in the context of overdose. *(Behrman, 1680–1682)*

64. (A) Given the history of travel to Mexico, hepatits A is the most likely etiology of this illness, and may be diagnosed by serology. The aspartate aminotransferase will be elevated but does not establish the etiology of the hepatitis. Twenty-four hour urinary copper excretion is useful in the diagnosis of Wilson disease which can present with hepatic dysfunction, but is not indicated in the clinical context presented here. Unless there is a suspicion of acetaminophen overdose, determination of serum level is not warranted. *(Behrman, 769–771)*

65. (D) Hepatitis A is a picornavirus spread via the oral-fecal route that has a mean incubation period of approximately 4 weeks. Most infected children are asymptomatic. In certain developing countries, prevalence of infection with this agent approaches 100%. After infection, protective antibodies persist for life. An effective vaccine currently is available and is in widespread use. Fortunately, most children completely recover from hepatitis A infection. Rarely, it will progress to fulminant hepatic failure. In patients with hepatitis B infection, coinfection with hepatitis D can lead to fulminant hepatic failure. Hepatitis B, C, and D are spread via exposure to blood products or via intimate sexual contact. Hepatitis A could theoretically be spread this way but that is not the most common manner. *(Behrman, 769–771)*

66. (B) Response to supplemental oxygen is helpful in the differential diagnosis of cyanosis in the neonate. The lack of response to increased oxygen suggests a right-to-left shunt, which in a newborn would most likely be due to cyanotic congenital heart disease. Hypoxemia associated with sepsis and pneumonia should respond to an increase in inspired oxygen. Because the PaO_2 is a measure of oxygen dissolved in plasma, it will be normal in patients with methemoglobinemia and will increase with administration of oxygen. However, cyanosis will persist as oxygen saturation of hemoglobin will remain impaired. While an arteriovenous fistula might produce right-to-left shunting and would not respond to increased oxygen, this is a much less likely entity than cyanotic congenital heart disease. *(Rudolph CD, 1824–1836)*

67. (A) Transposition of the great arteries (TGA) is the most likely cardiac malformation to present in the early newborn period with cyanosis and absence of heart murmur. TGA occurs in about 1/5000 live births and is more common in males and infants of diabetic mothers. The mediastinum often appears narrowed on chest radiographs. Tetralogy of Fallot usually presents slightly later in infancy with cyanosis and a systolic murmur from the associated ventricular septal defect. Total anomalous pulmonary venous return presents in a similar fashion but usually is associated with increased pulmonary vascular markings on chest radiography. *(Rudolph CD,1824–1836)*

68. (A) This infant is critically ill and immediate intervention is needed. The hypoxemia requires immediate cardiac catheterization for atrial septostomy to create a shunt and improve oxygenation. Antibiotics or pressors such as dobutamine may slightly improve the clinical state, but do nothing to correct the underlying problem. An arterial switch generally is deferred until the patient's electrolytes and medical status have stabilized. *(Rudolph CD,1824–1836)*

69. (B) The presence of anemia, jaundice, and dark urine suggests hemolysis as the most likely cause of the anemia. Evaluation should inquire about previous illnesses, episodes of pallor, and a list of all medicines taken, such as aspirin, antibiotics, or antimalarials. A family history of leukemia or sickle cell trait alone in a previously healthy child is unlikely to be relevant. Hepatitis A may cause jaundice but not pallor; also the cousin is described as healthy. Initial laboratory results to obtain include a smear to define red cell morphology, a reticulocyte count to determine marrow response, and the type of bilirubin made. A bone marrow may need to be performed at a later time. *(Behrman, 739, 2040–2042)*

70. (E) The unconjugated bilirubinemia is compatible with increased bilibrubin production resulting from hemolysis. Initial presentation of sickle cell disease at 6 years of life would be unusual. Absence of spherocytes on the peripheral smear weighs against the diagnosis of spherocytosis, although they may be absent in the face of acute hemolysis. Glucose-6-phosphate-dehydrogenase deficiency is the most likely etiology of those presented. Hemolysis associated with this disorder may be precipitated by sulfa-based antibiotics, antimalarials, aspirin, as well as organic solvents. Diagnosis depends on measurement of G6PD levels in older red cells. *(Behrman, 1474, 1489–1491)*

71. (C) The patient described has no evidence of cardiovascular instability; therefore, transfusion is not necessary or indicated. Close observation and serial hemoglobin determinations to monitor for continued hemolysis are sufficient. Removal of the offending agent usually results in cessation of hemolysis. Prednisone and other steroids have not been shown to change the course of the illness. *(Behrman, 1474, 1489–1491)*

72. (D) This is a classic presentation of Guillain-Barré syndrome (GBS), a postinfectious polyneuropathy. Illness is frequently preceded by a nonspecific viral illness. The patient experiences ascending paralysis with the bulbar muscles affected last, if at all. Deep tendon reflexes are lost, usually early in the course of the illness. Sensory function usually is spared. Nerve conduction velocity is decreased in Guillain-Barré syndrome. While there is no specific diagnostic test, the clinical picture combined with a cerebrospinal fluid showing an elevated protein and normal cell count is highly suggestive. Occasional cases of GBS can be associated with infection due to *M pneumonia* or *Campylobacter* species. The other laboratory abnormalities listed are not associated with Guillain-Barré syndrome. *(Behrman, 1200–1201, 2565–2566)*

73. (A) Patients in the early phase of the illness should be admitted for monitoring of their respiratory status as the muscles of respiration may become affected. Administration of IVIG has been shown to decrease the length of illness and lessen the associated long-term disability. Most patients will recover fully within 2–3 weeks and supportive care is all that is routinely needed. Other therapies that have been used for rapidly progressive courses include plasmapheresis, high-dose steroids, and immunosuppressive agents. Intravenous interferon-beta is a therapeutic agent that has shown promise in the treatment of multiple sclerosis but not GBS. *(Behrman, 1335–1336, 1892–1893)*

74. (D) The most likely cause of this patient's illness is diabetes mellitus with diabetic ketoacidosis (DKA). After assessing mental status and ensuring airway and breathing are intact, restoration of circulating volume using isotonic fluids is the first priority in the treatment of DKA. Diabetic ketoacidosis usually has an insidious onset as the body tries to compensate for the hyperglycemia and acidosis. The deficiency of insulin increases production of fatty acids and ketone bodies resulting in metabolic acidosis. Breathing becomes deep and rapid (Kussmaul respirations) as the respiratory centers increase ventilation to compensate for the metabolic acidosis. Additional lactic acidosis, when the osmotic diuresis is associated with hyperglycemia, results in increased urinary output (polyuria) and volume depletion. Dehydration and the caloric loss from glucosuria lead to weight loss. As thirst increases, patients will increase volume intake (polydipsia), but the acidosis and other metabolic derangements may lead to nausea, vomiting, and abdominal pain. Once these compensatory mechanisms are overwhelmed, DKA will become manifest as in this patient. Bicarbonate boluses have been associated with the development of cerebral edema. Although oral intake is not necessarily contraindicated in DKA, it is not the initial step in management. *(Berhman, 2415–2417)*

75. **(A)** A variety of metabolic derangements may result from the treatment of DKA. One of the more common is hypokalemia. Although serum potassium may be elevated in the untreated state, total body potassium is actually low. With insulin replacement and resolution of acidosis, hypokalemia may become manifest. Hypophosphatemia may also occur, as phosphate is transported intracellularly to restore adenosine triphosphate stores. Likewise, depletion of total body stores of magnesium and calcium occurs during DKA. *(Berhman, 1772–1777)*

76. **(E)** Parental requests for antibiotic therapy are frequent. A red eardrum alone is not diagnostic of otitis media. Diagnosis should be made only in the presence of a bulging tympanic membrane, opaque middle ear fluid, and abnormal membrane mobility on pneumatic otoscopy. For this child's likely viral illness, antipyretic therapy and fluids are all that is indicated at this time. The physician should take the time to discuss the development of a bacterial ear infection so the parents understand why antibiotics are not necessary at this time, but may become necessary over the course of the illness. *(Rudolph CD,1249–1255)*

77. **(A)** The child now has developed acute otitis media with effusion. Viral upper respiratory infections are the most frequent antecedent of otitis media in young children. They result in eustachian tube dysfunction that predisposes to middle ear bacterial superinfection, most commonly by *S pneumoniae*, nontypeable *Haemophilus influenzae*, or *Moraxella catarrhalis*. Amoxicillin is considered by many authorities to be first-line therapy for otitis media. Because of increasing pneumococcal penicillin resistance rates, high doses (ie, 80–90 mg/kg/day)

are appropriate. This is especially true in the context of day care attendance because of the increased risk for resistant pneumococci among children in this setting. Ceftriaxone has been demonstrated to be effective in the management of otitis media, but should generally be reserved for cases not responsive to initial antibiotic management. Erythromycin is not appropriate in the treatment of this infection because many of the offending organisms are resistant. An otorhinolaryngology consult is not routinely necessary in the management of acute otorrhea. *(Rudolph CD,1249–1255)*

78. **(D)** The physical findings described indicate that mastoiditis has developed as a complication of the otitis media. The organisms causing mastoiditis are the same as for otitis media. Computerized tomography of the mastoids permits delineation of the area of involvement. Intravenous antibiotic therapy including a third-generation cephalosporin and possibly additional gram-positive coverage are also indicated. Consultation with an otolaryngologist for drainage is appropriate. The other choices are inappropriate at this stage. *(Rudolph CD, 1249 –1255)*

79. **(E)** Diagnostic options for evaluating the etiology of this patient's problems are numerous. However, the first step is to interview the patient alone. Her symptoms and flat affect warrant a frank, private discussion with the patient regarding issues such as depression, suicidal ideation, abuse (physical, mental, and sexual), eating disorders, and drug abuse. It should be stressed that theses discussions will be kept in confidence. Although both organic and psychiatric conditions may cause the constellation of findings seen in this patient, the initial step in the evaluation of either is a careful history. The behavior described is not typical for a healthy adolescent and should not be ignored. *(Behrman, 122–123)*

80. **(D)** Psychiatric illness needs to be aggressively addressed. The health care professional needs to assess whether the patient poses a threat to herself or others; the rate of suicide in the 15–19-year-old age group is around 9/100,000.

If there is any indication of suicidal ideation, the patient should be evaluated emergently by a psychiatrist. Inpatient admission with close monitoring may be warranted in such cases. Collection of urine for drug screening against this patient's will increases barriers to establishing a therapeutic alliance. Although comorbidity with drug use is often seen in patients with psychiatric disorders, screening for drug use should only proceed with the patient's consent. Variation in mood is characteristic of adolescents, but the severity indicated here is outside the norm. Selective serotonin reuptake inhibitors are safe and possess minimal side effects. Initiation of this class of therapeutic agent along with counseling and close follow-up is appropriate in the case described. *(Behrman, 80, 92)*

81. **(B)** Bipolar disorder usually presents in the third decade of life but can present in late adolescence. Patients with this disorder vacillate from depression to mania or may present with mania alone. During manic spells the patient's behavior is characterized by high levels of activity, loquaciousness, insomnia, feelings of grandiosity, a tendency toward overspending, and an expansive mood that may persist for weeks. SSRIs can heighten energy but not to this extent. The lack of delusions and the ability to function well enough to purchase items make schizophrenia less likely. Sexual abuse can present in a variety of fashions but given her history, a bipolar disorder is more likely. Lithium carbonate, valproic acid, and/or carbamazepine along with intense psychiatric therapy may be necessary to control the symptoms of this illness. *(Behrman, 80, 92)*

82. **(C)** The findings indicate that this patient has leukemia and is presently neutropenic. Most infections in neutropenic patients arise from endogenous flora, primarily the gastrointestinal tract. Bacteria intermittently seed the blood stream by translocating across the mucosal surface due to impaired immune surveillance. Empiric antibiotics should be directed against gram-negative organisms, including *P aeruginosa*. Of the options presented, ceftazidime is the most appropriate, offering coverage of gram-negative organisms including *P aeruginosa*. Despite broad activity against gram-negative bacteria, including *P aeruginosa*, ciprofloxacin given orally is not appropriate in the situation described. *(Behrman, 1103–1104, 2116–2120)*

83. **(B)** Indicators of a more favorable prognosis in acute lymphocytic leukemia include age 1–10 years, hyperdiploidy over 50 chromosomes, absence of blasts in the CSF, initial white blood cell count of less than 50,000, absence of the 9:22 translocation (Philadelphia chromosome), and a TEL/AML-1 translocation. Poor prognostic factors include 11q23 or 4:11 translocations or lack of the previously described favorable conditions. *(Behrman, 785–787, 1543–1546)*

84. **(C)** Induction chemotherapy may produce the tumor lysis syndrome, a constellation of metabolic abnormalities resulting from destruction of large numbers of tumor cells with release of intracellular constituents. In particular, potassium, calcium, and phosphorus levels can rise precipitously. Hyperkalemia can lead to dangerous arrhythmias. Simultaneous development of hyperphosphatemia and hypercalcemia can lead to heterotopic calcifications in various organ systems; kidney involvement may result in renal failure. The release of uric acid can lead to nephrolithiasis. Preventative measures for these complications include aggressive hydration, alkalinization of the urine, and allopurinol administration. Dialysis may be needed if these preventative efforts fail. *(Behrman, 785–787, 1543–1546)*

85. **(E)** Colic typically begins prior to 3 months of age, and is characterized by 3 or more hours of unexplained crying at least three times a week. The cry is spontaneous and continuous, with the face appearing flushed, the legs drawn up, and the hands clenched. Bouts of crying associated with colic may resolve when the patient becomes exhausted or with the passage of flatus or belching. Without fever, ill appearance, vomiting, weight loss, or other abnormal signs or symptoms, reassurance and follow-up are the most appropriate initial steps. *(Rudolph CD, 414–417)*

86. **(B)** A wide variety of colic treatment modalities have been suggested. The most effective one remains time, as colic rarely persists over 3 months of age. Swaddling has been shown to calm some infants. Stress is a precipitant of colic, and subjecting a single caregiver to the unremitting crying associated with colic is likely to worsen the stress (of both caretaker and baby). Water has not been demonstrated to be effective in this condition and excessive amounts given to young infants may precipitate hyponatremia. Likewise, vigorous shaking obviously is very harmful to infants. Paregoric (morphine, alcohol, and anise oil) is ineffective and potentially harmful. *(Rudolph CD,414–417)*

87. **(E)** A preverbal child cries to express him- or herself, and this needs to be stressed to parents. A search for causes of discomfort needs to be performed by the physician. Potential causes include hair tourniquets, occult fractures or infection, corneal abrasions, and severe diaper rashes. Irritability can also be due to sepsis, intussusception, hernia, or feeding intolerance. Given this patient's appearance, and the associated bilious emesis, a prompt evaluation to exclude the diagnosis of volvulus is necessary. *(Rudolph CD,1410)*

88. **(C)** A history of constipation and the potential for an associated anal fissure would be useful, given the history of streaks of blood on the surface of the stools. Hemophilia rarely presents with gastrointestinal bleeding. Iron intake is irrelevant as iron (except in overdose) does not cause gastrointestinal bleeding. Rotavirus is unlikely in the absence of diarrhea and typically does not result in the presence of gross blood in the stools. Crohn disease would be rare in a patient of this age. *(Behrman, 1639)*

89. **(C)** Anal fissures are the most common cause of bloody stools in the pediatric population. Continued passage of hard stool may prevent healing, a fact that should be stressed to the parents. Initial treatment should be aimed at softening the stool. Increasing fiber intake is very useful but hard to do as it may require drastically altering the diet of the child (and the parents as well). A stool softener (such as lactulose or mineral oil) titrated to the desired consistency is usually needed as well. Infections of anal fissures are rare; parents should be taught what to look for, but routine antibiotics are not warranted. The use of rectal dilators, frequent rectal temperatures, or colonic manipulation should not be performed. *(Behrman, 1181)*

90. **(D)** Juvenile rheumatoid arthritis (now known as juvenile idiopathic arthritis or JIA) affects about 250,000 children in the United States with a yearly incidence of approximately 14/100,000 children under 16 years of age. Joint symptoms are typically more severe in the morning and improve through the day. Large joints are usually affected. Progression of disease may result in persistent joint effusion, arthritis, and fusion of wrist joints with loss of movement. JIA is classically divided into three types: polyarticular, pauciarticular (with two subtypes), and systemic onset. Of these, polyarticular, rheumatoid factor positive JIA tends to have the worst prognosis with respect to joint involvement. *(Behrman, 1001–1010)*

91. **(E)** Eye involvement can be seen in either polyarticular or pauciarticular type of JIA, but is more commonly seen in the pauciarticular type. Affected children complain of redness, pain, photophobia, and decreased visual acuity. Early detection by serial ophthamologic examinations is essential for prevention of blindness in these children. *(Behrman, 704–709)*

92. **(B)** The patient described is in shock which is characterized by inadequate end-organ perfusion. Evidence of inadequate perfusion in this patient includes tachycardia and delayed capillary refill time. Shock is considered to be compensated in the presence of a normal blood pressure. Hypotension is defined by a blood pressure less than the 5th percentile for age. For children aged 1–10 years, the lower limits of normal systolic blood pressure (in mm Hg) can be estimated using the following formula: 70 + (age in years X 2). Other causes of shock include cardiogenic (eg, due to myocarditis) and sepsis. However, the presence of sunken eyes and fontanelle, along with poor skin turgor and the history of fluid loss from vomiting and diarrhea

implicate hypovolemia as the most likely etiology of this patient's shock. *(McMillan, 63–64, 2582–2587)*

93. **(C)** Mild dehydration, that is, 3%–6% loss of body weight, is manifested by increased thirst and tachycardia but normal skin turgor and capillary refill time. Moderate dehydration in young infants such as this patient occurs when there is a fluid loss approximating 10% body weight, whereas older children have moderate dehydration with fluid losses of about 6%–9% body weight. Moderate dehydration is characterized by the signs and symptoms of mild dehydration together with weak peripheral pulses. Patients with severe dehydration (fluid loss > 10% body weight) frequently have associated hypotension, not present in the patient under discussion. Therefore, this child has an estimated fluid loss of 10% body weight (approximately 600–700 cc). *(McMillan, 63–64, 2582–2587)*

94. **(A)** The initial hydrating solution should have close to 130–155 meq/L of sodium so that it can expand the intravascular volume quickly. If the patient is hypernatremic, it will not decrease the serum sodium too quickly, and will also correct any hyponatremia slowly as well. Appropriate resuscitation fluid could be normal saline (154 meq/L) or lactated Ringer (130 meq/L). *(McMillan, 63–64, 2582–2587)*

95. **(E)** Onset of a vesicular exanthem and enanthem in the early neonatal period should suggest the possibility of herpes simplex infection. Most women giving birth to infected babies have no known history of herpes infection. Evaluation of babies with suspected herpes infection should include cultures of the lesions for virus. Examination of the CSF is also important to evaluate for concomitant central nervous system infection. Prompt initiation of acyclovir is important in reducing morbidity and mortality. Institution of antiviral therapy in patients with compatible signs and symptoms should not await culture confirmation. *(AAP:Red Book, 365–366)*

96. **(A)** The overall incidence of HSV infection is from 1/3000 to 1/20,000 of all live births. The

risk of vertical transmission in cases of primary maternal infection is 33%–50%. The risk of transmission is substantially lower (> 5%) in the setting of reactivated disease. *(AAP:Red Book, 362–363)*

97. **(C)** Risk factors for vertical transmission include prolonged rupture of membranes greater than 4–6 hours, primary maternal infection, presence of active lesions on the vaginal mucosal surface, and the use of scalp electrodes. Maternal coinfection with HSV type 1 or human immunodeficiency virus is not known to increase risk of transmission of HSV type 2. Peripartum administration of acyclovir has not been demonstrated effective in reducing the risk of transmission. *(A AAP:Red Book, 368–369)*

98. **(A)** This child has a healing clavicle fracture that likely occurred during childbirth. Large babies have an increased risk of this problem. Associated symptoms may be minimal or absent. Callus formation does not become apparent until about 2 weeks of age, so it is not surprising that this is when the parents brought the infant in for evaluation. Some infants will not display irritability despite this obvious fracture. Comparison views are not necessary in the evaluation. A fibroblast assay is not warranted as this fracture is most commonly seen in otherwise normal neonates. *(Behrman, 727)*

99. **(B)** Factors that increase the difficulty of delivery may increase the risk of clavicular fracture. These include maternal diabetes (because of the association with fetal macrosomia), cephalopelvic disproportion, shoulder dystocia, or extension of the arms in breech position. Congenital syphilis may be associated with skeletal abnormalities, but there is no increase in risk for clavicle fractures. Likewise, maternal drug use has not been implicated as a cause of this problem. Thanatophoric dysplasia, lethal form of chondrodysplasia with associated defects in bone growth, is a rare,. These infants have short limbs, narrow chests, and large heads, but do not have an increased risk of clavicle fractures. *(Behrman, 2877–2878)*

100. **(B)** The patient described has features typical of Down syndrome. Ninety-five percent of patients with Down syndrome have trisomy of chromosome 21, usually due to mitotic nondisjunction of maternal gonadal cells. About 4% of affected patients have a centromeric translocation of chromosome 21 onto another chromosome, usually 13, 14, 15, or 21. Translocations account for 9% of Down syndrome patients born to mothers under 30. *(Behrman, 507–509)*

101. **(B)** Down syndrome is the most common trisomy, occurring in about 1/600–1/800 births. For comparison, sickle trait occurs in approximately 1/12 of African Americans, trisomy 18 (Edwards syndrome) occurs in about 1/8000 births, and trisomy 13 (Patau syndrome) occurs in about 1/20,000 births. *(Behrman, 324–328)*

102. **(D)** Individuals with Down syndrome are at increased risk for a variety of disorders. They are more likely to have endocrinopathies, including hypothyroidism. Congenital heart disease (most commonly endocardial cushion defects) occurs in almost half of these children. They also have an increased likelihood of leukemia, but not solid tumors. Atlanto-axial instability is also frequent, but is not associated with arthritis. Streak gonads are a finding seen in Turner syndrome. *(Behrman, 507–509, 2122)*

103. **(E)** Neutropenia generally is defined as an absolute neutrophil count less than 1500/mm³. Neutropenia is one of the major risk factors for infection in patients undergoing chemotherapy for malignancy. Conversely, the previously healthy child with an acute undifferentiated febrile illness and a nontoxic appearance has a very low risk of serious infection. The fact that the other blood cell lines are normal is reassuring. The most likely cause of the neutropenia is transient bone marrow suppression from a viral infection. Antibiotic therapy is not routinely necessary. Observation and follow-up of the WBC count to document resolution of the neutropenia would be the most appropriate management. *(Behrman, 910–912)*

104. **(C)** The onset of hemiparesis most likely is due to a thrombotic stroke, a known complication of sickle cell disease. Rapid intervention is essential in order to minimize morbidity. Computerized tomography may not show evidence of ischemia for several hours after onset of symptoms. Exchange transfusion, which acts by decreasing the proportion of hemoglobin S, is the therapeutic intervention of choice. Unlike the situation in adults where strokes are primarily due to atherosclerosis and activation of the clotting cascade, heparinization or infusion of plasminogen activator provides no benefit in stroke associated with sickle cell. Hydroxyurea may be helpful in long-term treatment to increase hemoglobin F but is not useful in the acute management of stroke. *(Behrman, 2026–2031, 2509)*

105. **(D)** Patients with sickle cell disease have functional asplenia by 1–2 years of age and are particularly susceptible to infection by polysaccharide-encapsulated bacteria, including *S pneumoniae*, *Haemophilus influenzae*, and *N meningitidis*. Of these, the pneumococcus is the most frequent cause of bacteremia. *(Behrman, 1479–1483)*

106. **(E)** Sickle cell disease is an autosomal recessive disorder. Approximately 12% of African Americans are heterozygous for the abnormal gene. However, this risk varies in other ethnic/racial groups and the risk of this patient's children cannot be determined without knowing the risk of his future mate carrying the abnormal gene. However, the risk for future children of couples with an affected child is approximately 25%. *(Behrman, 1479–1483)*

107. **(C)** This boy has stigmata of Duchenne muscular dystrophy (DMD) including pseudohypertrophy of the calves and a waddling gait. Because of muscle weakness, patients with DMD may use their hands to "walk" up their legs when arising from a sitting position (Gower sign). Rovsing sign occurs in appendicitis when palpation of the left lower quadrant elicits pain in the right lower quadrant. Opisthotonus (hyperextension of the head, neck, and trunk) occurs in tetanus and kernicterus. Chvostek sign is present when tapping over the course of the facial nerve causes contraction of the muscles of the eye, mouth, or nose and occurs with hypocalcemia. Grey-Turner sign (bruising of the flanks) is associated with hemorrhagic pancreatitis. *(Behrman, 2540–2544)*

108. **(E)** As weakness progresses and difficulty handling oral secretions ensues, aspiration pneumonia becomes a problem for patients with Duchenne muscular dystrophy. Other complications seen include osteopenia and scoliosis due to the weakness and immobility. Scoliosis may become severe enough to contribute to impaired ventilation. Cardiomyopathy progressing to congestive heart failure may also occur. The myoglobinuria associated with this condition does not cause renal failure and the bulbar muscles are rarely affected. *(Behrman, 1966, 2540–2544)*

109. **(B)** DMD is primarily an X-linked recessive disorder, occurring in about 1/3600 male infants. As with other X-linked recessive diseases, approximately 50% of male offspring will be affected while 50% of female offspring will be carriers. Affected males will not pass the disease to their sons, but all of their daughters will be carriers. Although female carriers are generally not severely affected, Barr body inactivation can result in the expression of some stigmata of disease. Approximately 30% of cases result from new mutations. *(Behrman, 1432, 1797, 1873–1877)*

110. **(A)** Of the findings listed, pulsus parodoxus (decline in systolic BP > 10 mm Hg during inspiration) is the most suggestive of cardiac tamponade. This results from impeded left ventricular outflow and restricted left atrial filling during inspiration caused in part by the descent of the diaphragm exerting traction on the taut pericardium. Enlargement of the cardiac silhouette is neither sensitive nor specific for the diagnosis of tamponade. Neither bounding pulses nor egophany result from cardiac tamponade. Although the electrocardiogram may demonstrate low voltage, this finding can also be seen with myocarditis. *(Rudolph CD,1865–1866)*

111. **(D)** In the presence of symptoms, particularly hypotension, prompt intervention to remove the fluid can be lifesaving. Steroids, inotropes, diuretics, and/or pericardial window may be needed as part of further management, but immediate pericardiocentesis is needed to permit patient stabilization. *(McMillan, 2683; Rudolph CD,1865–1866)*

112. **(B)** Fractionation of the bilirubin will guide further workup of the jaundice. The history of acholic stools suggests the presence of an obstructive jaundice. The other tests listed may all be indicated, but it is the bilirubin determination that will provide the most immediately useful data. *(Behrman, 1671–1673)*

113. **(D)** The presence of an elevated conjugated bilirubin in a thriving infant makes an obstructive lesion such as bile duct paucity or a choledochal cyst within the liver most likely. The initial diagnostic study in the evaluation of this condition is ultrasound. Tyrosinemia, which is characterized by elevated urinary succinylacetone levels might present with conjugated hyperbilirubinemia but not acholic stools. Cystic fibrosis is less likely to present with jaundice alone, especially at this age. Finally, plain film radiography will not add specific information. *(Behrman, 1205–1206)*

114. **(E)** Biliary atresia affects about 1/10,000–1/15,000 infants and varies in severity. An exploratory laparotomy and cholangiography should be done to determine if a surgically correctable lesion is present. For those in whom none is seen, the Kasai hepatoportoenterostomy should be performed as soon as possible to prevent worsening of cholestasis and hepatic damage. The rationale is that minute channels may be present in the porta hepatis and permit reestablishment of some bile flow, particularly if the channels are greater than 150 mm in diameter. The rate of success with this procedure is greatest if performed prior to 8 weeks of age. Some patients can survive indefinitely with this procedure; for others it is palliative, permitting increased time for growth and location of a suitable liver for transplantation. Hepatocyte infusion has been performed on an experimental basis, but is not currently part of standard care for this condition. *(Behrman, 1205–1206)*

115. **(A)** The signs and symptoms presented are typical of pinworm infestation. Treatment includes antiparasitic agents and reassurance regarding the benign nature of the condition. Visualization of the worms establishes the diagnosis and obviates the need to perform stool ova and parasite examination. Pinworms are easily transmitted and lack of personal hygiene is not thought to be of primary importance in spread. Household pets do not harbor pinworms and are therefore not involved in perpetuation of transmission. Finally, the pruritis and perianal excoriations noted are common with pinworm infestation and are not suggestive of sexual abuse in this setting. *(Rudolph CD,1105–1106)*

116. **(A)** Appropriate choices for treatment of pinworms include mebendazole, albendazole, and pyrantel pamoate. An antipruritic agent such as hydroxyzine or diphenhydramine may be given for symptomatic relief. No special local hygiene is necessary. The other drugs listed are useful in a variety of other parasitic infections but not for pinworm infections. *(Rudolph CD,1105–1106)*

117. **(C)** The initial history in cases of accidental ingestion should include specific substance ingested, amount and concentration of ingested substance, potential for coingestants, and interventions (eg, induction of emesis) prior to emergency department evaluation. For this patient, it would be prudent to assume she drank the entire bottle of acetaminophen. This would be about 3000 mg (100 mg/cc ¥ 30 cc = 3000 mg). If so, the ingested dose would be approximately 230 mg/kg, a potentially toxic dose. Administration of activated charcoal with sorbitol to bind acetaminophen still within the gastrointestinal tract is the best option of those presented. There is no evidence of airway compromise, and acetaminophen is not associated with rapid loss of airway reflexes; therefore, intubation is not indicated. Gastric emptying by lavage or induced emesis is not recommended more than 1–2 hours following ingestion, unless the ingested substance is known to delay gastric emptying. Although an acetaminophen level should be obtained at 4 hour ingestion, administration of charcoal should not delay until the results are available. *(Rudolph CD,356–362)*

118. **(B)** The Rumack-Matthew nomogram is used to assess the risk of acetaminophen toxicity after an acute overdose. The initial serum level should be determined 4 hours after ingestion. At that time, levels over 150 µg/mL fall into the possible hepatic toxicity range, while levels over 200 µg/mL fall into the probable hepatic toxicity range.

    For patients with levels in the possible or probable toxic range, institution of N-acetylcysteine is indicated. Prompt initiation may be lifesaving, and long-term follow-up indicates that most patients receiving prompt treatment recover completely. *(Rudolph CD, 356–362)*

119. **(E)** Acetaminophen is metabolized primarily (94%) to the sulfate or glucoronide form within the liver. About 4% is metabolized via the cytochrome P-450 system and glutathione reductase to the mercapturic acid conjugate; the rest is secreted unchanged by the liver and, to a small amount, the kidney. When the load of acetaminophen depletes the glutathione to less than 70% of normal, the highly reactive P-450 metabolite generates significant amounts of free radicals, leading to hepatocyte destruction. NAC serves as a precursor for glutathione synthesis and prevents the free radical formation. *(Rudolph CD,356–362)*

120. **(D)** The first priority in this patient's management is to secure the airway. The deep depression of consciousness, reflected by lack of response to painful stimuli and absence of gag reflex, place the patient at risk for aspiration. In addition, ventilation is likely inadequate. Drug screen and determination of blood glucose will likely be indicated, but should not delay establishment of a secure airway. Flumazenil may be useful in benzodiazepine overdose, but is not the next step in this patient's management. *(Gunn, 19–20, 39–40, 748, 752, 894)*

121. **(C)** The toxidrome of bradycardia, hypopnea, marked lethargy, and miosis is most suggestive of a narcotic overdose. Clonidine ingestion can have bradycardia, hypotension, and respiratory depression but usually not miosis. Labetalol would cause bradycardia and hypotension but usually not the mental status changes. Diazepam can cause sleepiness but not usually miosis. *(Gunn, 19–20, 39–40, 748, 752, 894)*

SELECTED READINGS

American Academy of Pediatrics Policy Statement. Practice parameter: the neurodiagnostic evaluation of a child with a first simple febrile seizure. *Pediatrics* 1996;97(5):769–772.

Lang DM. An overview of EPR3 asthma guidelines: what's different? Allergy Asthma Proc. 2007 Nov-Dec; 28(6):620–627.

National Asthma Education and Prevention Program, National Heart, Lung, and Blood Institute. Expert panel report 2, guidelines for the diagnosis and management of asthma. NIH Publication no. 97-4051; July 1997.

Ruddy S, Harris ED, Sledge CB, et al. *Kelley's Textbook of Rheumatology*. 6th ed. Philadelphia, PA: WB Saunders; 2001.

CHAPTER 11

Practice Test

Mary Anne Jackson, MD

Sara S. Viessman, MD

This chapter is a 162-question sample examination that provides a final opportunity to review, evaluate, and improve your clinical knowledge in general pediatrics. You should be able to complete the sample examination within 4 hours. Good luck!

Questions

1. Among children, short stature and infertility are most commonly associated with which of the following?

   (A) Klinefelter syndrome
   (B) Beckwith-Wiedemann syndrome
   (C) Turner syndrome
   (D) Marfan syndrome
   (E) Pierre Robin sequence

2. Unilateral multicystic dysplastic kidney in an infant usually presents with which of the following?

   (A) an abdominal mass
   (B) hematuria
   (C) hypertension
   (D) nephrotic syndrome
   (E) oliguria

3. The Fanconi syndrome is characterized by which of the following?

   (A) azotemia, edema, and hypertension
   (B) glycosuria, aminoaciduria, and phosphaturia
   (C) hematuria, glycosuria, and proteinuria
   (D) hypoglycemia, glycosuria, hypoglycinemia, and glycinuria
   (E) uremia, phosphaturia, and albuminuria

4. Which of the following sets of values is most suggestive of proximal renal tubular acidosis?

	Urine (pH)	Serum bicarbonate (meq/L)	Serum chloride (meq/L)
(A)	8	22	98
(B)	8	15	115
(C)	7	22	115
(D)	6	22	98
(E)	6	15	115

5. The presence of bilateral renal masses and a midline suprapubic mass in a newborn male infant is most suggestive of which of the following?

   (A) bilateral Wilms tumor
   (B) congenital neuroblastoma
   (C) congenital rubella infection
   (D) rhabdomyosarcoma of the bladder
   (E) congenital urethral or bladder neck obstruction

6. Wilms tumor (nephroblastoma) is the most frequent malignant tumor of the genitourinary tract in childhood. The most common presenting sign of this neoplasm is which of the following?

   (A) abdominal mass
   (B) abdominal pain
   (C) edema
   (D) hematuria
   (E) hypertension

7. A newborn with abdominal distension is found to have a meconium ileus. Which of the following conditions is most likely present in this neonate?

   (A) trisomy 13
   (B) trisomy 21

(C) Tay-Sachs disease

(D) cystic fibrosis

(E) maple syrup urine disease

8. A 5-year-old male presents with a 48-hour history of headache, and meningismus. Evaluation of the CSF reveals clear fluid with normal protein and glucose content. The CSF cell count reveals 300 WBC/hpf, 90% lymphocytes. Which of the following is the most likely etiologic agent?

(A) *Streptococcus pneumoniae*

(B) *Haemophilus influenzae*

(C) *Neisseria meningitidis*

(D) adenovirus

(E) enterovirus

9. Compared to other methods of dialysis, peritoneal dialysis offers many advantages for children and their families including increased autonomy and flexibility, with resultant enhanced school attendance and peer interactions. Peritoneal dialysis is less costly than hemodialysis and can be used to treat even small infants. The major complication of peritoneal dialysis, either continuous ambulatory (CAPD) or continuous cycling (CCPD), is

(A) a high incidence of disequilibrium syndrome

(B) a high incidence of peritonitis

(C) a need for severe dietary restriction

(D) frequent electrolyte problems

(E) poor growth

10. Which of the following represents the occurrence of significant bilateral hearing loss in infants in well newborn nurseries in the United States?

(A) 1/100

(B) 1/1000

(C) 1/5000

(D) 1/10,000

(E) 1/100,000

11. The peak age of onset of childhood nephrotic syndrome associated with minimal-change morphology is which of the following?

(A) under 6 months of age

(B) between 12 and 18 months of age

(C) between 2 and 5 years of age

(D) between 5 and 10 years of age

(E) between 10 and 15 years of age

12. The finding of a low serum concentration of C3 component of complement in a child with nephrotic syndrome indicates which of the following?

(A) a high likelihood of spontaneous remission

(B) a high likelihood of good response to steroid therapy

(C) the presence of focal segmental sclerosis

(D) the presence of membranous glomerulonephritis

(E) the presence of membranoproliferative glomerulonephritis

13. A 4-year-old presents for a well-child visit. The parents state their family has practiced a strict vegan diet since the child was 2 years of age. Of the following, which is most likely to be deficient now or in the near future?

(A) vitamin C

(B) folic acid

(C) thiamine

(D) vitamin B_6

(E) vitamin B_{12}

14. The most common roentgenographic abnormality in a child with asthma is which of the following?

(A) bronchiectasis

(B) generalized hyperinflation

(C) lower lobe infiltrates

(D) pneumomediastinum

(E) right middle lobe atelectasis

15. The pattern of inheritance of achondroplasia is which of the following?

(A) autosomal recessive

(B) autosomal dominant

(C) X-linked recessive

(D) X-linked dominant

(E) polygenetic

16. The bacterial pathogens most commonly encountered in the lungs of patients with cystic fibrosis are which of the following?

    (A) *Escherichia coli* and alpha streptococcus
    (B) *Escherichia coli* and *Pseudomonas aeruginosa*
    (C) *Staphylococcus aureus* and *Proteus* species
    (D) *Staphylococcus aureus* and *P aeruginosa*
    (E) *Haemophilus influenzae* and *Streptococcus pneumoniae*

17. A 16-year-old male presents for a sports physical. Examination reveals hypermobile joints, pes planus, and a high-arched palate. Which of the following would be most appropriate at this time?

    (A) chromosomal analysis
    (B) cardiac ultrasound
    (C) urine for organic acids
    (D) cerebrospinal fluid for amino acids
    (E) urine for calcium to creatinine ratio

18. A 2-month-old infant presents with irritability and congestive heart failure. An ECG is interpreted as characteristic of myocardial infarction. Which of the following is the most likely explanation for these findings?

    (A) viral myocarditis
    (B) ventricular septal defect
    (C) endocardial fibroelastosis
    (D) anomalous origin of the left coronary artery
    (E) atherosclerotic heart disease secondary to a congenital lipid disorder

19. A 6-month-old infant is found to be lethargic and cyanotic. Blood obtained by venipuncture appears chocolate brown and does not become bright red when shaken in the presence of air. It is especially important to seek a history of exposure to which of the following?

    (A) automobile exhaust
    (B) fava beans
    (C) paint fumes
    (D) undercooked meat
    (E) well water

20. Peak height velocity for girls most often occurs around which sexual maturity rating (SMR)

    (A) zero
    (B) one
    (C) three
    (D) four
    (E) five

21. Which of the following is characteristic of a night terror?

    (A) most often occur during the first one-third of the night
    (B) onset usually is during the elementary school years
    (C) rarely persists until adolescence
    (D) occurs during REM sleep
    (E) the event is vividly recalled by the child

22. The primary lesion in acne is which of the following?

    (A) hyperplasia of the sweat gland
    (B) sterile inflammation of the sweat gland
    (C) plugging of the sebaceous gland
    (D) infection of the sebaceous gland
    (E) increased cornification of the epidermis

23. A 7-year-old child is brought to the office because of chronic nasal obstruction. Examination reveals bilateral, clear, serous discharge from the nose, but is otherwise unremarkable. Which of the following is the most likely diagnosis?

    (A) a defect in the cribriform plate
    (B) allergic rhinitis
    (C) choanal atresia
    (D) cystic fibrosis
    (E) immunodeficiency

24. Which of the following best describes atopic dermatitis in children?

    (A) it tends to spare the face and arms
    (B) it is frequently associated with uveitis
    (C) it rarely begins during the first 2 years of life

(D) it is characterized by pruritus and lichenification

(E) it is associated with elevated serum levels of IgA and IgM and decreased levels of IgE

25. A 15-year-old boy is bitten on the hand by a snake, which he then kills and brings to the emergency room. The snake is identified as a copperhead measuring 14 in. in length. The most likely complication to be expected in this child would be which of the following?

(A) fever

(B) local tissue necrosis

(C) paralysis

(D) renal failure

(E) shock

26. The major concern regarding chronic otitis media with effusion is the development of which of the following?

(A) meningitis

(B) mastoiditis

(C) permanent nerve deafness

(D) perforation of the tympanic membrane

(E) impaired speech and language development

27. Which of the following is the most common indication for surgical repair of pectus excavatum?

(A) thoracic scoliosis

(B) cardiac dysfunction

(C) pulmonary compromise

(D) cosmetic appearance

(E) cervical pain

28. Most nasal polyps in children are due to which of the following?

(A) allergy or immunodeficiency

(B) allergy or infection

(C) allergy or cancer

(D) cystic fibrosis or cancer

(E) cystic fibrosis or allergy

29. Which of the following is the most common manifestation of alpha$_1$-antitrypsin deficiency in infancy?

(A) pulmonary cysts

(B) myocarditis

(C) hepatic cirrhosis

(D) pancreatic insufficiency

(E) obstructive lung disease

30. The earliest indicators of Cushing syndrome (glucocorticoid excess) in children are which of the following?

(A) weight gain and growth arrest

(B) growth arrest and acne

(C) acne and hypertension

(D) hypertension and striae

(E) acne and striae

31. A 12-year-old girl presents with headache, visual changes, and papilledema. A CT scan reveals a mass lesion in the region of the anterior pituitary gland which of the following is the most likely diagnosis?

(A) chromophobe adenoma

(B) craniopharyngioma

(C) ganglioneuroma

(D) medulloblastoma

(E) neuroblastoma

32. An 8-year-old male with sickle cell disease presents with 2–3 days of runny nose and mild-to-moderate anterior chest pain. On chest x-ray a new infiltrate is noted in the right middle lobe. Which of the following diagnoses, is most likely?

(A) acute chest syndrome

(B) right middle lobe syndrome

(C) aspiration pneumonia

(D) foreign body

(E) RSV bronchiolitis

33. Which of the following is frequently seen in sickle cell patients with splenic sequestration?

(A) hyposplenism

(B) pneumonia

(C) polycythemia

(D) eosinophilia

(E) thrombocytopenia

34. Which of the following is the most common cause of deaths in infants under 12 months of age each year in the United States?

    (A) sudden infant death syndrome (SIDS)
    (B) RSV bronchiolitis
    (C) child abuse
    (D) infantile leukemia
    (E) congenital heart disease

35. Of the following, which is a significant risk factor for SIDS?

    (A) firm mattress
    (B) breastfeeding
    (C) early introduction of solid foods
    (D) pacifier use
    (E) maternal smoking during pregnancy

36. Which of the following in an 8-year-old child is most likely to indicate an underlying psychologic or behavioral problem?

    (A) enuresis
    (B) encopresis
    (C) motion illness
    (D) migraine headache
    (E) recurrent pharyngitis

37. A 4-year-old girl presents with a 1-year history of monthly episodes of fever and aphthous stomatitis. A CBC 6 months prior was reportedly normal, but a CBC now reveals a total neutrophil count of less than $200/mm^3$. The remainder of the CBC is normal. Physical examination reveals an inflamed pharynx and oral mucosa with several aphthous lesions on the gingival and buccal mucosa. There are bilateral, tender anterior cervical lymph nodes, the largest of which is about 4 cm in diameter. The remainder of the physical examination is normal. The most likely diagnosis is which of the following?

    (A) Chediak-Higashi syndrome
    (B) cyclic neutropenia
    (C) HIV infection
    (D) leukemia
    (E) Schwachman-Diamond syndrome

38. A 3-year-old male presents with random eye movements, ataxia, and developmental delay. Of the following, which is most likely the diagnosis?

    (A) acute cerebellar ataxia
    (B) migraine variant
    (C) neuroblastoma
    (D) retinoblastoma
    (E) rhabdomyosarcoma

39. An 11-week-old male presents with a 1-week history of poor feeding and constipation. On examination, you note poor head control and a weak cry. Though the infant's face is expressionless, he displays a paradoxical alertness and has normal features. The most likely condition of this infant is which of the following?

    (A) bacterial meningitis
    (B) infantile botulism
    (C) hypothyroidism
    (D) Hirschsprung disease
    (E) iron poisoning

40. Chronic upper airway obstruction from enlarged tonsils and adenoids in a child may cause which of the following?

    (A) convulsions
    (B) cor pulmonale
    (C) a pneumothorax
    (D) thymic hyperplasia
    (E) reactive airway disease

41. Febrile seizures occur most frequently at what age?

    (A) in the first month of life
    (B) in the first 6 months of life
    (C) between 6 months and 5 years of age
    (D) between 5 and 10 years of age
    (E) around the time of puberty

42. A mother calls to inform you that her previously well 4-year-old child has been complaining of headaches for about a month. For the past 2 weeks he has been keeping his head in a tilted position, and for the past few days he

has been vomiting in the morning. The most likely diagnosis is which of the following?

(A) acute torticollis
(B) brain abscess
(C) brain tumor
(D) degenerative brain disease
(E) meningitis

43. Episodes of cerebellar ataxia may be seen in which of the following?

(A) cystinuria
(B) Gaucher disease
(C) Hartnup disease
(D) oxalosis
(E) tyrosinosis

44. An 8-year-old child develops an intensely pruritic rash on the legs only. There are patches of erythematous papules and vesicles and several streaks of erythematous vesiculation. The child is afebrile and otherwise well. The most likely diagnosis is

(A) eczema
(B) Henoch-Schönlein purpura
(C) poison ivy dermatitis
(D) scabies
(E) varicella

45. A 2-day-old male presents with upper abdominal distension and bilious vomiting. He passed a normal meconium stool shortly after birth. Abdominal x-rays suggest duodenal obstruction. An upper gastrointestinal contrast study reveals a "bird's beak" appearance of the distal portion of the duodenum. Which of the following is most likely?

(A) malrotation with midgut volvulus
(B) infantile hypertrophic pyloric stenosis
(C) duodenal atresia
(D) intussusception
(E) Hirschsprung disease

46. The usual presentation of an annular pancreas in childhood is which of the following?

(A) hypoglycemia
(B) hyperglycemic acidosis
(C) jaundice
(D) vomiting
(E) steatorrhea

47. The classic radiologic finding in duodenal atresia is which of the following?

(A) a totally gasless abdomen
(B) free air below the diaphragm
(C) the double bubble sign
(D) the anchor sign
(E) the string sign

48. During the first year of life, birth length increases by what percent?

(A) 25%
(B) 50%
(C) 75%
(D) 100%
(E) 125%

49. Infants typically double their birth weight by what age?

(A) 2 weeks
(B) 2 months
(C) 4 months
(D) 8 months
(E) 12 months

50. A female-appearing infant is operated on for bilateral inguinal hernias only to have the surgeon discover that the masses are undescended testes. Chromosomal analysis reveals XY constitution. The patient's adolescent sister has primary amenorrhea. Chromosomal analysis of the sister also reveals XY constitution. The most likely cause of this syndrome in the patient and sister is which of the following?

(A) 20, 22-desmolase deficiency complex
(B) end-organ insensitivity to androgens
(C) congenital adrenal hyperplasia
(D) true hermaphrodism
(E) Turner syndrome

51. Which of the following is the normal, or average, hemoglobin concentration in a 12-month-old infant?

   (A) 8 g/dL
   (B) 10 g/dL
   (C) 12 g/dL
   (D) 15 g/dL
   (E) 17 g/dL

52. Breath-holding spells are best described by which of the following?

   (A) are most common between 4 and 6 years of age
   (B) are a common cause of sudden infant death
   (C) are a manifestation of infantile colic
   (D) represent a type of epilepsy
   (E) may terminate in cyanosis and loss of consciousness

53. Which of the following is the most common presentation of *Enterobius vermicularis* infection?

   (A) appendicitis
   (B) diarrhea
   (C) intussusception
   (D) perianal pruritus
   (E) vaginitis

54. A 10-day-old infant is evaluated for recurrent blisters and sores, mostly on the extremities at areas of friction or trauma. The child has been afebrile and well except for irritability. Examination is unremarkable except for blisters, varying in stage from fresh to ruptured and crusted, mostly on the extremities, especially the dorsal surfaces of the hands and feet. Which of the following would be highest on your differential diagnosis?

   (A) bullous impetigo
   (B) congenital syphilis
   (C) drug-induced toxic epidermal necrolysis
   (D) epidermolysis bullosa
   (E) staphylococcal scalded skin syndrome

55. Which of the following best describes juvenile gastrointestinal polyps?

   (A) they occur most commonly in the ileum
   (B) they rarely present in the first 5 years of life
   (C) they usually present as blood-streaked stools
   (D) they often already have malignant elements when first discovered
   (E) they have a significant risk of malignant transformation after puberty

56. A 2-week-old male presents with irritability, decreased feeding, and fever. Cerebrospinal fluid examination reveals cloudy fluid with 5500 WBC/mm^3 and a low glucose. Gram stain revealed no bacteria. Which of the following is the most likely causative agent?

   (A) *Treponema pallidum*
   (B) cytomegalovirus
   (C) *Mycobacterium tuberculosis*
   (D) group B streptococcus
   (E) *Staphylococcus epidermidis*

57. In comparison to cow milk, human milk contains more of what substance?

   (A) protein
   (B) sodium
   (C) casein
   (D) calcium
   (E) calories

58. On routine examination, a 2-month-old African-American male infant is noted to have a moderate size umbilical hernia. The contents of the hernia are easily reduced, and it is noted that the abdominal wall defect easily admits one examining finger but not quite two. The remainder of the examination is normal and the infant is asymptomatic. What is the most appropriate next step in management?

   (A) order thyroid function tests
   (B) refer the infant to a surgeon
   (C) instruct the parent in how to tape the defect
   (D) obtain an abdominal roentgenogram or ultrasound
   (E) advise the parent that the defect will probably close spontaneously

59. Which of the following best describes chylous ascites in infancy?

   (A) Congenital nephrosis is the most common cause.
   (B) Hypoalbuminemia and lymphopenia are common.
   (C) The condition usually is benign and transient.
   (D) Hypergammaglobulinemia is common.
   (E) Hepatic involvement is common.

60. A 12-year-old child presents with severe abdominal pain, nausea and vomiting, abdominal distension, and epigastric tenderness. Chest roentgenogram reveals a small pleural effusion. The child is afebrile but blood count reveals a marked leukocytosis. Which of the following is the most likely cause for this condition?

   (A) blunt abdominal trauma
   (B) systemic lupus erythematosis
   (C) hemolytic uremic syndrome
   (D) alcohol ingestion
   (E) Kawasaki disease

61. Which of the following best describes idiopathic scoliosis?

   (A) it is more common in boys than in girls
   (B) it is diagnosed by x-ray
   (C) it is generally associated with mental retardation
   (D) it is most commonly noted during preadolescence or adolescence
   (E) it is usually associated with considerable pain on motion of the back

62. A 6-month-old male presents with failure to thrive, eczema, and a history of recurrent bacterial infections. On evaluation, a thrombocyte count of 20,000/mm^3 is noted. The peripheral smear reveals microthrombocytes. Which of the following is the most likely condition causing these signs and symptoms?

   (A) Wiskott-Aldrich syndrome
   (B) 22q11 deletion syndrome
   (C) celiac disease

   (D) idiopathic thrombocytopenic purpura
   (E) leukemia

63. A 10-year-old male presents with an acute episode of nausea, vomiting, and severe testicular pain. On examination, scrotal edema and erythema with lack of cremasteric relex are noted. Color-flow Doppler ultrasonography confirms the suspected diagnosis. What is the initial treatment of choice?

   (A) observation for 24 hours
   (B) immediate surgical exploration
   (C) chemotherapy
   (D) intravenous antibiotics
   (E) intramuscular ceftriaxone

64. You examine a school-age child because of itchy scalp and note minute white-gray structures firmly attached to the hair shafts. You recommend which of the following?

   (A) a selenium-containing shampoo
   (B) a 1% permethrin cream rinse
   (C) oral tetracycline
   (D) oral and topical tetracycline
   (E) oral griseofulvin

65. A 2-year-old child drinks kerosene that had been left in a glass. After the first swallow, she cries and drops the glass. She is most likely to develop which of the following?

   (A) aplastic anemia
   (B) chemical pneumonitis
   (C) coma and/or convulsions
   (D) hepatitis
   (E) peripheral neuritis

66. Congenital hypothyroidism should be included in the differential diagnosis of a newborn with which of the following?

   (A) coma
   (B) prolonged jaundice
   (C) pulmonary edema
   (D) renal failure
   (E) severe anemia

67. A 2-month-old infant has had inspiratory stridor since the first month of life, but has been otherwise well. Physical examination is unremarkable except for moderate inspiratory stridor and retractions, which are worse when the infant is supine or agitated and better when he is prone and quiet. What is the most likely cause of these findings?

    (A) reactive airway disease
    (B) laryngomalacia
    (C) viral croup
    (D) an aspirated foreign body
    (E) a tracheoesophageal fistula

68. A significant number of children with recurrent gross or microscopic hematuria, normal renal ultrasound, and normal tests of renal function have which of the following?

    (A) hyperkaliuria
    (B) hypercalciuria
    (C) hypercalcemia
    (D) hyperphosphatemia
    (E) hemorrhagic urethritis

69. A 4-year-old child, previously well, presents with the rather sudden onset of wheezing which does not respond to treatment with aerosolized albuterol. An x-ray examination of the chest (see Figure 11–1) is obtained. What is the most likely diagnosis?

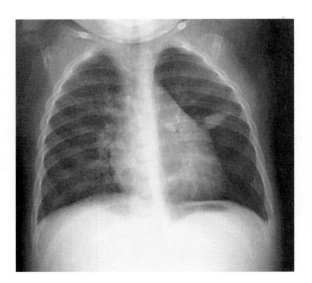

Figure 11-1
(*Courtesy of Doug Rivard, DO*)

    (A) asthma
    (B) foreign body
    (C) infantile lobar emphysema
    (D) pulmonary hypoplasia
    (E) right middle lobe syndrome

70. Physical examination of a 6-month-old child who does not walk reveals the findings shown below (Figures 11–2 and 11–3). What is the most likely diagnosis?

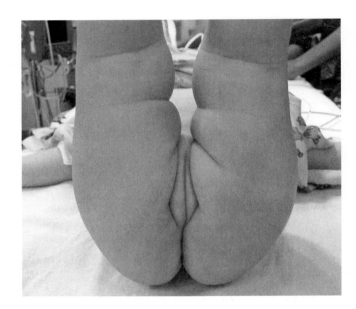

Figure 11-2
(*Courtesy of Mark R. Sinclair, MD*)

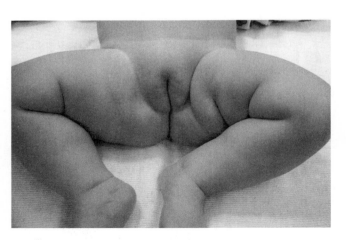

Figure 11-3
(*Courtesy of Mark R. Sinclair, MD*)

(A) arthrogryposis congenita
(B) congenital hip dislocation
(C) equinovarus deformity
(D) rickets
(E) tibial torsion

71. A 12-year-old girl complains of decreasing visual acuity and a slight feeling of discomfort in both eyes. Examination by an ophthalmologist reveals anterior uveitis. You suspect that the child may have which of the following?

(A) leukemia
(B) toxoplasmosis
(C) toxocara infection
(D) hypoparathyroidism
(E) juvenile idiopathic arthritis

72. A 5-year-old female presents with intoeing. Her mother states the child is very limber and has no complaints of pain. On examination, with the child in prone position and knees flexed 90 degrees the child can easily place her lateral malleoli on the table. What is the most likely condition described here?

(A) Perthes disease
(B) acute slipped femoral epiphysis
(C) metatarsus adductus
(D) tibial torsion
(E) femoral anteversion

73. For which of the following would laboratory testing for group A streptococcus (GAS) be recommended in the United States?

(A) an 18-month-old with pharyngitis
(B) a 5-year-old with pharyngitis and anterior stomatitis with discrete ulcerative lesions
(C) a 10-year-old with pharyngitis, conjunctivitis, and cough
(D) all household contacts of a child with documented GAS pharyngitis
(E) all household contacts of a child with documented poststreptococcal glomerulonephritis

74. The most consistent finding in lymphocytic thyroiditis (Hashimoto thyroiditis) is which of the following?

(A) enlargement of the thyroid gland
(B) hyperthyroidism
(C) hypothyroidism
(D) eosinophilia
(E) associated disturbances of the parathyroids

75. A 6-month-old male presents with diaper rash that is resistant to therapy. He has intermittent diarrhea. He is breastfeeding, and rarely seems interested in solid foods. Mother is a vegetarian. On examination, he is thin and listless. He has dry, plaque-like, sharply demarcated lesions around his mouth and eyes. His hair is coarse and scanty. A deficiency of which of the following could explain this condition?

(A) iron
(B) zinc
(C) vitamin A
(D) vitamin B_6
(E) vitamin D

76. A 2-year-old child has had recurrent episodes of fever, cough, and pulmonary infiltrates on chest roentgenograms. Diagnostic evaluation reveals a normal sweat test, barium swallow, and serum immunoglobulins, but a severe microcytic, hypochromic anemia. The child's diet is normal for age. Which of the following would be highest on your list of differential diagnoses?

(A) cystic fibrosis
(B) diffuse pulmonary hemangiomatosis
(C) extramedullary pulmonary erythropoiesis
(D) gastroesophageal reflux and hemorrhagic esophagitis
(E) primary pulmonary hemosiderosis

77. A 13-year-old female athlete presents with anterior knee pain of 2–3 weeks' duration. She has no history of trauma. On examination, she has good flexibility of lower extremities. There are no effussions. There is no tenderness over the tibial tubercle, or at the inferior pole of the patella. She has a positive patella glide test. Of the following causes of anterior knee pain, which is most likely in this patient?

(A) Osgood-Schlatter disease
(B) chondromalacia patellae
(C) Sinding-Larsen-Johansson disease
(D) osteochondritis dissecans
(E) slipped capital femoral epiphysis

78. On a 6-month well-child visit, you note a healthy well-grown male with a normal physical examination except for a closed anterior fontanelle. Which of the following should you consider?

(A) hypothyroidism
(B) trisomy 18
(C) hydrocephalus
(D) craniosynostosis
(E) hypophosphatasia

79. A previously well 9-year-old boy develops an intensely pruritic rash consisting of raised hive-like lesions with pink edges and pale centers. Lesions are well circumscribed and range in size from 2 to 6 cm in diameter. The history is unremarkable and physical examination is unrevealing except for the rash. Careful diagnostic workup probably will disclose which of the following?

(A) a food allergy
(B) an occult malignancy
(C) a collagen vascular disease
(D) C1-esterase inhibitor deficiency
(E) no specific cause for the rash

80. Most patients with XYY constitution are which of the following?

(A) short
(B) obese
(C) behaviorally normal

(D) impulsive and antisocial
(E) severely mentally retarded

81. A petechial rash is noted in a 10-hour-old newborn who is otherwise appearing normal and vigorous. There is no hepatosplenomegaly and radii are present. There are no risk factors for sepsis. A complete blood count reveals a normal WBC count with differential hemoglobin 17 g/dL; and platelet count 11,000/mm^3 with large platelets present. Which of the following would be the most appropriate next step?

(A) maternal platelet count
(B) abdominal ultrasound
(C) bone marrow aspiration
(D) chest x-ray
(E) PT and PTT

82. A 2-month-old male presents with a cough that has persisted for over 2 weeks. Mother has noted he coughs in spells and at the end of these spells, he vomits. She feels he has lost weight. On examination, you note a thin male infant who otherwise appears normal. Complete blood count reveals 30,000 white blood cells with 95% lymphocytes. Which of the following is the most likely diagnosis?

(A) respiratory syncitial virus bronchiolitis
(B) pneumococcal pneumonia
(C) pertussis
(D) laryngomalacia
(E) vascular ring

83. Pseudohypoparathyroidism is associated with which of the following?

(A) short stature
(B) renal failure
(C) long, spindly fingers
(D) generalized increased mineralization of bone
(E) decreased serum levels of parathyroid hormone

84. The most consistent abnormality in von Willebrand disease is which of the following?

(A) decreased platelet count

(B) prolonged bleeding time

(C) prolonged prothrombin time

(D) prolonged partial thromboplastin time

(E) decreased plasma level of factor XII

85. The most common cause of congenital hypothyroidism is which of the following?

(A) dysgenesis of the thyroid gland

(B) a defect in thyroid synthesis

(C) Hashimoto's thyroiditis

(D) maternal ingestion of iodides

(E) maternal iodine deficiency

86. A 6-year-old Hispanic male presents with a first-time generalized seizure lasting less than 5 minutes. There is no history of trauma or illness. The family recently immigrated to the United States from Mexico. The child is afebrile, and his examination is completely normal. Of the following, which would be the most likely cause for the seizure?

(A) herpes encephalitis

(B) cysticercosis

(C) lead poisoning

(D) vitamin B_{12} deficiency

(E) hypocalcemia

87. A 17-year-old boy with cystic fibrosis complains of a 5–10 lb weight loss over the past month, unaccompanied by changes in his pulmonary or gastrointestinal symptoms. You suspect that he has developed which of the following?

(A) a bronchogenic carcinoma

(B) an eating disorder

(C) biliary cirrhosis

(D) cor pulmonale

(E) diabetes mellitus

88. The diagnosis of cystic fibrosis is usually confirmed by the finding which of the following?

(A) elevated sweat chloride

(B) decreased sweat chloride

(C) elevated serum chloride

(D) decreased serum chloride

(E) elevated sweat and serum chloride

89. A 2-year-old male presents with upper respiratory symptoms for 3 days and 1 day of fever, irritability, and right ear pain. Examination reveals a temperature of 39°C, clear rhinorrhea, a bulging immobile right tympanic membrane with absent light reflex. What is the most appropriate initial therapy?

(A) antihistamines and ibuprofen

(B) antihistamines and acetaminophen

(C) penicillin

(D) amoxicillin

(E) erythromycin

90. Which of the following best describes an inguinal hernia in a 2-month-old girl?

(A) it may contain an ovary

(B) it is usually a direct hernia

(C) it does not require surgical repair

(D) it is a sign of pseudohermaphroditism

(E) it is generally associated with an imperforate anus

91. Which of the following would be expected in a 6-month-old child with a large ventricular septal defect?

(A) cyanosis

(B) an enlarged heart

(C) a continuous cardiac murmur

(D) decreased pulmonary vasculature on roentgenogram

(E) evidence of predominantly right ventricular hypertrophy on ECG

92. Which of the following is most common presentation of hypoparathyroidism beyond the neonatal period?

(A) syncope secondary to prolonged QT intervals

(B) tingling of extremities

(C) seizure

(D) bronchospasm

(E) laryngospasm

93. What is the most common cause of school absenteeism among adolescent females?

   (A) depression
   (B) asthma
   (C) headache
   (D) dysmenorrhea
   (E) drug overdose

94. An irritable 12-month-old male has a 1-week history of high fevers and macular truncal rash. Examination reveals bulbar conjuctivitis, bright red cracked lips, and cervical adenopathy. What is the most appropriate next step?

   (A) initiate airborne barrier precautions
   (B) intravenous antibiotics
   (C) intravenous antibiotics for the infant and oral antibiotics for all household members
   (D) intravenous gammaglobulin
   (E) intravenous corticosteroids

95. An 8-month-old female presents with failure to thrive, constipation, fevers, and polydipsia. On evaluation, you find hypokalemia and hyperchloremic metabolic acidosis and suspect Fanconi syndrome. Which of the following would be the most likely inherited cause?

   (A) cystinosis
   (B) cystic fibrosis
   (C) glycogen storage disease
   (D) Tay-Sachs disease
   (E) tyrosinemia

96. A 13-year-old male presents with a 3 cm annular scaling lesion on his right posterior trunk unresponsive to 2 weeks of a topical antifungal. On follow-up visit he presents with dozens of elliptical scaling lesions on his trunk. He has no palmoplantar or mucous membrane lesions and no adenopathy. What is the most likely diagnosis?

   (A) pityriasis rosea
   (B) secondary syphilis
   (C) lichen planus
   (D) tinea versicolor
   (E) Munchausen syndrome by proxy

97. An 18-month-old female presents for a well-child visit. On examination, there is an asymmetric red reflex, with the left appearing normal and the right appearing cream colored. Of the following, which is the most likely diagnosis?

   (A) rhabdomyosarcoma
   (B) retinoblastoma
   (C) neuroblastoma
   (D) leukemia
   (E) lymphoma

98. Which of the following represents the ethnic group with the highest neonatal and infant mortality rates in the United States?

   (A) American Indian
   (B) Asian and Pacific Island
   (C) African-American
   (D) Hispanic
   (E) Caucasian

99. Which of the following best describes patients with constitutional growth delay?

   (A) they will begin puberty at the same time as their peers
   (B) they have a bone age equal to their chronological age
   (C) they are usually obese
   (D) they will achieve normal adult height
   (E) they demonstrate height that is inappropriate for bone age

100. A 4-year-old male presents with a 1-day history of abdominal pain and vomiting. He is afebrile and has no diarrhea. He complains of knee pain bilaterally, and there is some tenderness of the knee joints but no effusions. Within 24 hours he develops a rash on his legs and buttocks which is petechial and purpuric, and his platelet count is normal. What is the most likely diagnosis?

   (A) hemolytic uremic syndrome
   (B) Henoch-Schönlein purpura
   (C) acute glomerulonephritis
   (D) Kawasaki disease
   (E) systemic lupus erythematosis

101. A 4-year-old female presents with a limp. The week prior she had an upper respiratory infection. There is no history of trauma. She has no history of fever. Examination reveals limitation of motion of the right hip joint, especially with internal rotation. X-ray reveals some swelling in soft tissues surrounding the hip joint. A complete blood count and sedimentation rate are normal. What would be the next most appropriate step?

(A) aspirate the hip joint
(B) begin nonsteroidal anti-inflammatory agents
(C) CT scan of the hip
(D) MRI of the hip
(E) begin intravenous antibiotics

102. A newborn is noted to have a large head and short limbs. On further examination, short broad fingers, a small face, and low-normal length are noted. The trunk appears long and narrow. What should be your first step to confirm the diagnosis?

(A) order an ophthalmologic examination
(B) obtain skeletal radiographs
(C) order chromosome analysis
(D) examine the parents
(E) perform the routine newborn screen

103. Infants fed exclusively goat milk are susceptible to which of the following?

(A) vitamin A deficiency
(B) vitamin B$_6$ deficiency
(C) vitamin E deficiency
(D) folate deficiency
(E) thiamine deficiency

104. A 5-month-old female presents in the winter with a 2-day history of vomiting, diarrhea, and fever. The diarrhea is without blood or mucus. On examination, she is moderately dehydrated and has a serum sodium of 152 meq/L. What is the most likely etiologic agent?

(A) *Giardia lamblia*
(B) *Salmonella*
(C) influenza

(D) enterovirus
(E) rotavirus

105. Among adolescents of 15–19 years of age, motor vehicle accidents cause the greatest number of deaths each year. Which of the following is the second leading cause of death in this age group?

(A) homicide and legal intervention
(B) suicide
(C) heart disease
(D) cancer
(E) cystic fibrosis

106. The most common congenital infection is infection with cytomegalovirus, affecting 3/1000–4/1000 livebirths. Of those babies infected, approximately what percent are normal at birth and develop normally?

(A) 5%
(B) 15%
(C) 25%
(D) 75%
(E) 90%

DIRECTIONS (Questions 107 through 128): The following group of questions is preceded by a list of lettered answer options. For each question, match the one lettered option that is most closely associated with the question. Each lettered option may be selected once, multiple times, or not at all.

Questions 107 through 110

On the second day of treatment for pneumococcal meningitis, a 10-month-old child who had been alert is noted to be lethargic. Serum electrolytes reveal: Na 120 meq/L; Cl 82 meq/L; K 3.1 meq/L; BUN 2 mg/dL.

107. What is the most likely cause of the lethargy and electrolyte disturbance in this patient?

(A) acute hepatic failure
(B) acute renal failure
(C) congestive heart failure
(D) inappropriate secretion of ADH
(E) subdural effusions

108. What is the most appropriate test to confirm this diagnosis?

(A) chest roentgenogram

(B) measurement of serum and urine osmolality

(C) determination of serum creatinine

(D) measurement of hepatic enzymes

(E) CT scan of the head

109. One would also expect this patient to exhibit which of the following?

(A) polyuria

(B) hypotension

(C) metabolic alkalosis

(D) high urine specific gravity

(E) high serum alkaline phosphatase

110. The most appropriate management of this problem would be which of the following?

(A) administration of hypertonic (3%) saline

(B) restriction of fluid intake to 70% of maintenance requirements

(C) restriction of sodium intake to about 10% of normal

(D) administration of a diuretic such as furosemide

(E) discontinue intravenous fluids and begin oral fluids as tolerated

Questions 111 through 113

A 12-year-old child is admitted because of the sudden onset of coma. The child had been well until about 6 hours prior to admission, when he began to complain of a headache. The headache became more severe and the child lapsed into coma. Physical examination reveals a temperature of 38.2°C. The child is flaccid and comatose. The remainder of the physical examination is unremarkable. A lumbar puncture reveals grossly bloody spinal fluid. After centrifugation, the fluid appears xanthochromic. There are 3000 RBCs and 7 WBCs/mm³. The protein concentration is 400 mg/dL and the glucose is 62 mg/dL.

111. Which of the following is the most likely etiology of the coma?

(A) intraventricular hemorrhage

(B) subarachnoid hemorrhage

(C) aqueductal stenosis

(D) viral encephalitis

(E) subdural effusion

112. Which of the following underlying structural abnormalities would most likely have led to the above event or condition?

(A) absence of the corpus callosum

(B) porencephalic cyst

(C) cerebral arteriovenous malformation

(D) cerebral aneurysm

(E) Arnold-Chiari malformation

113. What would the most appropriate next step at this time would be to

(A) obtain a CT of the head

(B) repeat the lumbar puncture

(C) administer fresh frozen plasma

(D) perform an exchange transfusion

(E) initiate a transfusion of packed red blood cells

Questions 114 through 116

A 21-day-old male infant is admitted because of vomiting for 12 days. Birth weight was 2925 g. The child had been normal at birth and did well for the first 9 days of life. He was initially begun on breastfeeding only, but on the eighth day of life, supplemental feeding with a commercially prepared cow milk formula was added. Vomiting began on the 10th day of life and persisted despite discontinuation of the prepared formula. On the 21st day of life, the child was hospitalized. Diarrhea had never been present. Several days prior to admission, the stools had become hard and infrequent. On admission, the anterior fontanel is sunken, the mucous membranes are dry, and skin turgor is poor. The diaper is dry and the mother cannot recall when the child last urinated. The child appears poorly nourished. Wt 2850 g, HR 152 beats per minute, RR 12 times per minute, T 37.5°C. Pulses and color are good. No abnormalities are palpated on examination.

114. Which of the following is the best diagnostic test for this condition?

(A) an unprepped barium enema

(B) a sweat test

(C) an abdominal ultrasound

(D) chromosomal analysis

(E) stool for *Giardia* antigen

115. One would expect the initial laboratory data to reveal which of the following?

(A) mixed metabolic and respiratory acidosis

(B) mixed metabolic and respiratory alkalosis

(C) normal acid-base status

(D) primary metabolic acidosis

(E) primary metabolic alkalosis

116. Which of the following intravenous solutions would be most appropriate as the initial hydrating fluid?

(A) 5% dextrose in water

(B) normal saline

(C) 140 meq/L of Na, 120 meq/L of Cl, 20 meq/L of bicarbonate

(D) 5% glucose, 40 meq/L of Na, 40 meq/L of K, 80 meq/L of Cl

(E) 3% dextrose plus 140 meq/L of Na, 115 meq/L of Cl, 20 meq/L of bicarbonate, and 5 meq/L of K

Questions 117 through 119

A 15-year-old male presents with a 2-day history of fever, chills, and cough. He complains of aching muscles. Today he noticed his urine was red. Examination revealed a tired-appearing adolescent with fever, pharyngitis, nasal congestion, and tender calf muscles.

117. Urine analysis reveals a positive test for hemoglobin with no red blood cells seen on microscopic examination. Which of the following is most likely to reveal the source of the red urine?

(A) detailed dietary history

(B) renal ultrasound

(C) intravenous pyelogram

(D) immunoglobulin levels

(E) serum creatine kinase

118. You obtain the above study and it is markedly abnormal. What is the most important next step?

(A) perform a lumbar puncture

(B) initiate intravenous antibiotics

(C) obtain a chest x-ray

(D) order serum electrolytes, BUN, and creatinine

(E) order liver function tests

119. Of the following infectious agents, which is most likely to cause this condition?

(A) influenza

(B) group A streptococcus

(C) group B streptococcus

(D) hepatitis A

(E) *Escherichia coli*

Questions 120 through 122

A 2-year-old child is hospitalized because of fever, abdominal pain, and hepatomegaly. The child lives in a poor, crowded home on a small farm. No one else at home is ill. Physical examination reveals a thin child with marked hepatomegaly. The spleen is not palpable and all lymph nodes are within normal limits. The remainder of the examination is within normal limits. Chest x-ray reveals bilateral scattered densities. White blood cell count is 14,000/mm^3 with 36% eosinophils.

120. Which of the following would be most likely to establish the diagnosis in this patient?

(A) bone marrow aspiration

(B) stool examination

(C) liver biopsy

(D) serum enzyme immunoassay

(E) duodenal aspiration

121. How did this child most likely acquire the disease?

(A) eating poorly cooked pork

(B) eating dirt

(C) kissing a dog

(D) contact with a sick bird

(E) contact with a sick rodent

122. This condition is which of the following?

    (A) more prevalent in the United States than in developing countries

    (B) more common in rural areas

    (C) nearly always symptomatic

    (D) most frequently present in school-aged children

    (E) transmitted only by mature dogs

Questions 123 through 125

A 6-month-old girl is admitted because of failure to thrive and persistent pneumonia. The child was well at birth but severe, recurrent diarrhea began at about 6 weeks of age. At 8 weeks the child developed pneumonia which responded only poorly to antibiotic therapy and since hospitalization, she continues to require oxygen by nasal cannula. Physical examination reveals a small, poorly nourished child with moderate respiratory distress. There are bilateral rales, oral thrush, and a monilial-appearing rash in the diaper area. The remainder of the examination is within normal limits. The total white blood cell count is 5200/mm^3 with 87% polymorphonuclear cells, 12% lymphocytes, and 1% eosinophils; hemoglobin and platelets are normal. Serum immunoglobulin levels are: IgA not detectable; IgG 280 mg/dL; IgM less than 5 mg/dL.

123. Which of the following diagnoses best explains the clinical picture?

    (A) chronic granulomatous disease

    (B) Wiskott-Aldrich syndrome

    (C) hereditary agammaglobulinemia

    (D) severe combined immunodeficiency

    (E) transient hypogammaglobulinemia of infancy

124. On further evaluation one would also expect to find which of the following?

    (A) increased numbers of plasma cells on bone marrow examination

    (B) enlarged superficial lymph nodes

    (C) absent thymic shadow on chest roentgenogram

    (D) positive intradermal reaction to *Candida* antigen

    (E) abnormal oxidative burst testing

125. Chest roentgenogram reveals bilateral patchy consolidations and diffuse granular densities with an almost ground-glass appearance to the lungs. Which of the following is the most likely cause of these x-ray findings?

    (A) pneumococcal pneumonia

    (B) *Pneumocystis jiroveci* pneumonia

    (C) pulmonary hemorrhage

    (D) pulmonary lymphangiectasia

    (E) miliary tuberculosis

Questions 126 through 128

A 4-month-old boy had been well until 4 weeks prior to admission, when vomiting and poor appetite were noted. Psychomotor development had been normal. The child was being fed whole cow milk and strained foods. Stools were normal. On the morning of admission, the child had a generalized convulsion and was brought to the emergency room where the seizure was controlled with intravenous medication. A second seizure occurred about 1 hour later and again responded to intravenous medication. Physical examination revealed a pale, listless infant, poorly nourished, but in no acute distress. The height was at the 25th percentile, the weight at the 3rd percentile, and the head circumference over the 97th percentile on a standard growth curve; T 38°C, RR 16 breaths per minute, HR 110 beats per minute, BP 76/50 mm Hg. The anterior fontanel is full, but not bulging. There are no focal neurologic signs. The remainder of the examination is within normal limits.

126. Which of the following diagnoses is most likely?

    (A) tuberculous meningitis

    (B) mastoiditis

    (C) subdural hematoma

    (D) congenital toxoplasmosis

    (E) pseudotumor cerebri

127. A funduscopic examination performed after one pupil is dilated with atropine reveals diffuse retinal hemorrhages. The most likely diagnosis now is which of the following?

    (A) tuberculous meningitis

    (B) mastoiditis

(C) subdural hematoma

(D) congenital toxoplasmosis

(E) pseudotumor cerebri

128. Of the following, what is the next most important step in diagnosis and management?

(A) lumbar puncture

(B) electroencephalography

(C) CT scan of the head

(D) bone marrow examination

(E) conjunctival biopsy

DIRECTIONS (Questions 129 through 162): The following group of questions is preceded by a list of lettered answer options. For each question, match the one lettered option that is most closely associated with the question. Each lettered option may be selected once, multiple times, or not at all.

Questions 129 through 137

(A) acetylcysteine

(B) atropine

(C) ammonium chloride

(D) calcium chloride

(E) deferoxamine

(F) digoxin

(G) EDTA

(H) ethanol

(I) fresh frozen plasma

(J) furosemide

(K) glucagon

(L) methionine

(M) methyldopa

(N) methylene blue

(O) naloxone

(P) nitroprusside

(Q) oxygen

(R) phenobarbital

(S) phenylephrine

(T) physostigmine

(U) potassium chloride

(V) potassium citrate

(W) propranolol

(X) sodium bicarbonate

(Y) sodium chloride

(Z) sodium nitrite

For each drug or poison, select the most specific and most important antidote.

129. Lead

130. Iron

131. Acetaminophen

132. Organophosphate

133. Jimsonweed

134. Ethylene glycol

135. Morphine

136. Cyclic antidepressants

137. Carbon monoxide

Questions 138 through 144

(A) 2 months

(B) 4 months

(C) 6 months

(D) 9 months

(E) 12 months

(F) 18 months

(G) 2 years

(H) 3–4 years

(I) 5 years

For each description of developmental accomplishments, select the earliest, most appropriate age.

138. Walks if led and is able to take a few steps unsupported, demonstrates a good pincer grip, drinks from a cup

139. Copies a circle, hops on one foot, recognizes colors

140. Smiles responsively, follows a moving object or face with turning of the head

141. Kicks a ball, builds a tower of six 1-in cubes, combines two different words

142. Sits without support, pulls to a stand, babbles loudly and happily, grabs a block with the entire hand

143. Startles at sudden noise

144. Draws a triangle, uses past and future tense in language

Questions 145 through 149

  (A) atrioventricular septal defect
  (B) mitral valve prolapse
  (C) supravalvular aortic stenosis
  (D) coarctation of the aorta
  (E) pulmonary stenosis

Choose the cardiovascular anomaly most closely associated with the condition below

145. Down syndrome

146. Williams syndrome

147. Marfan syndrome

148. Turner syndrome

149. Noonan syndrome

Questions 150 through 154

  (A) tongue fasciculations
  (B) Gower sign
  (C) heliotrope sign
  (D) nonthrombocytopenic purpura
  (E) thrombocytopenia

For each of the conditions below, choose the most closely associated finding from the list above.

150. Dermatomyositis

151. Werdnig-Hoffmann disease

152. Hemolytic uremic syndrome

153. Muscular dystrophy

154. Henoch-Schönlein purpura

Questions 155 through 160

  (A) adenovirus
  (B) *Borrelia burgdorferi*
  (C) *Ehrlichia chaffeensis*
  (D) *Eikenella corrodens*
  (E) *Escherichia coli*
  (F) group A coxsackievirus
  (G) human herpesvirus 6
  (H) *Pasteurella multocida*
  (I) parainfluenza virus
  (J) *Shigella*
  (K) *Spirillum minus*

For each of the following clinical scenarios, choose the most likely etiologic agent from the list above.

155. A 3-year-old presents 2 days after a cat bite to her face. She is febrile but not toxic and has three tubular shaped areas of induration approximately 1×3 cm each with surrounding warmth and erythema. The infected areas are very painful to touch.

156. A 4-year-old child presents in Missouri in late summer with a 3-day history of progressive vomiting and abdominal pain, fever, and petechial rash. He is obtunded and has multiple insect bites. He has leukopenia, elevated liver enzymes, and evidence of DIC on laboratory evaluation.

157. A 6-year-old presents with "pink eye," sore throat, and fever in the summer. His mother tells you that three or four of his friends have similar symptoms. Examination reveals pharyngitis with large tonsils and bilaterally erythematous conjunctiva.

158. A 6-month-old female presents with a 3-day history of fevers 39.5°C–40.0°C. On the fourth day, she developed an erythematous maculopapular rash and the fever resolved.

159. An 8-month-old with severe inspiratory stridor, fever, and a barking cough is admitted to the hospital for treatment with aerosolized racemic epinephrine and corticosteroids.

160. A 4-week-old presents with fever. She has a history of being well until 1 week prior when she was found screaming in her bed. Her mother noted she had a bite wound on her neck and suspected a rat to be the perpetrator. She watched the infant, who seemed to be doing well, until the past 24 hour when she developed fever. On examination, the infant is irritable and has mild erythema surrounding the bite wound.

Questions 161 through 162

(A) tuberous sclerosis

(B) neurofibromatosis type 1

(C) Sturge-Weber disease

(D) von Hippel-Lindau disease

(E) Albright syndrome

161. Facial port wine stain and intracranial angiomatosis

162. Axillary freckling, long arm of chromosome 17, autosomal dominant with 50% of cases associated with new mutation

Answers and Explanations

1. **(C)** Both Turner syndrome and Pierre Robin sequence are associated with short stature; however, Turner syndrome is also associated with gonadal dysgenesis and infertility. Children with Klinefelter syndrome and Marfan syndrome typically have long extremities, and children with Beckwith-Wiedemann syndrome typically have gigantism. *(Rudolph CD,745, 762, 2091)*

2. **(A)** Multicystic dysplastic kidney is one type of renal dysplasia, a group of disorders characterized by developmental abnormalities of kidney structure and differentiation. The entity is not related to polycystic kidney disease. Bilateral multicystic kidneys are rapidly fatal in the newborn period. The unilateral multicystic kidney usually presents in infancy as an abdominal mass. Hypertension has been noted, but is rare. In unilateral cases, renal function is preserved by the opposite normal kidney. *(Rudolph CD, 1704)*

3. **(B)** The term Fanconi syndrome currently is used to indicate a complex dysfunction of the proximal tubules, characterized by glycosuria, amino aciduria, and phosphaturia. Blood glucose as well as urea and creatinine levels usually are normal. It may be seen as an isolated finding (primary Fanconi syndrome) or secondary to disorders such as cystinosis or tyrosinemia. [Note: Fanconi syndrome is not related to Fanconi anemia, an autosomal recessive disorder characterized by pancytopenia and hypoplastic thumb and radius.] *(Rudolph CD,1709–1710)*

4. **(E)** The defect in proximal renal tubular acidosis is renal loss of bicarbonate due to an abnormally low threshold. Serum chloride is elevated and serum bicarbonate is low. Therefore, choices (A), (C), and (D) can be eliminated. A distinctive feature of these patients is their unimpaired ability to excrete adequate amounts of titratable acid and thereby lower urinary pH. The urine pH usually is acidic in these patients when the serum bicarbonate level is low. However, if they are given an infusion of bicarbonate to raise the serum level, urine pH will be alkaline during the infusion. *(Rudolph CD,1710)*

5. **(E)** The presence of bilateral renal masses and a midline suprapubic mass (the distended bladder) in a newborn infant is congenital urethral or bladder neck obstruction until proven otherwise. Posterior urethral valves are an especially important cause of such obstruction in the male infant. Early diagnosis is critical, as the renal parenchyma eventually will be destroyed by the resultant hydronephrosis. *(Rudolph CD, 1641)*

6. **(A)** An abdominal or flank mass is the most common presenting sign in children with Wilms tumor. Often, the mass is discovered on routine examination or during examination for a minor illness. This underscores the importance of a thorough examination at every physician visit. Occasionally, the parents will bring the child to the physician because they note an enlarging abdomen or feel the mass themselves. *(McMillan, 1775–1777)*

7. **(D)** Meconium ileus typically presents within the first 24–48 hours of life, and almost always occurs in neonates with cystic fibrosis. Of all

children with cystic fibrosis, 10%–20% have a history of meconium ileus as a neonate. The usual location of the obstruction is the distal ileum, resulting in a colon of small caliber referred to as a microcolon. Older patients with cystic fibrosis often develop obstruction of the distal ileum (typically in the ileocecal region) secondary to inspissated stool. This obstruction, termed meconium ileus equivalent or distal intestinal pseudo-obstruction syndrome, can be seen in cystic fibrosis patients of any age beyond the newborn period. *(Rudolph CD,1407)*

8. **(E)** Clearly this child's presentation suggests meningitis, a diagnosis which is confirmed by the CSF results. The relatively low number of total white blood cells, the predominance of lymphocytes, and the normal glucose and protein values are all suggestive of a viral illness. Therefore, the most likely etiologic agent is meningitis caused by enterovirus. *(Rudolph CD, 1021; Hay, 1113)*

9. **(B)** In most regards, chronic ambulatory peritoneal dialysis and chronic cycling peritoneal dialysis compare favorably to other methods of chronic dialysis. However, there is an increased risk of peritonitis. Usually diagnosed by a caretaker who notices cloudy effluent dialysate, the peritonitis most often is due to coagulase-negative *Staphylococcus* and is treated with intraperitoneal antibiotics, often at home. Frequent episodes of peritonitis may cause the nephrologist or patient to seek another form of dialysis. *(McMillan, 1846–1847)*

10. **(B)** In the past, evaluation of hearing was recommended for infants who met high-risk criteria such as birth weight less than 1500 g, family history of sensorineural hearing loss, and presence of congenital infections or craniofacial abnormalities. However, 50% of children with sensorineural deafness (1/1,000 infants in well newborn nurseries) did not meet these criteria for screening at birth. Many states have passed legislation which mandates universal newborn hearing screening programs. The American Academy of Pediatrics and the Joint Commissions on Infant Hearing recommend that the diagnosis of hearing impairment

be made before 3 months of age and the infant be receiving intervention services before 6 months of age. *(Hay, 474–475; Rudolph CD, 487–488)*

11. **(C)** Most cases of minimal-change nephrotic syndrome are diagnosed in children 2–5 years of age with a peak age of onset between 2 and 3 years of age. Older children presenting with nephrotic syndrome are more likely to have an underlying chronic nephritis (membranoproliferative glomerulonephritis, lupus nephritis, etc.) rather than minimal-change nephrotic syndrome. *(Rudolph CD,1678, 1691)*

12. **(E)** A low serum concentration of the C3 component of complement in a child with nephrotic syndrome almost always indicates the presence of membranoproliferative disease (assuming that the child does not have systemic lupus, endocarditis, or a shunt infection). Membranoproliferative glomerulonephritis is very unlikely either to respond to corticosteroids or to remit spontaneously. *(Rudolph CD,1681, 1694–1698)*

13. **(E)** Strict vegans eat exclusively foods of plant origin. Through education, strict vegans can have a diet balanced for most requirements. However, vitamin B_{12} is found only in products of animal origin. Therefore, strict vegans are at high risk for vitamin B_{12} deficiencies. Breastfed infants of strict vegan mothers are at marked risk of vitamin B_{12} deficiency. In children with vitamin B_{12} deficiency, irreversible neurologic damage can occur before the presence of anemia. *(Rudolph CD,1338, 1530)*

14. **(B)** Generalized or diffuse hyperinflation of the lungs, manifested by an increased anteroposterior diameter of the thorax and flattened diaphragms, is the earliest and most frequent roentgenographic abnormality in children with asthma. Infiltrates, atelectasis, and pneumomediastinum are seen occasionally during an acute attack. Bronchiectasis is a rare complication and would suggest the possibility of an underlying disorder such as cystic fibrosis, immunodeficiency, foreign body, or recurrent aspiration. *(Gershel, 309:336, 1983)*

15. (B) Achondroplasia, the most common form of short-limbed dwarfism, is an autosomal dominant disorder. Most cases, however, are the result of a sporadic mutation of FGFR3. Most patients have an identical missense mutation of codon 380 of FGFR3 causing an arginine residue to be replaced by glycine. The incidence of achondroplasia is approximately 1 in 26,000 live births. *(Hay, 791; Rudolph CD,759)*

16. (D) Chronic airway colonization and infection with *S aureus* and *P aeruginosa* is characteristic of patients with cystic fibrosis. Antibiotic therapy occasionally eliminates *S aureus* from the bronchial tree, but almost never eradicates *P aeruginosa* despite in vitro susceptibility to a variety of antibiotics. *(Rudolph CD,1975)*

17. (B) Marfan syndrome is a disorder of connective tissue affecting many organs. Affecting 1/5000 individuals without ethnic or gender predilection, this syndrome carries an increased risk of sudden death due to cardiovascular complications, primarily related to progressive dilation of the aortic root and ascending aorta. Ultrasound is a useful tool in diagnosing and following this potentially fatal manifestation of Marfan syndrome. *(Rudolph CD,762–763, 1897)*

18. (D) In the congenital abnormality of anomalous origin of the left coronary artery (LCA), the aberrant LCA arises from the pulmonary artery rather than from the aorta. This results in perfusion of the left ventricle by poorly oxygenated blood under low pressure. Myocardial ischemia can be severe. The presenting signs are irritability and congestive heart failure. The age at presentation is related to the degree of collateral circulation between the LCA and RCA. *(McMillan, 1612–1613)*

19. (E) The findings of cyanosis and blood which is chocolate brown and does not become red upon exposure to air are indicative of methemoglobinemia. One cause of methemoglobinemia is exposure to well water which has been contaminated with nitrites. In contrast, carbon monoxide poisoning (automobile exhaust) results in carboxyhemoglobin, which binds oxygen so tightly that it cannot be released to the tissues. In this situation the blood would be bright red, rather than dark brown. Fava beans are a cause of hemolysis in patients with glucose-6-phosphate dehydrogenase (G-6-PD) deficiency, but are not a cause of methemoglobinemia. *(Rudolph CD,371–372, 1544–1545)*

20. (C) Peak height velocity occurs typically during SMR 2–3 for girls, and during SMR 4 for boys. *(Rudolph CD,223–224)*

21. (A) Night terrors are partial arousals that occur during stage 4 non-REM sleep to near arousal transitions, which typically first present in the preschool-aged child. The child appears awake, but does not respond to surroundings, including the family members attempting to calm the child. Amnesia of the event is another one of the events distinguishing these from nightmares. Night terrors persist into adolescence in about one-third of the cases. *(Rudolph CD,418)*

22. (C) The primary lesion in acne is plugging of the duct of the sebaceous gland by dried or excessive sebum and keratin. The obstructed gland (comedo) eventually becomes inflamed. The relative roles of fatty acids, bacteria such as Propionibacterium acnes and S epidermidis, and the immunologic response in determining this inflammatory reaction are uncertain. *(McMillan, 875)*

23. (B) Although all the diseases listed can cause nasal obstruction and discharge, allergic rhinitis is by far the most common and the most likely in this child. Bilateral choanal atresia causes respiratory distress in the neonatal period; unilateral atresia causes persistent unilateral, purulent discharge. Immunodeficiency is most likely to cause chronic sinusitis and purulent discharge. Cystic fibrosis is much less common than allergy, and a defect in the cribriform plate is extremely rare. *(McMillan, 2428–2429)*

24. (D) Atopic dermatitis (eczema) is characterized by exudation, pruritus, and lichenification. Involvement in infancy is common, although the distribution and other features may be somewhat different than in older children. The classical adult distribution with predilection for popliteal and antecubital areas usually is not seen in infancy. Involvement of the face is common. Most patients have *elevated* serum IgE levels and normal levels of the other immunoglobulins. *(McMillan, 2424–2425)*

25. **(B)** The copperhead is a member of the group of poisonous snakes known as pit vipers or Crotalids. This group also includes the rattlesnake and the cottonmouth (water moccasin). All members of the group share similar toxins, the effects of which include local tissue injury and necrosis, neurologic manifestations, generalized bleeding, and shock. The severity of the reaction is related to the amount of venom injected (size of snake) and size of the victim. Local reactions are most common and are seen in almost all significant envenomations. Systemic reactions are less frequent and generally are seen only with severe envenomations. *(Rudolph CD,396–398)*

26. **(E)** The major concern for children with chronic otitis media with effusion (chronic OME) is that the associated conductive hearing loss will interfere with speech and language development during the critical early years of life. *(Rudolph CD,1253)*

27. **(D)** The most common indication for repair of pectus excavatum is to improve the appearance of the chest wall. *(Rudolph CD,2001)*

28. **(E)** Nasal polyps are uncommon in childhood. The two leading causes are allergy (allergic rhinitis) and cystic fibrosis. Although allergy is more common, any child with nasal polyps probably should have a sweat test, since allergic manifestations are not uncommon in children with cystic fibrosis. Benign (hemangioma, dermoid cyst) and malignant (rhabdomyosarcoma, nasal glioma) lesions are rare and can be mistaken for polyps. *(Rudolph CD,1262,1265; McMillan, 2428)*

29. **(C)** Unlike the situation in older children and adults, in infants the most frequent target organ of alpha$_1$-antitrypsin deficiency is the liver. This may take the form of prolonged neonatal cholestasis and/or cirrhosis and

portal hypertension. Obstructive lung disease can be seen in older children, but is rare in infancy. *(Rudolph CD,1490–1491)*

30. **(A)** Cushing syndrome (glucocorticoid excess) should be considered in any child with the combination of weight gain and growth arrest. In children younger than 7 years of age, glucocorticoid excess (noniatrogenic) is most often secondary to an adrenal tumor. In older children, the most common noniatrogenic cause of Cushing syndrome is true Cushing disease, adrenal hyperplasia caused by hypersecretion of pituitary ACTH. Over 80% of these older children have surgically identifiable pituitary microadenoma. *(Rudolph CD,2045–2046)*

31. **(B)** The most common tumor to cause destruction of the anterior pituitary gland in childhood is the craniopharyngioma. The diabetes insipidus that occurs as a result of the pituitary destruction can be very challenging to manage. The chromophobe adenoma is the most common destructive lesion in adults, but is rare in childhood. *(McMillan, 1771; Rudolph CD,2237)*

32. **(A)** Acute chest syndrome is a well described and potentially life-threatening complication of sickle cell disease. Early recognition and treatment are essential. Patients with acute chest syndrome can deteriorate rapidly and therefore require keen observation. *(AAP Section on Hematology/Oncology, 109:526–535, 2002; Rudolph CD, 1533)*

33. **(E)** Splenic sequestration is characterized by an acutely enlarging spleen and a decreasing (or decreased) hemoglobin, and frequently is associated with thrombocytopenia. Prompt recognition and treatment is necessary because some of the severe cases will rapidly progress to shock and death. Most of these acute splenic sequestration crises occur during infancy and early childhood and are uncommon after the fourth or fifth birthday, by which time autosplenectomy (due to recurrent infarctions) has occurred. In patients with sickle cell disease or sickle thalassemia, however, the spleen may remain large and sequestration crises can occur into the teens and adulthood. *(AAP Section on*

Hematology/Oncology, 109:526–535, 2002; Rudolph CD,1532)

34. **(A)** Since 1992 the American Academy of Pediatrics has recommended infants be placed on their backs to sleep in order to decrease the risk of SIDS. It has been called "The Back to Sleep" campaign, and has been very successful in helping to decrease SIDS by greater than 40%. Yet SIDS remains the leading cause of death in infants beyond the neonatal period. *(AAP Task Force on Sleep Position and Sudden Infant Death Syndrome, 105: 650–656, 2000)*

35. **(E)** Modifiable risk factors for SIDS that have been documented thus far include prone sleeping, soft sleep surfaces and loose bedding, overheating, maternal smoking during pregnancy, bed sharing (especially if the adults sharing the bed are smokers), and preterm birth and low birth weight. The factor most strongly associated with protection against SIDS is supine sleeping. Interestingly, studies recently have shown a substantially lower incidence of SIDS among pacifier-using infants compared to infants not using pacifiers. However, there is no proof that pacifier use prevents SIDS, and the use of pacifiers has other negative consequences. Therefore, a specific recommendation regarding pacifier use in SIDS prevention has not been made by the AAP. *(AAP Task Force on Sleep Position and Sudden Infant Death Syndrome, 105:650–656, 2000)*

36. **(B)** Although some cases of encopresis may be secondary to organic causes (spina bifida, Hirschsprung disease), the majority are psychologic or behavioral in nature. In contrast, the majority of cases of enuresis are most often due to a disturbance of bladder physiology or sleep mechanism, and generally are not considered to represent an emotional or behavioral disorder. If a child has been dry, then becomes enuretic (secondary enuresis), emotional factors may be involved in the process. Secondary enuresis may indicate sexual abuse. *(McMillan, 670–673,1920–1923)*

37. **(B)** This child probably has cyclic neutropenia, a defect in the production of granulocyte-macrophage colony-stimulating factor (GM-CSF). In these patients GM-CSF is produced in a cyclic rather than continuous manner. Episodes of neutropenia, often accompanied by fever, aphthous stomatitis, and cervical lymphadenitis recur at *regular* intervals, usually every 21–42 days. Few other conditions have such a remarkable periodicity. Schwachman-Diamond syndrome is the association of neutropenia with exocrine pancreatic insufficiency. Chediak-Higashi syndrome is an autosomal recessive disorder characterized by morphologically abnormal neutrophils, recurrent infections, partial albinism, mental retardation, and eventual pancytopenia. *(McMillan, 1713)*

38. **(C)** Random eye movements, ataxia, developmental delay, and abnormal behavior are found in the opsoclonus-myoclonus syndrome (otherwise called "dancing eyes, dancing feet" syndrome). This syndrome is associated with neuroblastoma. Though the associated tumors typically are small and resected, neurologic symptoms may persist. There may be an immune mechanism for these neurologic symptoms. *(McMillan, 1778; Rudolph CD,1618)*

39. **(B)** Infantile botulism should be considered in any infant with a history of progressive weakness, poor feeding, and constipation. Except for the insidious development of symptoms, the infants can be confused with those with sepsis or hypoglycemia. Their alertness with weakness resembles that seen in Werdnig-Hoffmann disease. However, infants with Werdnig-Hoffmann disease typically present before 6 months of age, lack lower limb deep tendon reflexes, and have very expressive faces. *(Rudolph CD,917–918, 2002, 2280)*

40. **(B)** Snoring is the hallmark of chronic upper airway obstruction from enlarged adenoids and tonsils in children. An infrequent but important complication of this is pulmonary hypertension with cor pulmonale. These children appear to hypoventilate, especially when asleep. The hypoxemia which results from the hypoventilation causes pulmonary arteriolar vasoconstriction, and this in turn results in cor pulmonale. *(Rudolph CD,1270)*

41. **(C)** Essentially all febrile seizures occur in children between 6 months and 5 years of age. Indeed, most authors incorporate this age range into the definition of febrile convulsions while some broaden the definition to between 3 months and 6 years. The peak age clearly is between 6 months and 3 years. In one study, the mean age was 23 months. *(Rudolph CD,2270–2271)*

42. **(C)** The clinical picture described is extremely suggestive of a brain tumor. Head tilt in these cases can be due to several mechanisms, including cranial nerve involvement with acute strabismus and secondary compensation by tilting the head. Head tilt is particularly common with posterior fossa tumors. Central nervous system tumors are now the most common neoplasms of childhood, accounting for 20%. The incidence of brain tumors is evenly distributed throughout childhood and adolescence. *(Rudolph CD,2207–2211)*

43. **(C)** Hartnup disease is an autosomal recessive disorder with a single defect in the transport of monoamino-monocarboxylic amino acids by the renal tubules and intestinal mucosa. There is increased loss of the involved amino acids (neutral amino acids). Most children remain asymptomatic, and the major clinical manifestation is cutaneous photosensitivity. Some children with this disorder will have attacks of cerebellar ataxia, which resolve spontaneously but also can be reversed by the administration of nicotinic acid. None of the other conditions listed are associated with ataxia. *(Behrman, 353)*

44. **(C)** The rash described is that of a contact dermatitis, most likely due to poison ivy. The lesions which are usually papules and vesicles are intensely pruritic. Restriction of the rash to the legs also is characteristic of poison ivy. Although the rash of Henoch-Schönlein purpura is usually restricted to below the waist, it is purpuric rather than pruritic. *(Rudolph CD,1180)*

45. **(A)** Bilious vomiting in the neonate can represent any gastrointestinal obstruction distal to the entry of the common duct into the duodenum and requires immediate evaluation and treatment. In this case, the "bird beak" appearance of the distal duodenum is diagnostic of midgut volvulus probably secondary to malrotation. The resultant strangulation of the superior mesenteric artery can lead to total destruction of the jejunoileum. *(Klaus, 185; Rudolph CD,1376)*

46. **(D)** Annular pancreas is a congenital malformation in which the pancreas encircles the duodenum. The condition may be asymptomatic or may cause partial or complete duodenal obstruction. The most frequent presenting complaint is vomiting. *(Rudolph CD,1464)*

47. **(C)** The classical radiologic finding in duodenal atresia is dilatation of the stomach and of the proximal duodenum—the so-called "double bubble" sign. The double bubble sign can also be seen with annular pancreas, and occasionally malrotation. Remember, 40% of all neonates with duodenal atresia have trisomy 21. *(Klaus, 185; Rudolph CD,1403)*

48. **(B)** During the first year of life, the average infant grows about 25 cm (10 in). That is, they grow from about 51 cm (20 in) at birth to about 75 cm (30 in) at the first birthday. Another way to phrase this is that by the end of the first year, birth length increases by 50%. *(Rudolph CD,5)*

49. **(C)** Infants typically double their birth weight by approximately 4 months of age, and triple their birth weight by approximately 12 months of age. Contrast this with height. A child doubles their birth length by 4 years of age and triples their birth length by 13 years of age. *(Rudolph CD,5)*

50. **(B)** The picture described is most suggestive of the X-linked recessive disorder of end-organ insensitivity to androgenic hormones (testicular feminization). Although the 20, 22-desmolase deficiency does cause male pseudohermaphrodism, the associated adrenal insufficiency is quickly fatal in infancy, unless diagnosed and treated. All other forms of congenital adrenal hyperplasia are virilizing rather than feminizing. True hermaphrodism is very rare and requires that both testicular and ovarian tissue be present. No evidence for this is presented in this case. *(Rudolph CD,2011, 2085)*

51. **(C)** At birth, the average hemoglobin is 17 g/dL in term babies. It then falls rapidly over the next 2–3 months to a low of about 11 g/dL. Hemoglobin values then gradually rise and eventually equal adult normal values in the early teen years. *(Rudolph CD,1519–1521)*

52. **(E)** Breath-holding spells always terminate spontaneously and are never fatal; they have no known relationship to sudden infant death syndrome. Breath-holding spells are common in early childhood, have a peak incidence between 12 and 18 months and usually disappear by about 5 years of age. The exact mechanism or etiology is not known but family pedigrees suggest they are associated with an autosomal dominant trait with reduced penetrance. Although many youngsters will hold their breath to the point of cyanosis and syncope or seizure, there is nothing to suggest that breath-holding is a type of epilepsy. Rather, the syncope and seizure are secondary to cerebral hypoxia. *(Rudolph CD,445)*

53. **(D)** The major manifestation of pinworm (*E vermicularis*) infection is rectal or perirectal itching. The female worms leave the rectum at night to lay their eggs in the perineal area and die shortly thereafter. Eggs remain viable and infective for 2–3 weeks in indoor environments. *(AAP:Red Book, 520–521)*

54. **(D)** Although all the conditions listed as possible answers are associated with bullous lesions, epidermolysis bullosa (EB) is the best fit and should be highest on the differential diagnosis. There are at least 15 known forms of EB, varying in severity and age of presentation. Many present in the newborn period, with lesions mostly at areas of friction or trauma as described in this patient. Both drug-induced toxic epidermal necrolysis (rare in neonates) and staphylococcal scalded skin syndrome (common in neonates) are associated with more generalized erythema and lesions than described in this patient. Neither the lesions of bullous impetigo nor the lesions of congenital syphilis are related to areas of trauma; the latter have a special predilection for the palms and soles. *(Rudolph CD,1173, 1187)*

55. **(C)** Juvenile polyps are most commonly found in the rectum. These are hamartomas with inflammatory infiltration. They are not adenomatous polyps and are neither malignant nor premalignant. They generally present in the first 5 years of life with the passage of red blood streaking on the stool. *(Rudolph CD,1453–1455)*

56. **(D)** The elevated white blood cell count and low glucose in the cerebrospinal fluid are most suggestive of a bacterial pathogen, of which group B streptococcus would be the most likely. Though a Gram stain of CSF provides presumptive evidence in the evaluation of meningitis, it frequently is misleading. The gold standard for diagnosis of a bacterial pathogen is the culture of the spinal fluid. *(AAP:Red Book, 620-624; Hay,1089)*

57. **(E)** Cow milk and human milk have many differences in composition. Cow milk has a higher protein content (32 vs. 10.6 g/L) and human milk has a higher fat (45 vs. 38 g/L) and carbohydrate (71 vs. 47 g/L) content. Cow milk also has higher sodium and calcium content. Except for colostrum—milk produced during the first few days following delivery of the baby—human milk has more calories (747 kcal/L) than does cow milk (701 kcal/L). *(Behrman, 156)*

58. **(E)** Umbilical hernias are quite common, especially in premature and in African-American infants. Although there is an increased incidence of umbilical hernias in infants with a variety of syndromes (eg, Beckwith-Wiedemann) and diseases (eg, hypothyroidism), the great majority occur in otherwise normal infants. Most resolve spontaneously and no therapy is required except for the rare case that incarcerates. An abdominal ultrasound examination should be done only if there is clinical evidence of an abdominal mass or ascites. Strapping or taping are ineffective and irritating and should not be advised. *(Behrman, 528)*

59. **(B)** Chylous ascites is characterized by a high concentration of lipids in the ascitic fluid. Most cases in infancy are due to congenital malformation of lymph channels; occasional cases are due to obstruction of the thoracic duct, tumor,

inflammation, or intestinal obstruction. Loss of albumin, gammaglobulin, and lymphocytes in the ascitic fluid leads to depletion of these elements from the blood. The prognosis is guarded, even with treatment. Spontaneous resolution has been reported, but is the exception rather than the rule. *(Rudolph CD,1497, 1515)*

60. **(A)** The clinical picture described is typical of acute pancreatitis, and can be the result of each condition listed. However, of these, blunt abdominal trauma (including child abuse) would be the most common cause. *(McMillan, 2010)*

61. **(D)** Although idiopathic scoliosis can present at any stage of growth, it is most commonly manifest during, or shortly before, adolescence. It is considerably more frequent in girls than in boys. These children are mentally and intellectually normal. The condition is never painful and is usually detected on routine physical examination. The diagnosis is made on clinical grounds using physical examination and an inclinometer. When the scoliosis exceeds 6 or 7 degrees with the use of the inclinometer, x-rays will be used for a more precise assessment. *(McMillan,2487–2491)*

62. **(A)** The Wiskott-Aldrich syndrome, an X-linked disorder, typically presents during the first 6 months of life with recurrent infections or bleeding episodes. The unusual aspect of the thrombocytopenia is that the thrombocytes are very small and thus called microthrombocytes. These small platelets are not common in any other thrombocytopenic disease. The treatment of choice is with HLA-matched bone marrow transplantation. *(McMillan, 2467)*

63. **(B)** Testicular torsion actually is torsion of the spermatic cord and is a true surgical emergency because irreversible change can occur in testes within 4–6 hours, and after 24 hours, infarction is the rule. This condition occurs in 1 in 4000 males 25 years of age and younger, with peak occurrence in the preadolescent age group. *(Rudolph CD,1740)*

64. **(B)** The minute structures attached to the hair are most likely nits, the eggs of the scalp louse (*pediculosis capitis*). The safest and most effective treatment of scalp lice is the topical application of a 1% permethrin cream rinse. Griseofulvin is useful for certain fungal infections such as tinea capitis, but is not effective against pediculosis. *(AAP:Red Book,488–492)*

65. **(B)** Chemical pneumonitis is the most common clinical manifestation of poisoning with hydrocarbons such as kerosene and may result from the aspiration of even minute amounts. Central nervous system changes are less common but can be seen. *(Rudolph CD,366–367, 1988)*

66. **(B)** Congenital hypothyroidism may be associated with prolonged neonatal hyperbilirubinemia, either indirect or mixed. The indirect hyperbilirubinemia is due to impaired hepatic glucuronidation of bilirubin and to enhanced enterohepatic circulation of bilirubin secondary to decreased intestinal motility. The mechanism of the mixed hyperbilirubinemia is uncertain. Hypothyroidism also can be associated with anemia and impaired renal function, but these are mild. *(Rudolph CD,2065)*

67. **(B)** Laryngomalacia is a condition of excessive compliance, or softness, of the cartilage of the larynx. It is presumed to be a problem of maturation rather than a congenital abnormality and is the most common cause of persistent inspiratory stridor in the young infant. Symptoms usually begin in the first month of life; are worse with agitation and in the supine position; and eventually resolve, usually by a year or so. Foreign body aspiration is an important cause of persistent stridor in the older infant and toddler but would be very unusual at this age. *(Rudolph CD,1271)*

68. **(B)** Hypercalciuria has been found in a very significant number of children with otherwise unexplained gross or microscopic hematuria. In most cases, the hematuria is not associated with renal stones or precedes the formation of stones by many years. The serum level of calcium is normal in these patients. *(Rudolph CD, 1663)*

69. **(B)** The chest roentgenogram reveals air trapping of the left lung with a shift of the heart and mediastinum to the right. This is most suggestive of a foreign body in the left mainstem bronchus. In the case of infantile lobar emphysema, the findings would be present in the first few months of life and would not cause the sudden onset of wheezing at 4 years of age. Also, in this condition, one lobe rather than an entire lung would be overdistended. Asthma is associated with bilateral, rather than unilateral, air trapping. *(McMillan, 1464–1466)*

70. **(B)** The unequal leg length and asymmetry of the inguinal (anterior) and thigh (posterior) skin creases are indicative of severe developmental dysplasia of the hip. Neither tibial torsion nor equinovarus deformity affect leg length or inguinal skin creases. Arthrogryposis is associated with severe joint contractures. *(Rudolph CD,2434–2436)*

71. **(E)** Any child with uveitis involving primarily the anterior structures of the eye should be suspected of having juvenile idiopathic arthritis (JIA). This association is strongest in girls with the pauciarticular form of JIA, especially those who are antinuclear antibody positive. Toxoplasmosis and toxocara are more likely to be associated with *posterior* uveitis. Neither leukemia nor hypoparathyroidism are associated with uveitis. *(Rudolph CD,837, 2382)*

72. **(E)** Intoeing is a very common pediatric issue and in most cases represents a developmental process which is self-limited. Femoral anteversion is seen in preschoolers and typically resolves around the age of 8 years. Tibial torsion typically is present in toddlers and is diagnosed with the toddler in a sitting position with legs dangling from the table at 90 degrees. Metatarsus adductus is seen more commonly in infants, and involves the foot. *(Rudolph CD,2422–2425)*

73. **(E)** There are many factors to be considered in the decision to obtain throat swab specimens for testing of GAS. Testing is not recommended in children with signs and symptoms such as coryza, conjunctivitis, hoarseness, anterior stomatitis, diarrhea, and discrete ulcerative lesions which are highly suggestive of viral syndromes. Testing generally is not recommended in children younger than 3 years of age because the risk of rheumatic fever is so remote. Testing is recommended only for symptomatic household contacts of patients with documented GAS pharyngitis, but is recommended for all household contacts of patients with documented rheumatic fever or poststreptococcal glomerulonephritis. *(AAP:Red Book,613–614)*

74. **(A)** Lymphocytic thyroiditis (Hashimoto thyroiditis) is an autoimmune disorder and circulating antithyroid antibodies can be demonstrated in most patients. However, other autoimmune disorders, including diabetes mellitus, adrenal insufficiency, hypoparathyroidism, and pernicious anemia, occur in only a *minority* of patients. The thyroid gland is *invariably enlarged*, often irregularly so. Most patients are euthyroid, some are hypothyroid, and a few are hyperthyroid. *(Rudolph CD,2070)*

75. **(B)** Before the 1970s, zinc deficiency was not known to be the cause of this devastating condition called acrodermatitis enteropathica. Breastfed infants are at risk of zinc deficiency when the maternal levels are low and vegetarians are at risk of zinc deficiency because the bioavailability of zinc in plant sources is low. Therefore, this infant was at risk. Patients receiving TPN also are prone to this condition, and should receive supplementation and monitoring. *(Rudolph CD,1338; McMillan, 175)*

76. **(E)** Primary pulmonary hemosiderosis is an uncommon disease of unknown origin characterized by repeated pulmonary hemorrhages. The clinical picture of recurrent episodes of fever, cough, and radiographic infiltrates is frequently misinterpreted as recurrent pneumonia, especially in infants and young children who do not expectorate and in whom hemoptysis may go undetected. The first clue often is a severe iron deficiency anemia. Some of these infants or children have improvement in pulmonary manifestations when cow milk is eliminated from their diet. Diffuse pulmonary hemangiomatosis and extramedullary pulmonary erythropoiesis are nonentities. *(Rudolph CD,1997–1998)*

77. **(B)** Chondromalacia patellae (also called patellofemoral pain and patellar compression syndrome) is a repetitive stress injury resulting from rubbing between the femoral groove and patella associated with high forces generated through sports and jumping. As with other conditions suffered from overuse or repetition, the pain remits with rest. Night pain or unremitting pain in this situation should always prompt further evaluation. *(Rudolph CD, 2432–2433)*

78. **(D)** The anterior fontanel normally closes between 9 and 18 months of age. Each of the choices, except for craniosynostosis, is associated with *delayed* closure of the anterior fontanelle. Craniosynostosis is the premature fusion of skull sutures which results in abnormalities of calvarial shape and occurs in about 1 in 2000 live births. The most common form of single suture fusion is sagital synostosis. Although most cases of craniosynostosis are diagnosed in the newborn period, early closure of the fontanelles should raise suspicion for this diagnosis, and with careful examination you should be able to palpate the ridging of the prematurely fused suture. *(Rudolph CD,755)*

79. **(E)** The rash described in this question sounds like urticaria, for which there are many causes. Although allergy to foods, drugs, or chemicals is high on the list, in most cases, no specific cause can be found. A few cases are associated with infections caused by hepatitis viruses or group A Streptococcus. A very few cases are due to collage vascular disease or malignancy. Hereditary deficiency of C1-esterase inhibitor (extremely rare) is usually associated with angioedema rather than urticaria. *(Rudolph, 1195)*

80. **(C)** The XYY karyotype is relatively common, occurring in about 1 in 1000 males. Patients with this karyotype generally are tall. It is debatable whether or not the XYY karyotype is associated with an increased risk of impulsivity, antisocial behavior, and psychopathic personality. But whether or not this is true, *most* XYY individuals are behaviorally normal, although IQ and language development tend to be below normal. *(Jones, 70–71, 707)*

81. **(A)** Thrombocytopenia with giant platelets in an otherwise well-appearing newborn most likely represents platelet destruction secondary to transplacental transmission of maternal antiplatelet IgG autoantibodies. Maternal thrombocytopenia would be expected if this were the case. If the maternal thrombocytes were normal and she had no history of autoimmune disease, alloimmune thrombocytopenia is the likely diagnosis. This would result from transplacental passage of a maternal antibody that specifically recognized an antigen on baby's platelets that baby inherited from the father. *(Klaus, 475)*

82. **(C)** Pertussis is most deadly for young infants. Complications include pneumonia, seizures, encephalopathy, and apnea. The case fatality rate in the United States is 1% for those infants less than 2 months of age. In adolescents, the illness more likely presents as a persistent cough. For those in between these age groups, the more classic picture is seen: paroxysms of 10–30 uninterrupted staccato coughs followed by a long loud gasping inspiration known as a "whoop," accompanied by an absolute lymphocytosis. Following implementation of pertussis immunization in the 1950s, the number of annual US cases fell dramatically. Pertussis incidence has increased since 1980 in the US and increase in incidence has been most notable for adolescents and adults. In 2005, pertussis containing vaccine (Tdap) for adolscents and adults has been available with hopes that implementation will reduce the large group of susceptibles and decrease the risk of disease in infants too young to immunize. *(AAP:Red Book,498–520)*

83. **(A)** The abnormality in pseudohypoparathyroidism is a defect in end-organ (kidney and bone) response to parathyroid hormone. Serum levels of parathyroid hormone are normal or elevated. Short stature and skeletal abnormalities, including demineralization, are common. Fingers are short and broad (brachymetacarpals). *(Rudolph CD,2011)*

84. **(B)** Also called pseudohemophilia, von Willebrand disease is characterized by a

prolonged bleeding time. There is a variable deficiency or molecular abnormality of factor VIII, giving rise to a variably abnormal PTT. The platelet count, factor XII level, and pro-thrombin time are all normal. The location for the encoding of the von Willebrand factor is on chromosome 12. Most commonly, children with von Willebrand disease will present with a history of nosebleeds and easy bruising. *(Rudolph CD,200)*

85. **(A)** Dysgenesis (aplasia, dysplasia, hypopla-sia) of the thyroid gland is the most common cause of congenital hypothyroidism. Inborn metabolic errors of thyroid synthesis are much less frequent. Maternal ingestion of iodides (as in expectorants) is a recognized cause of neona-tal hypothyroidism but is rare today. *(Rudolph CD, 2066, 2068–2069)*

86. **(B)** Cysticercosis is a condition of generalized tissue invasion by the larva of *T solium* and results from the ingestion of *T solium* eggs which have contaminated food or cooking utensils. Eating undercooked infected pork results in ingestion of an encysted worm which causes an intestinal tapeworm infestation, not cysticercosis. Cysticercosis is endemic in Mexico and is one of the most common causes of seizures in children in that population. In the United States it is seen primarily in areas with large Latin American immigrant popula-tions. The central nervous system is the most common target organ and seizures are the most frequent presenting complaint. *(AAP:Red Book, 644–646)*

87. **(E)** Approximately 40% of adults with cystic fibrosis have diabetes mellitus. It is thought to result from chronic obstruction of ductal flow from inspissated secretions which results in pancreatic fibrosis and beta-cell destruction. It behaves like maturity onset diabetes, with little tendency to ketoacidosis. Diabetes should always be considered when an older child with cystic fibrosis loses weight. *(Rudolph CD,2114)*

88. **(A)** Elevated sweat chloride concentration is an almost universal finding in patients with cystic fibrosis (CF). Even in this era of molecular diagnostics, the diagnosis of cystic fibrosis most often involves a sweat test. Normal children have sweat chloride concentrations less than 40 meq/L while CF patients have concentra-tions greater than 60 meq/L. It is strongly rec-ommended that sweat tests be performed only in established CF centers because tests per-formed outside these centers have unaccept-ably high rates of false positive and false negative results. *(Rudolph CD,1972)*

89. **(D)** Acute otitis media (AOM) resolves sponta-neously in about 80% of cases and 60% of chil-dren are pain free in 24 hours, with or without antibiotic treatment. The bacteria most com-monly involved in acute otitis media in child-hood in the United States is *Streptococcus pneumoniae* which accounts for 30–40% of AOM; 40% of which are resistant to penicillin and most do not spontaneously resolve. *H influenzae* (causes 25% of AOM, 25% are beta-lactamase producers), and *Moraxella catarrhalis* (causes 12% of AOM, 100% are beta-lactamase produc-ers) are more likely to resolve without therapy. Most experts agree that amoxicillin remains the initial drug of choice, and that an increased dose (80 mg/kg/day) is indicated given the pneu-mococcal resistance rates. *(Rudolph CD,1249–1252)*

90. **(A)** Inguinal hernias are not at all rare in female infants, and the great majority of these infants are genetically female and otherwise normal. Such hernias may contain intestine or an ovary, either of which can incarcerate. Prompt surgi-cal correction is indicated. Most inguinal her-nias in infants, males or females, are indirect. *(Rudolph CD,1742; McMillan, 1640–1642)*

91. **(B)** Large ventricular septal defects (VSD) usu-ally are associated with left deviation of the electrical axis and evidence of left ventricular hypertrophy on electrocardiogram, although signs of combined ventricular hypertrophy are not uncommon. An enlarged heart is common, but the pulmonary vasculature is increased, not decreased. The murmur of a VSD is systolic, rather than continuous. With large left-to-right shunts and a high pulmonary flow, there also may be a mid-diastolic rumble, but still not a continuous murmur. *(Rudolph CD,1354–1356)*

92. (C) All of the choices listed are manifestations of hypoparathyroidism, the hallmark of which is hypocalcemia and hyperphosphatemia with resultant neuromuscular instability. The most common presentation is seizure. *(Rudolph CD, 1768)*

93. (D) Nearly 60% of adolescent women will experience dysmenorrhea. It is the leading cause of school absenteeism among these young women. Most cases are primary dysmenorrhea (painful menses without pelvic pathology), and are associated with high levels of prostaglandins which correlate with the severity of the symptoms. For these young women, nonsteroidal anti-inflammatory agents are generally very effective. Oral contraceptives often are a good therapeutic option because they successfully treat the dysmenorrhea in 80%–90%. *(McMillan,565–566)*

94. (D) This child meets diagnostic criteria for Kawasaki disease. To establish the diagnosis the patient must have fever for at least 5 days, then have at least four of the following five criteria: (1) bilateral bulbar conjunctival injection without exudates; (2) changes in oral mucosa including erythematous mouth and pharynx, strawberry tongue, and red, cracked lips; (3) rash that is polymorphous, generalized, morbilliform, maculopapular or scarlatiniform, or erythema multiforme-like; (4) changes in peripheral extremities consisting of induration of hands and feet, palmoplantar erythema, or periungual desquamation; (5) acute, nonsuppurative cervical adenopathy with at least one node measuring 1.5 cm. The complication of coronary artery aneurysms occurs in about 25% of untreated patients. This declines to about 3%–6% with intravenous gammaglobulin treatment. Treatment should be initiated as soon as the diagnosis is made. *(AAP:Red Book,392–393; Rudolph CD,412–415)*

95. (A) Fanconi syndrome is a proximal tubule transport disorder which leads to hypophosphatemia, hypokalemia, and a hyperchloremic metabolic acidosis. The most common inherited cause in children is cystinosis, a disorder in which cystine accumulates in the lysosomes eventually leading to cell dysfunction. Children with this disorder typically are healthy for the first few months of life, then develop the symptoms described. Two other choices, tyrosinemia and glycogen storage disease also are associated with Fanconi syndrome. *(Rudolph CD,1708)*

96. (A) Pityriasis rosea (PR) is a common dermatosis. It is characterized by a progressive eruption of dozens of 2–10-mm, salmon-colored flat patches with a scaly perimeter. Lesions may be intensely pruritic. Characteristically the lesions follow skin lines and on the back create the so-called "Christmas tree" pattern. This generalized rash may be preceded by several weeks by a herald patch, a larger well-circumscribed lesion on the extremities or trunk. In any patient who also has palmoplantar or mucous membrane lesions or who is sexually active, serologic testing for syphilis is indicated. Epidemiologic evidence has long supported the idea this has an infectious etiology. Recently, PR has been described in patients with active human herpesvirus 6 and human herpesvirus 7 infection. *(Rudolph CD,1181; Watanabe, 119:779–780, 2002)*

97. (B) The presenting sign in over 60% of patients with retinoblastoma is leukocoria, or white pupil. Often, this is noted during a well-child examination. This patient represents the average age at diagnosis, 18 months. In 30%–35% of patients, tumors occur bilaterally. There is a 90% survival rate for patients with small, unilateral, promptly treated tumors. *(Rudolph CD,2396)*

98. (C) A grave disparity regarding neonatal and infant mortality rates exists between African American babies and babies of other races. Though preterm births are more common among African American mothers, this does not completely explain the nearly double rates for infant and neonatal mortality as compared to Caucasians. *(Rudolph CD,57)*

99. (D) Children with constitutional growth delay have no endocrine disease but lag behind their peers in both growth and physiologic maturation. Such children are small for their age. Bone age also is delayed and, therefore, is commensurate with height. Puberty is delayed, and, consequently, growth continues for a longer than normal period of time, resulting in ultimate adult height which is normal. *(Rudolph CD, 2103)*

100. **(B)** The most common form of systemic vasculitis in childhood is Henoch-Schönlein purpura. The most consistent sign is the presence of the purpuric rash on the lower extremities. Unfortunately, this rash does not necessarily develop at the beginning of the illness. Frequently a child is evaluated for arthritis or abdominal pain for 1–2 days before the onset of the rash makes the diagnosis apparent. The renal disease associated with HSP typically is variable, with most children having complete recovery. However, 3–4% of children will develop end-stage renal disease. *(Rudolph CD, 842, 1689)*

101. **(B)** This child most likely has transient synovitis of the hip, an acute inflammatory process that is generally self-limited. It is most important for this to be distinguished from a septic hip, which typically presents in younger patients and is accompanied by fever and laboratory evidence such as increased white blood cell count, increased platelets, or increased erythrocyte sedimentation rate. And, follow-up is your friend. This child should be closely observed and examined again within 24 hours; sooner if there are any parental concerns or worsening symptoms. *(Hay, 822)*

102. **(B)** The selective disturbance of skeletal growth in achondroplasia results in disproportionately short extremities. In the extremities the proximal bones are further disproportionately shortened in relation to the distal bones. The fingers are short and stubby. Hydrocephalus is seen occasionally, possibly related to a small foramen magnum. Overall height, of course, is markedly decreased. These patients characteristically have a relatively large head, bulging forehead, and depressed nasal bridge. The diagnosis is confirmed by skeletal radiographs. Most cases arise from a new mutation at *FGFR3* codon 380 to normal parents. However, achondroplasia, when inherited, behaves as an autosomal dominant trait. *(Lissauer, 288)*

103. **(D)** Goat milk, compared to human milk and cow milk, is low in folate and iron. Babies exclusively fed goat milk are susceptible to megaloblastic anemia from folate and B_{12} deficiency. Additionally, if the goat milk is fresh and not boiled, the infants are at risk of brucellosis. *(Behrman, 156–157)*

104. **(E)** Rotavirus is the most common cause of winter diarrhea in the United States and is a leading cause of death among children in developing countries. Hypernatremic dehydration (serum sodium > 150 meq/L with dehydration) is frequently seen in hospitalized infants with rotavirus infection. A significant decrease in hospitalizations for rotavirus enteritis has followed the implementation in 2006 of live attenuated rotavirus vaccine. There are currently 2 preparations on the market which differ in number of required doses but both appear to be equally efficacious at this time. *(AAP:Red Book,572–574)*

105. **(A)** Motor vehicle accidents lead to approximately 5500 adolescent deaths each year in the United States. Homicides result in the death of nearly 3000 adolescents per year, making this the second most common cause of death in this age group. Of these 3000 deaths, 2500 are associated with firearms. The importance of firearms in these deaths is evident. An additional 1200 suicidal deaths are associated with firearms each year. *(McMillan, 140)*

106. **(E)** Despite the devastating effect congenital infection with cytomegalovirus can have on the fetus and newborn, most congenital infections are asymptomatic. If however, symptoms of infection are present at birth, most will have severe neurodevelopmental disabilities such as cerebral palsy, epilepsy, sensorineural hearing loss, and learning difficulties. Most severe effects are seen in infants whose fetal infection occurred during the first half of pregnancy. *(Lissauer, 73–74; AAP:Red Book,273–277)*

107. **(D)** The syndrome of inappropriate secretion of antidiuretic hormone (SIADH) is a common complication of a variety of central nervous system problems, including bacterial meningitis.

Usually the SIADH resolves as the meningitis is treated, even if a subdural effusion is present. (*McMillan, 2603–2605*)

108. **(B)** Theoretically, the syndrome of inappropriate ADH secretion would be most accurately diagnosed by measurement of serum ADH levels. However, the assay for antidiuretic hormone is not readily available. Therefore, the diagnosis usually is confirmed by demonstrating a low urine output and inappropriate high urine osmolality in the presence of low serum osmolality. (*McMillan, 2605*)

109. **(D)** Patients with inappropriate secretion of ADH have a decreased urine output and are hypervolemic. They are neither hypotensive nor alkalotic. High urine specific gravity is one of the criteria for the diagnosis of SIADH. (*McMillan, 2605*)

110. **(B)** Therapy of inappropriate ADH secretion consists primarily of fluid restriction and, of course, treatment of the underlying condition, in this case, bacterial meningitis. Attempts to correct the hyponatremia by administration of sodium usually result in more retention of water and further hypervolemia and edema. Intravenous administration of hypertonic saline would be indicated only if the hyponatremia were life-threatening. Maintenance amounts of sodium should be administered. Diuretics are not very effective in this condition. (*McMillan, 2605*)

111. **(B)** The cerebrospinal fluid findings, especially the xanthochromic appearance after centrifugation, indicate an intracranial hemorrhage. The bleeding is primarily subarachnoid or, at least, there has been extension of the bleeding into the subarachnoid space. Intraventricular hemorrhage is uncommon except in the small, premature infant. Fever is seen in patients with intracranial hemorrhage. (*Rudolph CD,2196, 2238*)

112. **(C)** Of the abnormalities listed, only cerebral arteriovenous malformation (AVM) and aneurysm predispose to hemorrhagic disasters. In children, cerebral AVMs are the most common cause of spontaneous intracranial hemorrhage.

Unlike the situation in adults, intracranial hemorrhage in children is rarely due to a ruptured aneurysm. (*Rudolph CD,2196, 2238*)

113. **(A)** The most appropriate management at this time would be to perform a CT scan, followed, *if necessary*, by further imaging. It would not have been unreasonable to have performed the CT prior to the lumbar puncture. It is a question of judgment as to the likelihood of meningitis in this child with only a slight fever. Intracranial hemorrhage rarely is associated with volume depletion or the need for transfusion. In the absence of evidence of a bleeding disorder, there is no indication for administration of fresh frozen plasma. (*Rudolph CD,2196, 2238*)

114. **(C)** The clinical picture described is almost pathognomonic for infantile hypertrophic pyloric stenosis, which would best be confirmed with abdominal ultrasound. (*McMillan, 371–373*)

115. **(E)** Most infants with hypertrophic pyloric stenosis develop a hypochloremic metabolic alkalosis secondary to the loss of hydrogen and chloride ions in the vomitus, which in this condition is essentially pure gastric secretion. Hypochloremic metabolic alkalosis occurs so regularly in this disorder, that it often is used as a diagnostic feature. (*McMillan, 371–373*)

116. **(B)** The physical findings suggest that the child is moderately dehydrated. Glucose and water alone is never the appropriate hydrating or maintenance solution for an infant or a child. Bicarbonate should be withheld from this child who is not described as appearing clinically acidotic and who is very likely to have a metabolic alkalosis secondary to the prolonged vomiting. Indeed, the respiratory rate of 12 is rather slow for an infant of this age and could be explained on the basis of respiratory compensation for a metabolic alkalosis. Although the child might be hypokalemic secondary to prolonged alkalosis, there also is the possibility of hyperkalemia secondary to dehydration and prerenal azotemia. Normal saline is the most appropriate initial rehydrating fluid until the serum electrolytes are documented. (*Behrman, 1131*)

117. **(E)** In this clinical scenario, urine positive for hemoglobin on dipstick but negative for red blood cells on microscopic examination probably represents myoglobinuria. This would be presumptively confirmed with an elevated serum creatine kinase. *(McMillan, 1214–1215)*

118. **(D)** Acute myoglobinuria can lead to tubular injury and acute renal failure. Serum electrolytes and renal function should be evaluated. *(Rudolph CD,1660)*

119. **(A)** Acute myoglobinuria is caused by influenza viruses A and B, some enteroviruses, and less commonly, adenovirus, herpes simplex virus, and Epstein-Barr virus. This patient most likely has influenza virus infection. *(AAP:Red Book, 401)*

120. **(D)** This child most likely has visceral larva migrans, which in this country usually is caused by *Toxocara canis*, or *Toxocara cati*, the dog and cat ascarids, respectively. Diagnosis can be established by biopsy of the liver but negative biopsy does not exclude the diagnosis. Since the human is an unnatural host, the parasite does not complete its life cycle and ova or worms do not appear in the stool or in duodenal fluid. The diagnosis cannot be established by examination of the bone marrow or a blood smear. An enzyme immunoassay for Toxocara antibodies in serum can confirm the diagnosis. Most patients, if not blood type AB, have markedly elevated anti-A and anti-B isohemagglutinin antibody titers. Often the diagnosis is made on the basis of the clinical, hematologic, and serologic data, without liver biopsy. *(Rudolph CD, 1110–1111; AAP:Red Book,665)*

121. **(B)** *Toxocara canis* infection usually is acquired by eating soil contaminated by dog stool. The *T canis* eggs which are passed in the dog's stool are not directly infective, but in the soil the eggs develop into infective ova containing second-stage larva. Infection, therefore, is probably not acquired by direct contact with the animal, but only by contact with infected soil; usually a history of pica is obtained. *(Rudolph CD, 1110–1111)*

122. **(A)** If you keep a mental picture of preschoolers playing in the dirt around puppies all over the United States, you can begin to remember the epidemiology of this infection. This parasitic infection is more common in the United States than in developing countries and is equally prevalent in urban and rural populations. In humans, this infection is most frequently reported in children of 1–4 years of age. The vast majority of newborn puppies are infected. *(Rudolph CD,1110–1111)*

123. **(D)** The most likely diagnosis is severe combined immunodeficiency syndrome (SCIDS). Both Wiskott-Aldrich syndrome and hereditary agammaglobulinemia are X-linked recessive conditions and, therefore, are unlikely in this female child. Most 3-month-old infants have low, but detectable, levels of IgA and IgM (normal range for 3-month-old: 3–90 and 115–120 mg/dL, respectively). The IgG is maternally derived. HIV infection is a consideration but is not included in the differential diagnosis listed. Patients with transient hypogammaglobulinemia of infancy usually are not as sick as this patient and infection generally does not start as early as 6 weeks. Patients with chronic granulomatous disease are generally boys and primary pathogens include *S aureus*, *Serratia marcescens*, and *Aspergillus fumigatus*. Of the diagnoses listed, only SCIDS explains all the findings including lymphopenia. *(Rudolph CD,793–796, 799)*

124. **(C)** Severe combined immunodeficiency is associated with an absence or paucity of plasma cells in the bone marrow, absence or paucity of superficial lymphoid tissue, and an absent thymic shadow on chest roentgenogram. Cutaneous reactivity to various common antigens is absent. In an immunologically normal child with *Candida* infection, one would expect to find a positive reaction to intradermal testing with *Candida* antigen. In a child with severe combined immunodeficiency, there is global anergy and all skin tests are nonreactive. *(Rudolph CD, 793–796, 799)*

125. **(B)** The roentgenographic picture described is typical of *Pneumocystis jiroveci* infection

(previously known as *Pneumocystis carinii*), to which these infants are unduly susceptible. Viruses such as cytomegalovirus could produce a similar picture, but it is not listed as a choice. Lymphangiectasia is a congenital lesion of the lung, unrelated to immunologic disorders. Neither pneumococcal pneumonia nor pulmonary hemorrhage is likely to be so protracted or indolent. Miliary tuberculosis is a possibility, but usually does not produce such extensive bilateral disease or a ground-glass appearance radiographically. It also is uncommon in patients this young. *(Rudolph CD,793–796; AAP:Red Book,537–542)*

126. **(C)** Of the conditions listed, subdural hematoma is the most likely and would best explain all the clinical findings. Tuberculous meningitis can cause obstructive hydrocephalus and a large head, but fever and cranial nerve abnormalities usually are evident on physical examination. Mastoiditis is generally associated with fever, and, by itself, would not explain the neurologic findings. Pseudotumor cerebri is relatively benign and is not associated with convulsions. All three conditions—tuberculous meningitis, mastoiditis, and pseudotumor are uncommon in the first few months of life. With congenital toxoplasmosis, other findings and delayed psychomotor development would likely be present. *(Rudolph CD,465, 953, 2398)*

127. **(C)** Retinal hemorrhages may be found in up to 40% of cases of subdural hematoma and usually are indicative of the shaking injury as a form of child abuse now termed abusive head trauma baby syndrome (rather than the old name, abusive head trauma syndrome). The forceful shaking of the infant creates shearing forces in the brain and retina, resulting in bleeding in both organs. Congenital toxoplasmosis is associated with chorioretinitis rather than hemorrhage. *(Behrman, 1937; Rudolph CD,465)*

128. **(C)** The presentation of this infant necessitates CT scan of the head to begin to define the extent of the intracranial injuries. Head injuries remain the most common cause of death to children who have been abused. *(Rudolph CD, 469)*

129. **(G)** The most important intervention in any child with an elevated lead level is to stop further exposure of the child to the source of the lead. Children with blood lead levels of 45–69 mg/dL should receive chelation therapy. Chelation with oral meso-1,3-dimercaptosuccinic acid (DMSA) should be considered for children who have no signs of symptomatic lead poisoning. EDTA is the chelation agent of choice for children with symptomatic lead poisoning or severe lead poisoning involving the central nervous system or any child with a blood lead level of greater than or equal to 70 mg/dL. *(Rudolph CD,370)*

130. **(E)** Children with either acute iron poisoning or chronic iron overload from repeated transfusions should be treated with the iron chelating agent deferoxamine. For acute ingestion, the drug usually is administered intravenously. *(Rudolph CD,368)*

131. **(A)** If treatment is begun early (ideally within 24 hours of ingestion), acetylcysteine may prevent hepatic injury from acetaminophen ingestion. Acetaminophen itself is not hepatotoxic, but some of its metabolites are. These hepatotoxic metabolites ordinarily are inactivated by glutathione as soon as they are formed. Large overdoses of acetaminophen deplete the liver's stores of glutathione, permitting the toxic metabolite to accumulate. Acetylcysteine replenishes hepatic glutathione, protecting the liver from the toxic by-products of acetaminophen metabolism. *(Rudolph CD,360; Hay, 341)*

132. **(B)** Atropine is an important part of the treatment of organophosphate poisoning. Although it has little effect on the central nervous system effects of organophosphate, atropine will control respiratory secretions and other cholinergic effects. Pralidoxime, a cholinesterase-regenerating oxime may be needed to reverse muscle weakness. *(Rudolph CD,373–374)*

133. **(T)** Jimsonweed is ingested, typically by adolescents, for its hallucinogenic properties. The anticholinergic symptoms this chemical causes include the classic "red as a beet, mad as a hatter, hot as a hare, blind as a bat, and dry as

a bone." Physostigmine, which binds competitively to acetylcholinesterase in the synapse, can reverse the anticholinergic symptoms. *(Tobias, 424; Rudolph CD,359)*

134. **(H)** Ethylene glycol is the primary component of antifreeze. Organic acids formed by metabolism of ethylene glycol are more toxic than the parent compound and are responsible for most of the major toxicity. Ethanol, an effective antidote, works by competing for the enzyme alcohol dehydrogenase which catalyzes the first step in the metabolism of ethylene glycol. The same enzyme initiates the metabolic pathway for methanol and isopropyl alcohol, and therefore, ethanol is also useful in treating poisoning with these substances. Some prefer fomepizole as an alternative. *(Rudolph CD,359; Tobias, 423)*

135. **(O)** Naloxone is a competitive antagonist to the opiates, including morphine. The drug is best administered intravenously. The usual dose is 0.03 mg/kg, but a second, larger dose (0.1 mg/kg) may be given if there is no response. Naloxone is not itself a depressant, and is a very safe drug. *(Rudolph CD,359, 372)*

136. **(X)** Cyclic antidepressants remain a leading cause of death from ingestions of pharmaceutical agents. These deaths occur principally in two age groups: toddlers who are unaware and adolescents who are attempting self-harm. The treatment of the cardiovascular toxicity seen in this overdose is the administration of sodium bicarbonate. The therapeutic effect of alkalinization most likely is multifactorial. *(Nichols,1375–1377; Rudolph CD,359)*

137. **(Q)** The most common cause of poisoning death is carbon monoxide inhalation. The sources most often are home fires and exposure to incomplete combustion of carbon fuels. When the source is smoke inhalation, most victims of fatal CO poisoning will die before arrival to the hospital. However, CO poisoning is treated with the antidote 100% oxygen. Hyperbaric oxygen is used in many centers. *(Rudolph CD,359, 363)*

138. **(E)** Most 1-year-old children are able to perform the tasks described. The pincer grip is

developed on average at 10.5 months of age. *(Lissauer, 15)*

139. **(H)** Children typically are able to copy a circle at 3 years of age, and copy a cross at 4 years of age. Hopping on one foot generally is accomplished at 4 years of age. *(Lissauer, 17)*

140. **(A)** These are expected findings in the evaluation of the supine infant (6–8 weeks of age). An 8-week-old infant who does not demonstrate responsive smiling should be further evaluated. *(Lissauer, 14)*

141. **(G)** The 2-year-old is at the end of the mobile toddler phase and is expected to walk will with normal gait, and to be able to kick a ball. Though most 20-month-old toddlers are able to combine two different words, toddlers are more likely closer to 24 months of age before they are able to build a tower of six 1-in cubes. *(Lissauer, :16)*

142. **(D)** The sitting child, 6–9 months of age, typically develops the ability to pull to a stand by age of 9 months, and babbles nonspecifically, but quite happily, by 9–10 months. The palmar grasp is predominant at 6 months of age and the pincer grasp develops between 10 and 11 months of age. *(Lissauer, 15)*

143. **(A)** Newborns should startle to sudden loud noise, so the best choice is the 2-month-old. *(Lissauer, 14)*

144. **(I)** Most 5-year olds are able to copy a triangle. (Remember, most children are able to copy a circle by 3 years of age, a cross by 4 years of age, and a triangle by 5 years of age. The ability to copy a square is demonstrated between 4 and 5 years of age. Past tense typically is used in language by 4 years of age, and future tense by 5 years of age. *(Lissauer, 17; Behrman, 43)*

145. **(A)** Among children with Down syndrome and congenital heart disease, 40% will have atrioventricular defect, 30% ventricular septal defect, and 20% atrial septal defect. Approximately 5% will have tetralogy of Fallot. *(Lissauer, 174)*

146. **(C)** Williams syndrome, also known as idiopathic infantile hypercalcemia, features growth delay, mental retardation, characteristic facial features, stellate iris, and supravalvular aortic stenosis. A very interesting characteristic of children with Williams syndrome is their unique chatter ability, referred to as "cocktail chatter." *(Rudolph CD,740, 1805)*

147. **(B)** Mitral valve prolapse can be demonstrated by echocardiography in about 80% of patients with Marfan syndrome. The most important cardiovascular manifestation, progressive dilation of the aortic root and ascending aorta, was not listed as a choice. *(Rudolph CD,1797)*

148. **(D)** Turner syndrome (45X) occurs in about 1/2500 live newborns. Clinical features include short stature, neck webbing, ovarian dysgenesis with infertility, cardiac defects, and normal intellectual development. The most common cardiac defect in this syndrome is coarctation of the aorta. One-third of girls with Turner syndrome have bicuspid aortic valves. *(Lissauer, 56; Rudolph CD,1781)*

149. **(E)** Children with Noonan syndrome have a high incidence of valvular pulmonary stenosis. *(Jones, 122; Rudolph CD,1810)*

150. **(C)** The heliotrope sign is a purplish discoloration of the periorbital skin which is frequently found in children (typically school-aged children) with dermatomyositis. Dermatomyositis is a chronic inflammatory disease affecting primarily the skin and skeletal muscles. *(Rudolph CD, 1109)*

151. **(A)** Profound muscle weakness, hypotonia, tongue fasciculations, and swallowing dysfunction are characteristic of Werdnig-Hoffmann disease, or spinal muscular atrophy type 1. This disease *typically* presents before 6 months of age and is fatal by 2 years of age. The infants involved are of normal intelligence and normal social ability, making their slow demise all the more difficult for the loved ones involved. *(Rudolph CD,2002, 2279)*

152. **(E)** Hemolytic uremic syndrome is diagnosed by the presence of microangiopathic hemolytic anemia, thrombocytopenia, and renal insufficiency. Most affected children will have a preceding gastrointestinal infection with *E coli* that produces a *Shigella*-like toxin. *(Rudolph CD,1696; AAP:Red Book,291–292)*

153. **(B)** Gower sign, or Gower maneuver, reflects hip-girdle weakness and most commonly is associated with Duchenne muscular dystrophy, although it can also be seen in spinal muscular atrophy and in some cases of dermatomyositis. The Gower maneuver enables children with proximal muscle weakness to move from a prone to standing position and involves first moving the feet close to the hands, then walking hands up the legs to push the trunk upright. *(Rudolph CD,2278, 2289)*

154. **(D)** The most common form of systemic vasculitis in children is HSP. Nearly 100% of children with this disorder will develop purpura with a normal platelet count. The purpuric rash is generally noted on the legs and buttocks and the arthritis, and abdominal pain complete the classic triad. *(Rudolph CD,842)*

155. **(H)** This scenario most likely represents bacterial infection following the cat bite. Cat bites are particularly prone to infection because the very long narrow teeth of the cat inoculate the cat's oral flora deep into the tissue. Of the choices given, the most likely causative agent is *P multocida*. The drug of choice for treatment is penicillin. However, because of the possibility of a polymicrobial infection including anaerobes and *S aureus*, the drug most often chosen in this scenario is oral amoxicillin-clavulanate or intravenous ampicillin-sulbactam sodium. *(AAP:Red Book,487)*

156. **(C)** This clinical picture is most consistent with human monocytic ehrlichiosis, most commonly seen in the southeastern and south central United States. The clinical findings closely resemble Rocky Mountain spotted fever, another tick-borne infection though the rash is seen less commonly. Leukopenia, hyponatremia, and liver dysfunction can be seen. Both are treated with doxycycline even in those less than 8 years of age. *(AAP:Red Book, 281–283)*

157. **(A)** Pharyngoconjunctival fever is an acute viral illness typically seen in summer-time pool outbreaks and manifests with fever, conjunctivitis, and pharyngitis. The most likely etiologic agent is adenovirus. *(AAP:Red Book,202–203)*

158. **(G)** Roseola (sixth disease) typically presents in children less than 24 months of age. Fever is characteristically high and persists 3–6 days. Frequently, the fever abates with the onset of the rash. Febrile seizures occur in 10–15% of cases. Human herpes virus 6 is the most common etiologic agent. *(AAP:Red Book,375–377)*

159. **(I)** Most cases of croup (laryngotracheobronchitis) are due to infection with parainfluenza. Among other viruses, adenovirus, influenza virus, and measles virus infections can also cause croup. *(AAP:Red Book,478–479)*

160. **(K)** Rat bite fever is caused by *Streptobacillus moniliformis* or *S minus*. The causative agent colonizes the upper respiratory tract of most rodents. Typically the fever does not begin at the time of the bite but develops a few days later as the wound appear to be healing. Fever occurs along with rash and migraotory polyarthritis in 50% of patients. In as many as 1/3 of cases, close contact with rats without a bite is noted, so history remains key to making this diagnosis. *(AAP:Red Book,559–560)*

161. **(C)** Sturge-Weber disease, also called encephalofacial angiomatosis, is the most unique of the neurocutaneous conditions listed. It does not have a clear inheritance pattern, lacks cutaneous pigmentation, and does not carry an increased risk of tumors. It is a progressive disorder and may be associated with mental retardation, seizures, hemiparesis, and visual problems. For children less severely affected, deterioration after age of 5 years is unusual, but learning difficulties and seizures may persist. The nevus flammeus (port wine stain) generally is in the distribution of the trigeminal nerve. *(McMillan, 2025; Lissauer, 310)*

162. **(B)** Neurofibromatosis type 1 (von Recklinghausen disease) is an autosomal dominant neurocutaneous condition with cafe au lait spots as the hallmark. Typically, the cafe au lait spots develop during the first year of life and increase in size and number for the first few years of life. Axillary freckling is closely associated with neurofibromatosis. Cutaneous neurofibromas often are not apparent until puberty. Though inheritance is autosomal dominant, one-half of all cases are the result of new mutation. *(McMillan, 2019–2021)*

Bibliography

AAP Committee on Injury and Poison Prevention, 2001–2002. Bicycle helmets. *Pediatrics*. 2001; 108:1030–1032.

AAP Committee on Injury, Violence and Poison Prevention. Poison treatment in the home. *Pediatrics*. 2003;112:1182–1185.

American Academy of Pediatrics (AAP) Committee on Environmental Health. Lead exposure in children: Prevention, detection, and management. *Pediatrics*. October 2005;116(4):1036–1046(doi:10.1542/peds.2005-1947).

American Academy of Pediatrics (AAP) Committee on Nutrition. Use of whole cow milk in infancy. *Pediatrics*. 1983;72:253–255.

American Academy of Pediatrics (AAP) Section on Hematology/Oncology, Committee on Genetics. Health supervision for children with sickle cell disease. *Pediatrics*. 2002;109:526–535.

American Academy of Pediatrics (AAP) Task Force on Sleep Position and Sudden Infant Death Syndrome. Changing concepts of sudden infant death syndrome. *Pediatrics*. 2000;105: 650–656.

American Academy of Pediatrics (AAP). *Pediatric Nutrition Handbook*. 5th ed. Elk Grove, IL: American Academy of Pediatrics; 2004.

American Academy of Pediatrics Committee on Sports Medicine and Fitness. Athletic participation by children and adolescents who have systemic hypertension policy statement. *Pediatrics*. 1997;99: 637–638.

American Academy of Pediatrics Section on Radiology. Diagnostic imaging of child abuse policy statement. *Pediatrics*. 2000;105:1345–1348.

American Academy of Pediatrics. *Red Book: 2006 Report of the Committee on Infectious Diseases*. 27th ed. Elk Grove Village, IL: American Academy of Pediatrics; 2006.

Ballard JL, Khoury JC, Wedig K, et al. New Ballard score, expanded to include extremely premature infants. *J Pediatr*. 1991;119:417–423.

Behrman RE, Kliegman RM, Jenson HB. *Nelson Textbook of Pediatrics*. 17th ed. Philadelphia, PA: Saunders; 2004.

Block SL, Harrison CJ. *Diagnosis and Management of Acute Otitis Media*. 3rd ed. Caddo, OK: Professional Communications, Inc.; 2005.

Brodsky D, Martin C. *Neonatology Review*. Philadelphia, PA: Hanley & Belfus Inc.; 2003.

Brunton LL, Lazo JS, Parker KL. *Goodman and Gilman's: The Pharmacological Basis of Therapeutics*. 10th ed. New York, NY: McGraw-Hill; 2006.

Burg FD, Ingelfinger JR, Polin RA, Gershon A. *Gellis & Kagan's Current Pediatric Therapy*. 17th ed. Philadelphia, PA: WB Saunders Co.; 2002.

Caffey J. The whiplash shaken infant syndrome. *Pediatrics*. 1974;54:396–403.

Cassidy JT, Petty RE, Laxer RM, Lindsley CB. *Textbook of Pediatric Rheumatology*. 5th ed. Saunders 2005.

Chase PH, Martin HP. Undernutrition and child development. *N Engl J Med*. 1970;282:933–939.

Committee on Injury, Violence, and Poison Prevention. Poison treatment in the home. *Pediatrics*. 2003;112: 1182–1185.

Dahshan A, Donovan GK. Severe methemoglobinemia complicating topical benzocaine use during endoscopy in a toddler: Case report and review of the literature. Pediatrics. 2006;117(4):e806–e809.

Davies D. *Child Development: A Practitioner's Guide*. New York, NY: Guilford Press; 1999.

Dietary Reference Intakes at Institute of Medicine website: http://www.iom.edu.

Dixon SD, Stein MT, eds. *Encounters with Children: Pediatric Behavior and Development*. 4th ed. Philadelphia, PA: Mosby Elsevier; 2006.

Dorland WAN. *Dorland's Illustrated Medical Dictionary*. 30th ed. Philadelphia, PA: Saunders; 2003.

Eichenfield LF, Frieden IJ, Esterly NB. *Textbook of Neonatal Dermatology*. Philadelphia, PA: WB Saunders Co.; 2001.

English R. Cat-scratch disease. *Pediatr Rev.* 2006;27: 123–127.

Fanaroff AA, Martin RJ. *Neonatal-Perinatal Medicine*. 7th ed. St. Louis, MO: Mosby; 2002.

Feigin RD, Cherry, JD, Demmler GJ, et al. *Textbook of Pediatric Infectious Diseases*. 5th ed. Philadelphia, PA: Saunders; 2004.

Finberg L, Kravath RE, Hellerstein S. *Water and Electrolytes in Pediatrics: Physiology, Pathology, and Treatment*. 2nd ed. Philadelphia, PA: Saunders; 1993.

Fleisher GR, Ludwig S, Henretig FM, et al. *Textbook of Pediatric Emergency Medicine*. 5th ed. Philadelphia, PA: Lippincott Williams & Wilkins; 2006.

Flomenbaum NE, Goldrank LR, Hoffman RS, et al. *Goldfrank's Toxicologic Emergencies*. 8th ed. New York, NY: McGraw-Hill Companies; 2006.

Gaudreault P, Temple AR, Lovejoy FH. The relative severity of acute versus chronic salicylate poisoning in children. *Pediatrics.* 1982;70: 566–572.

Gershel JD, Goldman HS, Stein RE, et al. The usefulness of chest radiographs in first asthma attacks. *N Engl J Med.* 1983;309:336–339.

Hay WW, Hayward AR, Levin MJ, et al. *Current Pediatric Diagnosis & Treatment*. 16th ed. New York, NY: McGraw-Hill; 2003.

Jones KL, Smith DW. *Smith's Recognizable Patterns of Human Malformation*. 6th ed. Philadelphia, PA: Elsevier Saunders; 2006.

Kattwinkel J. *Neonatal Resuscitation Textbook*. 5th ed. American Academy of Pediatrics and American Heart Association; 2006.

Katz M, Stiehm ER. Host defenses in malnutrition. *Pediatrics.* 1977;59:490–494.

Kelly LF. Pediatric cough and cold preparations. *Pediatr Rev.* 2004;25:115–123.

Klaus MH, Fanaroff AA. *Care of the High-Risk Neonate*. 5th ed. Philadelphia, PA: W.B. Saunders; 2001.

Kliegman RM., Behman RE, Jenson HB, Stanton B.. *Nelson's Textbook of Pediatrics*. 18th ed. 2007, Saunders, Philadelphia, PA: Saunders; 2007.

Klish WJ. Childhood obesity. *Pediatr Rev.* 1998;19: 312–315.

Knight ME, Roberts RJ. Phenothiazine and butyrophenone intoxication in children. *Pediatr Clin North Am.* 1986;33:299–309.

Levine MD, Carey WB, Crocker AC. *Developmental-Behavioral Pediatrics*. 3rd ed. Philadelphia, PA: Saunders; 1999.

Lissauer T, Clayden G. *Illustrated Textbook of Pediatrics*. 2nd ed. Edinburgh; New York, NY: Mosby; 2001.

Lissauer T, Clayden G. *Illustrated Textbook of Pediatrics*. London, England: Times Mirror International Publishers Ltd.; 1997.

Long SS, Pickering LK, Prober CG, eds. *Principles and Practice of Pediatric Infectious Diseases*. 3rd ed. New York, NY: Churchill Livingstone; 2008.

Lowry JA. Use of activated charcoal in pediatric populations. Second Meeting of the Subcommittee of the Expert Committee on the Selection and Use of Essential Medicines Geneva. 29, September to 3 October 2008.

MacDorman MF, Arialdi MM, Strobino DM, et al. Annual summary of vital statistics—2001. *Pediatrics.* 2002;110:1037–1052.

Maraffa JM, Hui A, Stork CM. Severe hyperphosphatemia and hypocalcemia following the rectal administration of a phosphate-containing fleet (R) pediatric enema. *Pediatr Emerg Care.* 2004 Jul;20(7): 453–456.

McMillan JA, DeAngelis CD, Feigin RD, et al. *Oski's Pediatrics: Principles and Practice*. 4th ed. Philadelphia, PA: Lippincott Williams & Wilkins; 2006.

Merenstein GB, Gardner SL. *Handbook of Neonatal Intensive Care*. 6th ed. Philadelphia, PA: Mosby Elsevier; 2006.

Miller D. *Seals & Sea Lions*. Stillwater, MN: Voyager Press Inc.; 1998.

Nichols DG. *Rogers Textbook of Pediatric Intensive Care*. 4th ed. Baltimore, MD: Lipincott, Williams & Wilkins; 2008.

Norwood VF. Hypertension. *Pediatr Rev.* 2002;23:197–208.

Parker S, Zuckerman B, Augustyn M, eds. *Developmental and Behavioral Pediatrics: A Handbook for Primary Care*. 2nd ed. Philadelphia, PA: Lippincott, Williams and Wilkins; 2004.

Poirier MP. Care of the female adolescent rape victim. *Pediatr Emerg Care.* 2002;18:53–59.

Polin RA, Spitzer AR. *Fetal and Neonatal Secrets*. Philadelphia, PA: Hanley & Belfus, Inc.; 2001.

Robertson J, Shilkofski N. *The Harriet Lane Handbook: A Manual for Pediatric House Officers*. 17th ed. Philadelphia, PA: Mosby; 2005.

Rose SR, Vogiatzi MG, Copeland KC. A general pediatric approach to evaluating a short child. *Pediatr Rev.* 2005;26(92):404–413.

Roth KS, Amaker BH, Chan JCM. Nephrotic syndrome: Pathogenesis and management. *Pediatr Rev.* 2002;23:237–247.

Rudolph AM, Kamei RK, Overby KJ. *Rudolph's Fundamentals of Pediatrics.* 3rd ed. New York, NY: McGraw-Hill; 2002.

Rudolph CD, Rudolph AM, Hostetter MK, et al. *Rudolph's Pediatrics.* 21st ed. New York, NY: McGraw-Hill; 2003.

Schmitt BD. Nocturnal enuresis. *Pediatr Rev.* 1997;18:183–191.

Shinwell ED, Gorodischer R. Totally vegetarian diets and infant nutrition. *Pediatrics.* 1982;70: 582–586.

Singer HS, Freeman JM. Head trauma for the pediatrician. *Pediatrics.* 1978;62:819–825.

Snedeker JD, Kaplan SL, Dodge PR, et al. Subdural effusion and its relationship with neurologic sequelae of bacterial meningitis in infancy: A prospective study. *Pediatrics.* 1990 Aug;86(2): 163–170.

Stellwagen L, Boies E. Care of the well newborn. *Pediatr Rev.* 2006;27:89–97.

Tobias JD. *Pediatric Critical Care: The Essentials.* Armonk, NY: Futura Publishing Co.; 1999.

Tsang RC, Zlotkin SH, Nichols BL, et al. *Nutrition During Infancy, Principles and Practice.* 2nd ed. Cincinnati, OH: Digital Educational Publishers; 1997.

UNICEF Statistics: http://www.childinfo.org.

UNICEF. *The State of the World's Children 2008.* New York, NY: Hatteras Press, Inc.; 2007.

United Nations Millennium Development Goals. http://www.un.org/millenniumgoals/.

Volpe JJ. *Neurology of the Newborn.* 4th ed. Philadelphia, PA: Saunders; 2001.

Watanabe T, Kawamura T, Jacob SE, et al. Pityriasis rosea is associated with systemic active infection with both human herpesvirus 7 and human herpesvirus 6. *J Investig Dermatol.* 2002;119(4):793–797.

Wolraich ML, Lindgren SD, Stumbo PJ, et al. Effects of diets high in sucrose or aspartamine on the behavior and cognitive performance of children. *N Engl J Med.* 1994;330:301–307.

Zitelli BJ, Davis HW. *Atlas of Pediatric Physical Diagnosis.* 4th ed. Philadelphia, PA: Mosby; 2002.

Index

Note: Page numbers referencing figures are followed by an "*f.*"